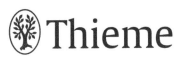

# Cost-Effective Evaluation and Management of Cranial Neuropathy

**Seilesh C. Babu, MD**
Neurotologist and Skull Base Surgeon
Department of Otology, Neurotology and Skull Base Surgery
Michigan Ear Institute
Farmington Hills, Michigan;
Program Director
Ascension Macomb Otolaryngology Residency
Macomb, Michigan;
Assistant Professor
Department of Otolaryngology and Neurosurgery
Wayne State University
Detroit, Michigan

**Neal M. Jackson, MD**
Chief of Neurotology
Department of Otolaryngology and Neurosurgery
Tulane University School of Medicine
New Orleans, Louisiana

136 illustrations

Thieme
New York • Stuttgart • Delhi • Rio de Janeiro

**Library of Congress Cataloging-in-Publication Data**

Names: Babu, Seilesh C., editor. | Jackson, Neal M., editor.
Title: Cost-effective evaluation and management of cranial neuropathy/[edited by] Seilesh C. Babu, Neal M. Jackson.
Description: New York : Thieme, [2020] | Includes bibliographical references and index.
Identifiers: LCCN 2019042673 (print) | LCCN 2019042674 (ebook) | ISBN 9781684200191 (hardcover) | ISBN 9781684200207 (ebook)
Subjects: MESH: Cranial Nerve Diseases—diagnosis | Cranial Nerve Diseases—therapy | Cranial Nerves
Classification: LCC RC410 (print) | LCC RC410 (ebook) | NLM WL 330 | DDC 616.85/6–dc23
LC record available at https://lccn.loc.gov/2019042673
LC ebook record available at https://lccn.loc.gov/2019042674

©2020. Thieme. All rights reserved.

Thieme Publishers New York
333 Seventh Avenue, New York, NY 10001 USA
+1 800 782 3488, customerservice@thieme.com

Georg Thieme Verlag KG
Rüdigerstrasse 14, 70469 Stuttgart, Germany
+49 [0]711 8931 421, customerservice@thieme.de

Thieme Publishers Delhi
A-12, Second Floor, Sector-2, Noida-201301
Uttar Pradesh, India
+91 120 45 566 00, customerservice@thieme.in

Thieme Publishers Rio de Janeiro,
Thieme Publicações Ltda.
Edifício Rodolpho de Paoli, 25º andar
Av. Nilo Peçanha, 50 – Sala 2508,
Rio de Janeiro 20020-906 Brasil
+55 21 3172-2297

Cover design: Thieme Publishing Group
Cover illustration: Karl Wesker
Typesetting by DiTech Process Solutions, India

Printed in USA by King Printing Company, Inc.          5 4 3 2 1

ISBN 978-1-68420-019-1

Also available as an e-book:
eISBN 978-1-68420-020-7

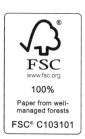

We sincerely appreciate the guidance and support offered by our mentors, colleagues, and family throughout the development of this book.

*Seilesh C. Babu, MD*
*Neal M. Jackson, MD*

# Contents

Contents

Contents

# Foreword

It is with great enthusiasm that I am writing this foreword. The authors have cleverly "isolated and yet combined" the signs and symptoms of this conglomeration of diseases. Well done! In this environment of ever escalating cost of health care, it is timely that we also teach the cost effectiveness of health care.

We currently spend $3 trillion in health care. It is predicted that if left unchecked, the United States will be spending $6 trillion in 2028.

The editors and authors are to be complimented for putting together this valuable book.

*K. J. Lee, MD*
*Emeritus Chief of Otolaryngology–Head and Neck Surgery*
*Hospital of St. Raphael Campus, Yale New Haven Hospital*
*New Haven, Connecticut;*
*Associate Clinical Professor*
*Yale University School of Medicine*
*New Haven, Connecticut;*
*Associate Clinical Professor*
*Zucker School of Medicine*
*Hofstra/Northwell Hempstead, New York;*
*Director, Business Service Line Development*
*Northwell Health*
*System Manhattan, New York;*
*Past President*
*American Academy of Otolaryngology–Head*
*and Neck Surgery/Foundation*
*Alexandria, Virginia*

# Preface

This textbook is the result of many conversations around the country in clinics, on hospital rounds, and at professional conferences. Patients with cranial neuropathy can be clinically challenging. Sometimes a missed diagnosis can be life threatening. Nowadays more and more payers, such as governments and insurance companies, are concerned with cost effectiveness of diagnostic and treatment steps. Therefore, physicians are often put in a challenging position between being good stewards of financial resources and being good providers of quality medical care. As the reader will observe in the subsequent chapters, cranial nerve issues are inherently complex and require expert clinical and radiographic evaluation. The primary aim of this textbook is to guide clinicians during these difficult situations.

We are indebted to the authors who contributed to the chapters. The diverse expertise of authors include neurosurgeons, ophthalmologists, speech language pathologists, radiologists, and otolaryngologists of various subspecialty fields including neurotology, laryngology, rhinology, and head and neck cancer.

It must be acknowledged that the recommendations in this book may require modification as new technologies and evidence are made available. The astute physician is encouraged to remain informed.

*Seilesh C. Babu, MD*
*Neal M. Jackson, MD*

# Contributors

**Lacey Adkins, MD**
Assistant Professor
Department of Otolaryngology–Head and Neck Surgery
Louisiana State University Health Science Center-New Orleans
Baton Rouge, Louisiana

**Eric N. Appelbaum, MD**
Otology, Neurotology, and Skull Base Fellow
Bobby R. Alford Department of Otolaryngology–Head
    and Neck Surgery
Baylor College of Medicine
Houston, Texas

**Rizwan Aslam, DO, MScEd, MBA, FACS**
Associate Professor
Department of Otolaryngology and Neurosurgery
Tulane University School of Medicine
New Orleans, Louisiana

**Seilesh C. Babu, MD**
Neurotologist and Skull Base Surgeon
Department of Otology, Neurotology and Skull Base Surgery
Michigan Ear Institute
Farmington Hills, Michigan;
Program Director
Ascension Macomb Otolaryngology Residency
Macomb, Michigan;
Assistant Professor
Department of Otolaryngology and Neurosurgery
Wayne State University
Detroit, Michigan

**Marc L. Bennett, MD, FACS**
Associate Professor
Department of Otology and Neuro-otology;
Quality Officer QSRP
Department of Otolaryngology–Head and Neck Surgery
Vanderbilt University Medical Center
Nashville, Tennessee

**Daniel H. Coelho, MD, FACS**
G. Douglas Hayden Professor
Department of Otolaryngology–Head & Neck Surgery
Virginia Commonwealth University School of Medicine
Richmond, Virginia

**Matthew M. Dedmon, MD, PhD**
Assistant Professor
Department of Otolaryngology–Head and Neck Surgery
University of North Carolina School of Medicine
Chapel Hill, North Carolina

**Michael Duan, BA**
Medical Student
Baylor College of Medicine
Houston, Texas

**Wissam Elfallal, DO**
Neurosurgery Resident
Department of Neurosurgery
William Beaumont Royal Oak
Oakland university
Royal Oak, Michigan

**Adam Folbe, MD**
Vice Chair, Academic Affairs
Department of Otolaryngology
William Beaumont Hospital
Royal Oak, Michigan

**Richard K. Gurgel, MD**
Associate Professor
Department of Otolaryngology–Head and Neck Surgery
University of Utah School of Medicine
Salt Lake City, Utah

**Erica E. Jackson, MD**
Fellow
Department of Otolaryngology
Louisiana State University School of Medicine
New Orleans, Louisiana

**Neal M. Jackson, MD**
Chief of Neurotology
Department of Otolaryngology and Neurosurgery
Tulane University School of Medicine
New Orleans, Louisiana

**Jeff Jacob, MD**
Neurosurgery/Skull Base Surgeon
Department of Neurosurgery
William Beaumont Royal Oak, MHSI, and  Mayo Clinic
Royal Oak, Michigan

**Nicolas-George Katsantonis, MD**
Otolaryngologist Head and Neck Surgeon
Raleigh Capitol Ear nose and Throat
UNC Rex Hospital
Raleigh, North Carolina

**Matthew Kircher, MD**
Associate Professor
Department of Otolaryngology–Head and Neck Surgery
Loyola University Medical Center
Maywood, Illinois

**Gavriel D. Kohlberg, MD**
Assistant Professor
Department of Otolaryngology–Head and Neck Surgery
University of Washington School of Medicine
Seattle, Washington

**Melda Kunduk, PhD, CCC-SLP**
Professor
Department of Communication Sciences and Disorders
Louisiana State University Health Science Center-New Orleans
Baton Rouge, Louisiana

**Andrew G. Lee, MD**
Chair, Blanton Eye Institute
Houston Methodist Hospital
Houston, Texas;
Professor of Ophthalmology, Neurology, and Neurosurgery
Weill Cornell Medicine
New York, New York;
Professor of Ophthalmology
UTMB and UT MD Anderson Cancer Center and Texas A and M
   College of Medicine (Adjunct)
College Station, Texas;
Adjunct Professor
Baylor College of Medicine and the Center for Space Medicine
The University of Iowa Hospitals and Clinics, and the University
   of Buffalo
Iowa City, Iowa

**John Leonetti, MD**
Professor and Vice Chair
Department of Otolaryngology–Head and Neck Surgery
Loyola University Medical Center
Maywood, Illinois

**Andrew J. McWhorter, MD**
Professor
Department of Otolaryngology–Head and Neck Surgery
Louisiana State University Health Science Center-New Orleans
Baton Rouge, Louisiana

**Anna M. Pou, MD**
Senior Surgeon
Department of Otolaryngology–Head and Neck Surgery
Ochsner Health System;
Interim Medical Director
St. Tammany Cancer Center
Covington, Louisiana

**Claudia M. Prospero Ponce, MD**
Fellow
Department of Ophthalmology
Blanton Eye Institute
Houston Methodist Hospital
Houston, Texas

**Ravi N. Samy, MD, FACS**
Chief, Division of Otology and Neurotology
Program Director, Neurotology Fellowship
University of Cincinnati and Cincinnati Children's Hospital
Cincinnati, Ohio

**Brendan Smith, MS**
Medical Student
Department of Otolaryngology–Head and Neck Surgery
Rutgers New Jersey Medical School
Newark, New Jersey

**Peter Svider, MD**
Rhinology Fellow
Department of Otolaryngology–Head and Neck Surgery
Rutgers New Jersey Medical School
Newark, New Jersey

**Abigail Thomas, MD**
Residency Physician
Department of Otolaryngology–Head and Neck Surgery
Medical College of Wisconsin
Milwaukee, Wisconsin

**Vanessa Torrecillas, MD**
Resident Physician
Department of Otolaryngology–Head and Neck Surgery
The University of Utah School of Medicine
Salt Lake City, Utah

**Aroucha Vickers, DO**
Fellow
Department of Ophthalmology
Blanton Eye Institute
Houston Methodist Hospital
Houston, Texas

**Robert Wayne Jr., MBS**
Medical Student
Department of Otolaryngology–Head and Neck Surgery
Rutgers New Jersey Medical School
Newark, New Jersey

**Richard H. Wiggins, III, MD, CIIP, FSIIM**
Professor
Department of Radiology and Imaging Sciences, Otolaryngology,
   Head and Neck Surgery
University of Utah Health Sciences Center
Salt Lake City, Utah

**Junru Yan, BA**
Medical Student
Baylor College of Medicine
Houston, Texas

**David Young, MD**
Clinical Instructor
Department of Otolaryngology
Vanderbilt University Medical Center
Nashville, Tennessee

# 1 Introduction to Cost-Effective Evaluation of Cranial Neuropathy

*Seilesh C. Babu and Neal M. Jackson*

## 1.1 Introduction

Cranial neuropathy may be an indication of a devastating, life-threatening condition or it may be a simple benign disease for which spontaneous, complete recovery is expected. In the evaluation of cranial neuropathy, the clinician must make decisions in order to determine the significance and permanency of the diagnosis. While there are numerous testing options available, cost containment and necessity of these tests need to be taken into account. Because of this, the authors of this book recruited a team of experts from various disciplines to provide their expert interpretations of available literature combined with their informed opinions to discuss a cost-effective evaluation and management of cranial neuropathy.

## 1.2 Cranial Nerves

A cranial nerve is defined as a nerve that leaves the brain and innervates an organ, muscle, gland, or sensory receptor. There are 12 paired cranial nerves which are presented in ▶ Table 1.1.

Cranial nerve functions are vital to human existence, from airway protection to communication and sensing the environment. All of our life functions occur via the cranial nerves. Actions such as tasting, smelling, swallowing, speaking, visualizing, and hearing are critical to our survival as well as enjoyment.

Although the 12 pairs of cranial nerves are grouped as such, they are heterogenous in their nerve fiber types. Some cranial nerves are purely motor (e.g., CN IV, CN VI, and CN XII) and some are purely sensory (e.g., CN II, and CN VIII). Many nerves perform mixed functions (e.g., CN III carries motor efferents and parasympathetics, while CN V has sensory and motor branches).

## 1.3 Neuropathy

Neuropathy can be defined in many ways. Clinically, a neuropathy is when there is dysfunction of the cranial nerve (e.g., facial droop with facial nerve weakness, facial numbness with trigeminal nerve weakness). This could be due to a problem with the nerve itself or an issue with the nucleus or ganglion more centrally located. Histologically, peripheral neuropathy can be categorized based on degree of nerve injury to the axons and connective tissues. The most popular classification is Sunderland's five classes: ranging from simple compression neuropraxia to complete transection of all axons and connective tissue. The causes of nerve injury can include iatrogenic transection, mass compression, viral swelling, infection, tumor invasion, and many others.

**Table 1.1** Names and functions of cranial nerves

| Nerve number | Name | Fiber types | Function |
|---|---|---|---|
| I | Olfactory | Purely sensory | Transmits smell sense from the nasal cavity |
| II | Optic | Sensory | Transmits vision information from the retina to the brain |
| III | Oculomotor | Mainly motor | Innervates most eye muscles (levator palpebrae superioris, superior rectus, medial rectus, inferior rectus, and inferior oblique) and muscles of the ciliary body and sphincter pupillae |
| IV | Trochlear | Motor | Innervates the superior oblique muscle, which depresses, rotates laterally, and intorts the eyeball |
| V | Trigeminal | Both sensory and motor | Receives sensation from the face and innervates the muscles of mastication |
| VI | Abducens | Mainly motor | Innervates the lateral rectus muscle, which abducts the eye |
| VII | Facial | Both sensory and motor | Provides motor innervation to the muscles of facial expression, posterior belly of the digastric muscle, stylohyoid muscle, and stapedius muscle. Also receives the special sense of taste from the anterior two-thirds of the tongue and carries secretomotor fibers to most salivary glands (not the parotid) and the lacrimal gland |
| VIII | Vestibulocochlear | Mostly sensory | Transmits sensation of sound and head movement |
| IX | Glossopharyngeal | Both sensory and motor | Carries taste sensation from the posterior one-third of the tongue, provides secretomotor innervation to the parotid gland, provides motor innervation to the stylopharyngeus, and contributes to pharyngeal plexus |
| X | Vagus | Both sensory and motor | Supplies sensory and motor innervation to most laryngeal and pharyngeal muscles and provides parasympathetic fibers to nearly all thoracic and abdominal viscera down to the splenic flexure |
| XI | Accessory | Mainly motor | Innervates the sternocleidomastoid and trapezius muscles |
| XII | Hypoglossal | Mainly motor | Provides motor innervation to most of the muscles of the tongue |

## 1.4 The Clinical Challenge of Cranial Neuropathy

Because cranial nerves enable so many of our daily functions, patients are often aware of even the slightest changes. Some cranial neuropathies are obvious after sudden events like trauma, stroke, or severe infection. Others present insidiously as subtle changes over a protracted time course, and the patient may not notice this gradual change. Sometimes patients are aware of the change (e.g., hearing loss), but assume it is "normal." Therefore, a team of clinicians in various specialties may be called upon for diagnosis and management.

Patients with cranial neuropathy can present at any clinical setting: emergency room, primary care physician, otolaryngology, or neurology office. The evaluation and workup can range from obtaining a clinical history and physical examination (e.g., Bell's palsy) to extensive functional testing and multiple imaging modalities (audiovestibular disorders).

Part of the challenge with cranial neuropathy is the complex anatomy involved. Evaluating the pathway from the central brain nucleus to the end organ innervated by the nerve may be complex in certain situations. While some nerves are short (e.g., cochlear nerve), others are lengthy (e.g., spinal accessory nerve) with tortuous pathways. Each chapter includes a discussion of the anatomy. Additionally, there is a chapter dedicated to radiology of cranial neuropathy.

For each given sense, there are multiple nerves working in conjunction to provide a coherent sense. When one of the two paired nerves is diseased, there is a discordant combination of signals to the brain and the neuropathy is thus symptomatic. Examples include diplopia from oculomotor nerve dysfunction or vertigo from vestibular nerve dysfunction. There is also a bilaterality to cranial nerves that can make diagnosis difficult. Taste or smell disturbance is nearly impossible for the patient to indicate laterality. The same is true with dysphonia or dysphagia due to unilateral vocal cord dysfunction.

There is a spectrum of complexity dysfunction of cranial nerves. For example, a clinically observed dysfunction could be central (brain) or peripheral (the nerve itself). For example, a patient's face can be weak due to stroke or due to Bell's palsy.

## 1.5 An Increased Interest in Cost-Effectiveness

Medical care has become costly. With third-party payers (government, insurance companies) playing a larger role in reimbursement of certain tests and procedures, there has been more emphasis on cost-effective evaluation and management of disease processes. Cost-effectiveness can be defined in multiple ways. In general, the value of the care provided is compared to the costs of that care. While this ratio may at first appear simple, it can be quite complex to accurately define value and cost to an individual or at a larger scale. Oftentimes, the calculation of value of medical care includes multiple intangibles for which there are no metrics.

Many of these assigned values are based on what society deems acceptable and may differ from culture to culture and depending on the attitudes of time era. With respect to cranial neuropathy, there are definitely relative values of disease morbidity (e.g., blindness is generally considered worse than anosmia). Sometimes a cranial nerve weakness may be the sign of a much larger problem (e.g., brain tumor or demyelinating disease) and therefore warrants prompt and thorough evaluation.

True costs of medical care are often difficult to predict and tabulate. The costs can vary from patient to patient based on insurance provider, clinician fees, facility fees, and negotiated rates. There are also frequent new diagnostic and therapeutic options that can obfuscate financial considerations.

## 1.6 Cost-Effectiveness in Cranial Neuropathy

Cost-effectiveness in cranial neuropathy can be complex. While some disorders are straightforward and benign, others may be complex and involve any number of specialists such as otolaryngologists, neurotologists, neurologists, ophthalmologists, neurosurgeons, neuroradiologists, radiation oncologists, physical therapists, laryngologists, speech-language pathologists, audiologists, and others. The authors assembled for this textbook reflect a broad spectrum of clinical roles in the hope of demonstrating a clinical pathway to assist in the evaluation and management of cranial neuropathy.

# 2 Cranial Nerve I: Olfactory Nerve Disorders

*Brendan Smith, Peter Svider, Robert Wayne Jr., and Adam Folbe*

**Abstract**

Smell loss is a common presenting symptom seen in clinics. There are a number of potential etiologies for olfactory dysfunction, but upper respiratory tract infections, sinonasal disease, and head trauma cause the majority of cases. A careful history and physical examination including nasal endoscopy are able to differentiate between the most common causes of olfactory dysfunction, thereby minimizing the need for costly and potentially unhelpful diagnostic tools such as imaging. Inexpensive smell tests can help confirm the diagnosis of olfactory dysfunction and allow monitoring of response to treatment. There is limited data on treatment options for olfactory dysfunction, and the treatment tends to depend on the etiology. Smell training has also showed promise for treating olfactory dysfunction due to multiple etiologies and may be the most effective treatment for patients who have anosmia and hyposmia that do not respond to initial treatments. This chapter will cover the epidemiology, anatomy, diagnosis, and management of anosmia and hyposmia, with a focus on delivering cost-effective health care.

*Keywords:* anosmia, olfactory dysfunction, nasal polyps, skull base tumors, smell and taste disorders

## 2.1 Introduction

A properly functioning sense of smell is an important part of the human experience. Smell plays a role in the enjoyment of food, perception of memories, and avoidance of potential dangers (e.g., smoke from fire, spoiled food that should not be eaten, etc.). Therefore, disorders of olfaction (anosmia and hyposmia) impact patients in multiple areas of life. Anosmia is defined as a total loss of smell, while hyposmia is defined as a reduced ability to detect smells and odors. The relationship between anosmia and decreased quality of life has been illustrated throughout the literature, as a loss of smell and the consequent inability to taste can have significant impact on one's well-being, including an association with mental illness and depression.[1,2]

## 2.2 Epidemiology

The prevalence of smell disturbances in the overall U.S. population has not been well studied. In recent years, the National Health and Nutrition Examination Survey (NHANES) added questions encompassing chemosensory disturbances (including anosmia/hyposmia).[3] Subsequent cross-sectional studies on results of this analysis provide some of the best available data on the prevalence of anosmia/hyposmia in the adult U.S. population; importantly, 23.3% of adults older than 40 years self-reported a history of smell disturbance at any point in their life.[4] The severity of dysfunction has also been studied, and between 12.4 and 13.5% have olfactory disturbance, defined as correctly identifying less than six of eight NHANES pocket smell test items, while 3.2% had anosmia/severe hyposmia (less than three odors correctly identified).[3,5]

While the causes of anosmia/hyposmia are diverse, certain risk factors such as older age and male sex may predispose to development. For example, the incidence of olfactory dysfunction increases with age, and has a prevalence of 4.2% in people aged 40 to 49 years, 12.7% in people aged 50 to 59 years, and 39.4% in those aged 80 years and older.[3] Additionally, males appear to be at increased risk as compared to females. Of the 3.2% of people who had anosmia/severe hyposmia in the NHANES database, 74% were males.[3] Further complicating this task is the fact that the length and severity of olfactory dysfunction varies by etiology.

The most common causes of olfactory dysfunction are post upper respiratory tract infection (URI), sinonasal disease including chronic rhinosinusitis (CRS) or obstructing lesions, and a history of head trauma.[2,6] Collectively, these three entities account for approximately 75% of cases of olfactory dysfunction.[2,6] Less common causes include sinonasal surgery, congenital anosmia, xerostomia, toxin exposure (e.g., smoking), certain medications (e.g., angiotensin-converting enzyme [ACE] inhibitors, calcium channel blockers, etc.), intracranial tumors, chronic diseases including hepatic or renal failure, endocrine disorders, autoimmune disorders, nutritional deficiencies, and neurologic dysfunction such as stroke or Parkinson's disease.[2,6,7,8] Around 18% of cases have no immediately identifiable cause.[2,6] A differential diagnosis is detailed in ▸ Table 2.1.

The primary impact of olfactory dysfunction on patients is a decrease in quality of life. Of patients experiencing taste or smell disturbance within the prior year, 5.8% felt it affected their quality of life.[9] In a separate study, patients with olfactory

**Table 2.1** Etiologies of olfactory dysfunction

| | |
|---|---|
| Sinonasal disease | Chronic rhinosinusitis, allergic rhinitis, nasoseptal deviation, nasal polyposis |
| Postviral | Upper respiratory tract infections |
| Head trauma | |
| Neurodegenerative diseases | Parkinson's disease, Alzheimer's disease, multiple sclerosis |
| Toxins | Cigarette smoke, volatile chemicals, radiation/chemotherapy |
| Medications | Many including ACE inhibitors, calcium channel blockers, and diuretics |
| Cerebrovascular disease | Ischemic stroke, subarachnoid hemorrhage, intracerebral hemorrhage |
| Tumors | Sinonasal tumors, olfactory meningiomas |
| Congenital syndromes | Kallmann's syndrome |
| Malnutrition | Vitamin B12 and B6, zinc |
| Chronic medical conditions | Renal disease, hepatic disease, endocrinopathies (hypothyroidism, diabetes, Addison's disease, Cushing's syndrome), autoimmune disorders |

*Abbreviation:* ACE, angiotensin-converting enzyme.
*Source:* Malaty and Malaty 2013.[7]

dysfunction reported a 20% decrease in quality of life on a survey measuring effects on daily functioning and dissatisfaction.[2] Overall, the high prevalence of olfactory disorders as well as the psychosocial impact these have makes this an important condition for clinicians to understand and manage.

## 2.3 Anatomy and Physiology of Olfaction

Signaling for the olfactory system begins with the nasal mucosa, and the nasal passages represent the first component. One function of the nasal passages is to transport air to the cribriform plate, superior septum, and superior and middle turbinates, where odor molecules dissolve in mucus. Once solubilized, odorants can then be sampled by chemoreceptors buried within the mucosa at these sites. Olfactory neurons express 1 of up to 350 different individual chemoreceptor proteins expressed by humans.[10] When chemoreceptors on an olfactory neuron bind its specific substrate, the neurons are depolarized, and signals travel up the branches of the olfactory nerve in the mucosal epithelium through perforations in the cribriform plate to reach the olfactory nerve (cranial nerve I). The olfactory nerve then projects to the olfactory cortex, which has multiple functional areas (▶Fig. 2.1). These include the piriform cortex, amygdala, and entorhinal cortex, which function in concert to provide odor discrimination.

In addition to smell discrimination, the olfactory system is critical for the function of taste experience as well. During chewing of food, retrograde air movement from the pharynx to the olfactory epithelium in the superior nasal cavity allows food odors to be appreciated, which allows for a depth of taste not possible from taste buds alone. While humans are able to taste five broad categories (sweet, salty, bitter, sour, or savory), the ability to identify up to 350 separate odors helps explain the variety of taste experiences possible.[10]

Odor discrimination is essential to overall olfactory function. Because air movement is required to bring odorant molecules in proximity with chemoreceptors in the superior nasal cavity, any airflow obstruction (e.g., sinonasal masses or nasal congestion) can cause olfactory dysfunction. Trauma, mass effect, or demyelinating disorders that affect the olfactory nerve can also result in olfactory dysfunction. Due to their location in the nasal mucosa, olfactory nerve endings are readily exposed to toxic inhalants (e.g., tobacco smoke), which can affect odor discrimination. Finally, because an intact sense of smell is important to food taste, patients may initially report loss of taste (ageusia/hypogeusia) even though the primary issue is olfactory dysfunction.[7] Since each of these etiologies present similarly, a thorough history and physical examination is critical to identifying the causative pathology.

## 2.4 Diagnostic Evaluation

### 2.4.1 History of Present Illness

A thorough patient history is low cost and essential for an accurate diagnosis for patients with olfactory dysfunction. The severity, duration, and abruptness of symptom onset should be ascertained.[7,8,11,12] A diagnostic algorithm based on history is shown in ▶Fig. 2.2. Abrupt onset of anosmia/hyposmia without prior history is most commonly due to post-URI, open or closed head trauma, or iatrogenic causes (e.g., sinonasal surgery). Follow-up questions for patients with abrupt onset should therefore include history of head trauma, recent surgical procedures, and review of systems for URI symptoms such as fever, nasal congestion, rhinitis, sore throat, or cough.[7,8,11,12]

Progressive or intermittent olfactory dysfunction is most likely due to chronic sinonasal disease (CRS, nasal septal deviation, allergic rhinitis, vasomotor rhinitis), toxin exposure (e.g., heavy metals, acids), advanced age, neurodegenerative diseases, medications, or tumors.[7,8,11,12] CRS with or without nasal polyposis is a common cause of progressive olfactory loss.[13] If the patient also has mucopurulent nasal drainage, facial pressure, or nasal obstruction for at least 12 weeks, the diagnosis of CRS is strongly considered.

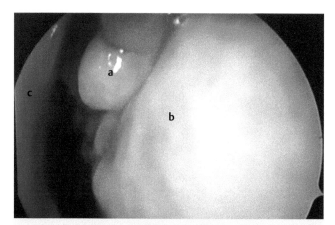

**Fig. 2.1** Endoscopic exam of left nasal cavity. **(a)** Nasal polyp. **(b)** Inferior turbinate. **(c)** Nasal septum.

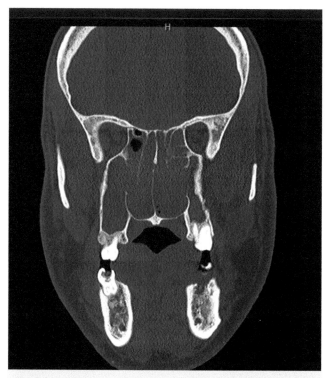

**Fig. 2.2** CT scan, coronal view with bone window showing sinus disease involving the ethmoid and maxillary sinuses.

Patients with congenital causes of olfactory dysfunction will not report a change in smell, and therefore may instead have deficiencies in sense of smell pointed out by others. The most common example of this includes Kallmann's syndrome, which results from the lack of gonadotropin-releasing hormone (GnRH) leading to infertility and absent smell.

Additional reports of nasal obstruction, sinusitis, rhinitis, problems with memory, and neurologic deficits will help elucidate the most probable etiology. Family history of atopy or neurodegenerative disorders may also be revealing. Social history of cigarette smoking, illicit drug use, or environmental toxin exposure and a review of medications will help rule in or rule out most remaining potential causes.[7,8,11,12]

## 2.4.2 Physical Examination Findings

The physical examination of patients with suspected hyposmia/anosmia should begin with a full head and neck examination with particular attention to the head, nasal cavity, and nasopharynx.[7,8,11,12] Among the acute causes of olfactory dysfunction, supporting evidence of URI (rhinitis, nasopharyngeal erythema) or trauma (lacerations, ecchymosis) may be found in this portion of the examination.

Patients with progressive olfactory dysfunction should be closely evaluated for evidence of CRS, sinonasal disease, or allergic/nonallergic rhinitis. When inspecting the external nose, signs of the allergic salute (a transverse nasal crease resulting from excessive scratching of the external nose) and allergic shiners (defined as discoloration below the eyes resulting from venous congestion and stasis associated with histamine release and vasodilation) suggest allergic rhinitis. Rhinoscopy with nasal speculum focuses on visualization of the vestibule, anterior septum, and inferior turbinates for nasal cavity lesions. Nasal endoscopy allows visualization of the posterior nasal septum, turbinates, middle meatus, as well as sinus ostia. Patients with allergic/vasomotor rhinitis may present with rhinitis and cobblestoning of the nasopharynx. Visible causes of olfactory dysfunction include nasal cavity lesions, inferior turbinate hypertrophy, and nasal polyps.

After inspection of the nasal cavity and nasopharynx is completed, cranial nerve testing should be performed. Attention should be paid to cranial nerves V, VII, IX, and X, as these cranial nerves are all involved in gustatory sensation and deficits may indicate a primary neurologic disorder or taste dysfunction, rather than smell dysfunction.[7,8,11,12] The remainder of the neurologic examination should be completed to assess for focal neurologic deficits or tremor, which could indicate intracranial pathology or other neurodegenerative diseases that can cause anosmia such as multiple sclerosis and Parkinson's disease.[7,8,11,12] Cognitive testing can be undertaken at this time to diagnose mild cognitive impairment and dementia, which may be caused by neurodegenerative disease that also causes olfactory dysfunction.[7,12]

## 2.4.3 Olfactory Testing

Olfactory testing serves to confirm the diagnosis of hyposmia/anosmia and should be undertaken after completion of the history and physical examination. Olfactory domains tested include identification, threshold, intensity, and discrimination.

Confirming that hyposmia or anosmia is the cause of the patient's symptoms is important to differentiate it from primary taste disorders and dysosmia (diminished smell) or phantosmia (smelling phantom odors). Examples of commonly used olfactory tests include the University of Pennsylvania Smell Identification Test (UPSIT), San Diego Odor Identification Test (SDOIT), Sniffin' Sticks, Connecticut Chemosensory Clinical Research Center (CCCRC) Test, and Briner and Simmen Diskette.[8,11]

The UPSIT is a 40-odor scratch and sniff test that can be administered in approximately 15 minutes. It is the most commonly used test for olfactory dysfunction in the clinic due to its ease of administration (can be self-administered) and test–retest reliability in detecting anosmia and hyposmia.[14] Patients are asked to identify each of the odors; the number of correctly identified odors are then scored and compared to a database of controls. Using normative data allows clinicians to account for normal variations in smell discrimination based on age and gender.[8,11] An abbreviated version of this test called the Cross-Cultural Smell Identification Test (CC-SIT; also known as the Brief Smell Identification Test [B-SIT]) uses 12 scratch and sniff items and is also a subjective forced answer test.[14] While this abbreviated test format is quicker to administer, the test–retest reliability is lower than the full-length UPSIT test.[14] UPSIT testing is usually covered by insurance, and the test packet costs $26.95.[15]

The SDOIT test uses eight odors in opaque jars along with illustrations of scent items from which patients must choose the correct odor. In adults between the ages of 50 and 70 years, this test has a reliability of 0.85 and test–retest reliability of 96%.[16] Generally, a new scent is administered every 45 seconds to reduce the risk of adaptation.[16] Therefore, the SDOIT can be administered in a similar amount of time as the B-SIT. This test kit is not currently available commercially.

In the olfactory evaluation with Sniffin' Sticks, felt-tip pens loaded with solutions containing different scents are held approximately 2 cm from the patient's nose.[17] Unlike some of the other olfactory tests that are limited to identification alone (e.g., UPSIT), Sniffin' Sticks can be used to test threshold, identification of odors from a forced choice four-item list, and discrimination.[17] Normosmia is defined as answering at least 75% of the total forced choice answers correctly.[8,17] Threshold is tested using $n$-butorphanol at different concentrations and asking patients to identify the pen with $n$-butorphanol from two other pens with solvent alone.[17] To test discrimination, patients are asked to identify which of three Sniffin' Sticks is different from the other two.[17] This test takes approximately 25 minutes to complete, and has good test–retest reliability ($r$ = 0.730).[8] The initial cost for Sniffin' Sticks is much higher than for single UPSIT kits, with most retailers charging a few 100 dollars for the 16 odor identification set. However, these are stable for a long time and can be used on multiple patients, and therefore may be a better choice than UPSIT for physicians who frequently perform olfactory dysfunction testing.

The CCCRC developed an olfactory test for threshold and odor identification in 1988.[18] Threshold testing is similar to Sniffin' Sticks, and aqueous solutions of $n$-butorphanol at varying concentrations in squeeze bottles are tested in each nostril until the patient can correctly detect four $n$-butorphanol-containing solutions from two blank solutions.[18] Odor identification testing features a panel of 10 odorant solutions in opaque jars and patients must then choose correctly from a panel of 20 answer choices.[18] Scoring is a composite of performance scores on both subtests, and a composite score over 6 is considered normosmia. The test–retest reliability is not well studied for CCCRC testing. One of the disadvantages is the lack of commercial availability.[17]

Smell Diskettes Test was developed by Briner and Simmen, and uses eight odorant-impregnated diskettes to test scent discrimination via a forced-choice question format.[19] For this test, normosmia is defined as greater than six correct identifications.[19] Anything less than three correct answers is considered anosmia, and this result can then be confirmed using olfactometry, an instrument used to evaluate concentration of odors, to determine threshold.[19] The test takes approximately 5 minutes to complete and has high test–retest reliability ($r = 0.999$).[8] The sensitivity and specificity of this test is not well studied. It is commercially available, though pricing information is unclear.

Although this section covers some of the most commonly used olfactory tests, it is certainly not exhaustive. There are other olfactory tests that have however they are not as well studied as the ones presented here.

## 2.4.4 Diagnostic Imaging

After confirming the diagnosis of olfactory dysfunction, imaging studies can be considered based upon history and physical examination findings and targeted at the most likely etiologies. Since the lifetime prevalence of olfactory dysfunction in the general population is high, a cost-effective approach should consider potential etiologies before ordering imaging studies.

Most patients presenting with olfactory dysfunction as their primary complaint do not require imaging studies. In a recent study of 100 patients with anosmia or hyposmia, MRI yielded an important finding in 7%; however, these findings only affected management in 1% of cases.[20] This study excluded patients with CRS and nasal polyposis, which are obstructive lesions more typically diagnosed by history and physical examination.[20]

In the cases where obstructive lesions have been confirmed by nasal endoscopy, imaging may be warranted as surgery may be needed to address these. When structural lesions are seen on endoscopy, the first imaging test should be noncontrast thin-slice computed tomography (CT) scan to detail bony anatomy and facilitate surgical planning. MRI should be utilized primarily in patients with nasal lesions found on endoscopy that are suspicious for cancer,[21] as it can help delineate whether the nasal lesion has any intracranial extension or is entirely extracranial. MRI is also typically done in patients with head trauma, and may show changes to the olfactory bulb; however, this does not affect management. Imaging should also be considered for patients who present with other neurologic deficits or seizures suggestive of intracranial pathology.

# 2.5 Cost-Effective Evaluation of Olfactory Dysfunction

## 2.5.1 Olfactory Testing

The most commonly used olfactory testing kit is the UPSIT test. The testing kit costs $26.95 and takes approximately 15 minutes to perform. For these reasons, it is a good screening test in patients with suspected olfactory dysfunction.

## 2.5.2 Diagnostic Imaging Cost-Effectiveness

Diagnostic imaging, such as CT and MRI, is controversial as cost-effective methods of evaluation. As stated previously, most patients with olfactory dysfunction can be diagnosed with history, physical examination, and confirmatory smell testing.

Patients with acute onset of olfactory dysfunction and sinonasal or obstructive disease can have nasal endoscopy performed to diagnose most causes such as nasal polyposis or deviated nasal septum. CT imaging of the head and sinuses is another option for detailing the anatomy in these patients, especially when surgery is being considered. In patients with head trauma, MRI may typically show changes to the olfactory bulb, and management is unchanged based on these findings. Patients with progressive olfactory dysfunction with unremarkable nasal endoscopy may undergo MRI.[22] Imaging studies are not required when post-URI is the suspected etiology.

According to the 2018 Center for Medicare and Medicaid Services (CMS) reimbursement database, the cost of a CT of the head with and without contrast is $195.12, the cost of MRI of the head with and without contrast is $385.56, and the cost of nasal endoscopy is $214.56.

For patients with confirmed olfactory dysfunction but no obvious cause by history and physical examination, the literature regarding cost-effectiveness of imaging is mixed.

In a recent study on 122 patients with olfactory loss, MRI revealed pathology related to olfactory dysfunction in 25.4% of patients.[23] Of the MRI series that revealed pathology related to olfactory dysfunction, about three-quarters revealed occult frontoethmoidal sinusitis.[23] The remainder of patients with findings related to olfactory dysfunction were due to central causes such as olfactory meningioma, olfactory atrophy, olfactory trauma, or infarcts within the olfactory system.[23] Of the entire series of 122 patients, 6 patients (4.9%) had benign tumors on MRI. Only 2 had olfactory meningiomas related to olfactory dysfunction, and the remaining lesions were deemed to be unrelated to dysosmia.[23] The authors of this study argue that the cost of MRI is appropriate when weighed against the average malpractice payout for a missed intracranial tumor.[23] Finding a single intracranial tumor that was related to olfactory dysfunction required 61 MRI to be performed, at an estimated cost of $146,400.[23] This is compared to the average medical malpractice costs of around $600,000 per misdiagnosis or delayed time to treatment suit.[23]

However, a recent economic analysis using the probability of finding an intracranial neoplasm from this study found that the incremental cost-effectiveness ratio of using MRI in patients with idiopathic olfactory dysfunction was $115,669.50.[22] This is much higher than the most commonly used willingness to pay threshold of $50,000. A subsequent sensitivity analysis was performed that showed the "no-MRI" method was cost-effective at a willingness to pay threshold of $50,000 with a certainty of 81%.[22]

Another recent study on 100 patients suggests routine MRI in patients with olfactory dysfunction has a low clinical yield.[20] In this study, seven patients (7%) had evidence of pathology related to olfactory dysfunction on MRI.[20] However, six of the seven patients had poorly developed or absent olfactory organs for which there is no treatment.[20] Only one patient had an intracranial tumor (neuroblastoma) that caused olfactory dysfunction, meaning that only 1% of the total study group had their management plan changed based upon MRI findings.[20] Importantly, all of the studies excluded patients with more apparent causes of olfactory dysfunction such as CRS.

Ultimately, these findings suggest that the routing use of imaging in olfactory dysfunction is not cost-effective in patients with idiopathic olfactory dysfunction. Therefore, the history and physical examination are of paramount importance for patients with a chief complaint of loss of smell. Most patients can be diagnosed and managed without imaging, and imaging infrequently affects management even when intracranial findings are present.[20,22,23]

## 2.6 Management

### 2.6.1 Post-Viral Olfactory Dysfunction

One of the most commonly cited treatments for post-viral olfactory dysfunction is intranasal or oral glucocorticoids.[24] In contemporary practice, both oral steroids and many commonly used intranasal steroids harbor modest costs and are generally covered by insurance providers. There are a number of studies that compare different formulations of steroids in treating post-viral olfactory dysfunction. One study found significantly higher CC-SIT smell test scores after 4 weeks of treatment ($p < 0.001$) with oral prednisolone for 2 weeks (30 mg daily for 3 days, 20 mg daily for 4 days, 10 mg daily for 7 days) plus mometasone twice daily for 1 month.[25] However, this study looked at the effect of *Ginkgo biloba* on improvement of olfactory dysfunction, and therefore did not have a true negative control group.[25]

A double-blind placebo-controlled study showed that patients with various causes of anosmia/hyposmia all showed significantly higher CCCRC threshold test scores following a 10-day course of oral steroids combined with intranasal steroids.[26] There was no significant difference of CCCRC scores between treatment, placebo, and control groups at any point during the remainder of the study period.[26]

Finally, Schriever et al found that 26.6% of patients with olfactory dysfunction who were treated with a 14-day course of systemic steroids improved their Sniffin' Sticks composite score by more than 6 points.[27] However, although this study included patients with post-viral olfactory dysfunction, it does not contain a performance analysis for this subgroup, making it difficult to draw conclusions.

Other treatments including vitamin A, minocycline, caroverine, and alpha lipoic acid have been studied; however, there is insufficient evidence for their efficacy at this time.[24]

In summary, there is low-level evidence that supports the use of steroids in patients with post-viral olfactory dysfunction. In the senior author's practice, a 2-week steroid taper is generally prescribed for these patients; however, there is clearly not an evidence-based consensus in our field. However, more studies are required both to test the use of steroids versus observation and to better delineate the natural course of the disease.

### 2.6.2 Sinonasal Disease

Like post-viral olfactory dysfunction, steroids are commonly used in the treatment of sinonasal etiologies of smell loss.

In particular, allergic rhinitis, chronic rhinitis, and nasal polyposis have all been shown to respond to systemic glucocorticoids.[27]

In one study treating patients with various etiologies of olfactory dysfunction, there was improved performance in Sniffin' Sticks scores after treatment.[27] Interestingly, subgroup analysis revealed that patients with sinonasal disease had significantly higher Sniffin' Sticks scores than any other subgroup.[27] A total of 36.7% of patients with sinonasal disease showed an increase in the Odor Threshold, Discrimination, and Identification (TDI) score of greater than 6 points over the 14-day treatment.[27] Allergic rhinitis is another sinonasal cause of olfactory dysfunction, which responds well to intranasal steroids, showing significantly higher Sniffin' Sticks scores after 1 month of treatment.[28] In addition to intranasal steroid management, patients with nasal polyposis or CRS and olfactory dysfunction respond well to appropriate surgical management, with significantly higher B-SIT scores postoperatively compared to baseline.[29]

### 2.6.3 Trauma

Treatment options for posttraumatic olfactory dysfunction are limited. Most patients can be observed for spontaneous recovery. Unless damage or scarring of the olfactory tract is severe, olfactory neuron regeneration should provide some restoration of olfaction. In a small, retrospective study on 14 patients, 4 patients showed improvement in olfactory function testing by olfactometry.[30] More studies are required before steroids can be recommended for management of posttraumatic olfactory dysfunction.

### 2.6.4 Neurodegenerative Conditions

Since neurodegenerative conditions such as Parkinson's disease, Alzheimer's dementia, and multiple sclerosis are progressive and irreversible, there are no reliable treatment options for olfactory dysfunction in these patients. Treating the underlying disease process may be the best option for prolonging olfactory function in these patients, although further study is needed to better characterize the evidence for this.

### 2.6.5 Smell Training

Smell training in patients with olfactory dysfunction is a treatment choice for multiple causes of smell loss.[31] Smell training includes repeated daily exposures to different odorants during a treatment course of a few weeks.[31] It has been shown to improve the TDI performance by multiple studies.[31] In a recent meta-analysis, smell training showed a mean increase in TDI score of 3.77 (95% confidence interval [CI]: 2.28–5.26).[31]

## 2.7 Conclusion

Olfactory dysfunction is common and the most frequent causes are post-viral olfactory dysfunction, head trauma, and sinonasal disease. A thorough history and physical examination including nasal endoscopy by an otolaryngologist is essential. The diagnosis of anosmia or hyposmia can be confirmed with well-validated and inexpensive tests such as the UPSIT or Sniffin'

Sticks. For patients with confirmed smell loss but otherwise negative examination findings, costly tests such as CT and MRI are controversial as the vast majority of results are negative, and the positive findings are frequently not amenable to clinical intervention. Treatment options are based on the underlying pathology, and usually include topical intranasal and/or systemic steroid therapy. Smell training has been shown to improve TDI scores in patients with olfactory dysfunction. Well-designed randomized controlled clinical trials are needed to determine the most effective treatment of post-viral and neurodegenerative olfactory dysfunction.

# References

[1] Kohli P, Soler ZM, Nguyen SA, Muus JS, Schlosser RJ. The association between olfaction and depression: a systematic review. Chem Senses 2016;41(6):479–486

[2] Temmel AFP, Quint C, Schickinger-Fischer B, Klimek L, Stoller E, Hummel T. Characteristics of olfactory disorders in relation to major causes of olfactory loss. Arch Otolaryngol Head Neck Surg 2002;128(6):635–641

[3] Hoffman HJ, Rawal S, Li C-M, Duffy VB. New chemosensory component in the U.S. National Health and Nutrition Examination Survey (NHANES): first-year results for measured olfactory dysfunction. Rev Endocr Metab Disord 2016;17(2):221–240

[4] Rawal S, Hoffman HJ, Bainbridge KE, Huedo-Medina TB, Duffy VB. Prevalence and risk factors of self-reported smell and taste alterations: results from the 2011–2012 US National Health and Nutrition Examination Survey (NHANES). Chem Senses 2016;41(1):69–76

[5] Liu G, Zong G, Doty RL, Sun Q. Prevalence and risk factors of taste and smell impairment in a nationwide representative sample of the US population: a cross-sectional study. BMJ Open 2016;6(11):e013246

[6] Kim DH, Kim SW, Hwang SH, et al. Prognosis of olfactory dysfunction according to etiology and timing of treatment. Otolaryngol Head Neck Surg 2017;156(2):371–377

[7] Malaty J, Malaty IAC. Smell and taste disorders in primary care. Am Fam Physician 2013;88(12):852–859

[8] Enriquez K, Lehrer E, Mullol J. The optimal evaluation and management of patients with a gradual onset of olfactory loss. Curr Opin Otolaryngol Head Neck Surg 2014;22(1):34–41

[9] Bhattacharyya N, Kepnes LJ. Contemporary assessment of the prevalence of smell and taste problems in adults. Laryngoscope 2015;125(5):1102–1106

[10] DeVere R. Disorders of taste and smell. Continuum (Minneap Minn) 2017;23(2, Selected Topics in Outpatient Neurology):421–446

[11] Daramola OO, Becker SS. An algorithmic approach to the evaluation and treatment of olfactory disorders. Curr Opin Otolaryngol Head Neck Surg 2015;23(1):8–14

[12] Boesveldt S, Postma EM, Boak D, et al. Anosmia: a clinical review. Chem Senses 2017;42(7):513–523

[13] Alt JA, Mace JC, Buniel MCF, Soler ZM, Smith TL. Predictors of olfactory dysfunction in rhinosinusitis using the brief smell identification test. Laryngoscope 2014;124(7):E259–E266

[14] Doty RL, McKeown DA, Lee WW, Shaman P. A study of the test-retest reliability of ten olfactory tests. Chem Senses 1995;20(6):645–656

[15] Sensonics International. https://sensonics.com/smell-identification-test-international-versions-available.html

[16] Krantz EM, Schubert CR, Dalton DS, et al. Test-retest reliability of the San Diego Odor Identification Test and comparison with the brief smell identification test. Chem Senses 2009;34(5):435–440

[17] Hummel T, Sekinger B, Wolf SR, Pauli E, Kobal G. "Sniffin' sticks": olfactory performance assessed by the combined testing of odor identification, odor discrimination and olfactory threshold. Chem Senses 1997;22(1):39–52

[18] Cain WS, Gent JF, Goodspeed RB, Leonard G. Evaluation of olfactory dysfunction in the Connecticut Chemosensory Clinical Research Center. Laryngoscope 1988;98(1):83–88

[19] Briner HR, Simmen D, Jones N. Impaired sense of smell in patients with nasal surgery. Clin Otolaryngol Allied Sci 2003;28(5):417–419

[20] Powell J, Elbadawey MR, Zammit-Maempel I. Does imaging of the olfactory tract change the clinical management of patients with olfactory disturbance? A case series of 100 consecutive patients. J Laryngol Otol 2014;128(9):810–813

[21] Holbrook EH, Leopold DA. Anosmia: diagnosis and management. Curr Opin Otolaryngol Head Neck Surg 2003;11(1):54–60

[22] Rudmik L, Smith KA, Soler ZM, Schlosser RJ, Smith TL. Routine magnetic resonance imaging for idiopathic olfactory loss: a modeling-based economic evaluation. JAMA Otolaryngol Head Neck Surg 2014;140(10):911–917

[23] Decker JR, Meen EK, Kern RC, Chandra RK. Cost effectiveness of magnetic resonance imaging in the workup of the dysosmia patient. Int Forum Allergy Rhinol 2013;3(1):56–61

[24] Harless L, Liang J. Pharmacologic treatment for postviral olfactory dysfunction: a systematic review. Int Forum Allergy Rhinol 2016;6(7):760–767

[25] Seo BS, Lee HJ, Mo J-H, Lee CH, Rhee C-S, Kim J-W. Treatment of postviral olfactory loss with glucocorticoids, Ginkgo biloba, and mometasone nasal spray. Arch Otolaryngol Head Neck Surg 2009;135(10):1000–1004

[26] Blomqvist EH, Lundblad L, Bergstedt H, Stjärne P. Placebo-controlled, randomized, double-blind study evaluating the efficacy of fluticasone propionate nasal spray for the treatment of patients with hyposmia/anosmia. Acta Otolaryngol 2003;123(7):862–868

[27] Schriever VA, Merkonidis C, Gupta N, Hummel C, Hummel T. Treatment of smell loss with systemic methylprednisolone. Rhinology 2012;50(3):284–289

[28] Dalgic A, Dinc ME, Ulusoy S, Dizdar D, Is A, Topak M. Comparison of the effects of nasal steroids and montelukast on olfactory functions in patients with allergic rhinitis. Eur Ann Otorhinolaryngol Head Neck Dis 2017;134(4):213–216

[29] Levy JM, Mace JC, Bodner TE, Alt JA, Smith TL. Defining the minimal clinically important difference for olfactory outcomes in the surgical treatment of chronic rhinosinusitis. Int Forum Allergy Rhinol 2017;7(8):821–826

[30] Ikeda K, Sakurada T, Takasaka T, Okitsu T, Yoshida S. Anosmia following head trauma: preliminary study of steroid treatment. Tohoku J Exp Med 1995;177(4):343–351

[31] Pekala K, Chandra RK, Turner JH. Efficacy of olfactory training in patients with olfactory loss: a systematic review and meta-analysis. Int Forum Allergy Rhinol 2016;6(3):299–307

# 3 Cranial Nerve II: Visual Disorders

*Junru Yan, Michael Duan, Aroucha Vickers, Claudia M. Prospero Ponce, and Andrew G. Lee*

**Abstract**

This chapter focuses on the different types of optic nerve (cranial nerve II) disorders; how optic neuropathies may present to the general physician; and recommendations regarding diagnosis, referrals, and some cost considerations. It may be important to take into consideration the limitations on care imposed by the presence of insurance coverage, the type of insurance, the types of procedures covered under various insurance plans, and a general sense of the average cost of various procedures. For the purposes of this chapter, average estimated costs will be used, but geographic and other variations may occur locally, and prices may vary significantly based on local, regional, and state market differences. Ophthalmology consultation is recommended for each of the visual disorders discussed. Some procedures that are performed frequently for patients with CN II disorders include magnetic resonance imaging, computed tomography scans, orbital ultrasound, fluorescein angiography, Humphrey visual field and other automated perimetry, optical coherence tomography, electroretinography, and visual evoked response. Some sample, estimated costs for these procedures are listed in the text.

*Keywords:* optic nerve, optic neuropathy, optic neuritis, papilledema, optic disc

## 3.1 Initial Evaluation and General Considerations

### 3.1.1 History

The clinical history and physical examination are important aspects of the clinical workup that provide useful insight for reaching an accurate diagnosis. Clinicians should note the following when eliciting the history: presence of existing eye defects including but not limited to glaucoma or cataracts; age of the patient; medical history with special attention to diabetes, hypertension, or visual changes; use of corrective eyewear and if this is up to date; notable changes pertaining to the eye including but not limited to pain, redness, tearing; diplopia, specifying monocular versus binocular diplopia; and other changes in vision including hyperopia, myopia, scotomas, or flashes/specks/spots in the visual field. If blurry vision is the main complaint, careful attention should be placed for onset, duration, triggers, time of day, bilaterality, and whether central or peripheral vision is affected. Additionally, it is important to note whether the blurry vision is more pronounced at a given distance (far vs. near).

### 3.1.2 Physical Examination

Comfort and familiarity with techniques for physical examination of the visual and oculomotor systems are essential. An example script for how a basic ocular examination may be performed by the front-line provider is as follows:

1. Assess visual acuity: ask the patient to read the lowest line they are able to read from any vision testing chart (from the appropriate distance) with one eye and then the other and with and without corrective prescription. Near cards should be held at approximately 14 inches from the patient or at a normal reading distance. Patients may have blurry vision secondary to ocular dryness, which may be improved simply by administering an artificial tear solution. If a pinhole mask is available and utilized, the blurry vision from a refractive error is expected to improve. If not available, an easy way to test for refractive error is by making a hole with a pencil tip on a card and asking the patient to read through it.
2. Assess visual fields: facing the patient at an arm's length, ask the patient to cover one eye and look toward the physician's nose without moving. Cover your contralateral eye (the one in front of the patient's covered eye) and move your free hand to all corners of visual quadrants and extend any number of fingers, asking the patient to state the number of fingers shown. Repeat in all four quadrants and in both eyes.
3. Assess extraocular movements: facing the patient, ask the patient to look directly at the physician and hold their head steady. Have the patient follow your extended finger (about 1 ft away) with only the eyes as you slowly move in an "H" pattern. Conclude by bringing your finger toward the patient's nasal bridge to test convergence. Evaluate for smooth pursuit, nystagmus, and difficulty in completing movements.
4. Examine eyes: look at the color and fullness of the eyelids and the periorbital skin. Observe any asymmetry of the eyelids and their distance from the center of the pupil. Examine the light reflex position for alignment. Spread the eyelids to examine the eye surface for discharge or hemorrhage, and assess the corneal surface for abrasion.
5. Test orbicularis oculi: ask the patient to close their eyes tightly. Have them resist as you attempt to open the eyelids with your fingers.
6. Test intraocular pressure (rough approximation): ask the patient to close their eyes and gently press over the eyelids toward the center of the eyeball. Compare this to the tip of your nose—the eyeball should be softer or equally soft to the tip of your nose.
7. Examine pupils: note the size of the pupils and presence of red reflex. Test pupillary responses (both direct and indirect) by first decreasing the room light and then asking the patient to look into the distance as you shine light into the pupils, waiting a few seconds between eyes. Also note for the presence of a relative afferent pupillary defect.

8. Fundoscopic examination: decrease the room light and ask the patient to look into the distance. Hold ophthalmoscope in the right hand for examination of the right eye and vice versa. Check for red reflex from 12 to 18 inches away and approach to within 2 to 3 inches. Evaluate any opacity of the cornea or vitreous. Examine the retina and retinal vasculature. Examine the optic disc for color, contour, edema, and cupping.

## 3.1.3 Indications for Urgent Referral and Diagnostic Testing

Patients presenting with the following symptoms should be referred immediately to an ophthalmologist:

1. Physical wound of the eye including a scratch, cut, puncture, or concern that something is stuck in the eye.
2. If the patient uses contacts and reports they may be "stuck" underneath their lids.
3. Sudden acute loss of vision with or without pain.
4. Painful binocular diplopia.
5. Presence of flashing light or floaters even if only part of the visual field is affected.
6. Acute and unexplained pain or redness of the eye. Chronic symptoms may be referred as a routine visit to the ophthalmologist.
7. Eye pain that is concurrent with nausea, headache, or vomiting.
8. Exposure of chemicals to the eye.
9. Infectious conditions, such as herpes simplex or zoster or acute dacryocystitis.

Other changes in vision may not be emergent but may still warrant referral to an ophthalmologist for observation. When referring or ordering diagnostic testing, physicians should consider the cost of common procedures and imaging as summarized in ▸Table 3.1. These estimated prices are for reference only, as actual prices may vary significantly based on insurance coverage and market differences.

Table 3.1 Medicare allowables of some common procedures in testing for an optic neuropathy

| Test (CPT code) | Cost: Medicare allowables ($) |
| --- | --- |
| Brain MRI (70553) | 400 |
| Head MR angiography with and without dye (70546) | 510 |
| Head CT with and without contrast (70470) | 201 |
| Orbital ultrasound (76510) | 150 per eye |
| MRI orbit with and without contrast (70543) | 460 |
| Fluorescein angiography (92242) | 241 |
| Electroretinography (92275) | 160 |
| Visual evoked response (95930) | 74 |
| Optical coherence tomography (92134) | 44 |
| Humphrey visual field (92083) | 68 |

Note: Genetic testing may be indicated for some patients with CN II disorders. The price for these tests may vary, but it is important to note that such testing is often not covered by insurance.

# 3.2 Vascular

## 3.2.1 Anterior Ischemic Optic Neuropathy

### Nonarteritic

#### Etiology and Pathophysiology

Nonarteritic anterior ischemic optic neuropathy (NAION) is the most common acute, unilateral optic neuropathy in adults. Proposed risk factors include hypertension, diabetes, atherosclerosis, past surgeries with major blood loss, prothrombotic conditions, obstructive sleep apnea, nocturnal hypotension, use of amiodarone derivatives, and erectile dysfunction drugs.[1,2]

#### Presenting Symptoms and Signs

The presentation is usually an acute, unilateral, painless vision loss. Patients with NAION usually have a small cup-to-disc (C:D) ratio, which is a proposed predisposing structural risk factor. The visual acuity loss is variable. Ophthalmoscopy reveals optic disc edema in the acute phase.[3] Optic atrophy (sector or diffuse) may develop over time (▸Fig. 3.1).

#### Clinical Considerations

##### Diagnosis

The diagnosis of NAION is primarily clinical because there is no diagnostic laboratory or imaging finding for NAION. The diagnosis is made based on older age, the presence of vasculopathic risk factors, visual loss patterns, optic disc edema, and a small C:D ratio. Patients with NAION typically do not require neuroimaging. In older patients (e.g., older than 50 y), giant cell arteritis (GCA) may need to be ruled out with clinical examination and laboratory testing (see below).

#### Current Treatment

Eliminating or adjusting the risk factors listed earlier may be beneficial. There is currently no evidence-based treatment for NAION. Optic nerve decompression and aspirin have not been shown to improve vision and the use of corticosteroids remains controversial (http://quarkpharma.com/?p=12476).[4,5] Clinical trials are currently underway for NAION (http://quarkpharma.com/?p=12476).

| Cost considerations[a] | |
| --- | --- |
| Not recommended | MRI, lumbar puncture not indicated for typical NAION |
| Recommended | ESR/C-reactive protein (CRP) if GCA is suspected |
| Practice option | Complete blood count (CBC) and platelet count |

[a] Authors' opinions, not consensus statement.

### Giant Cell Arteritis/Arteritic

#### Etiology and Pathophysiology

Arteritic anterior ischemic optic neuropathy (AAION), or GCA, is a systemic granulomatous vasculitis, affecting medium to large-sized arteries. GCA is considered an ophthalmic emergency due to its aggressive course.[4]

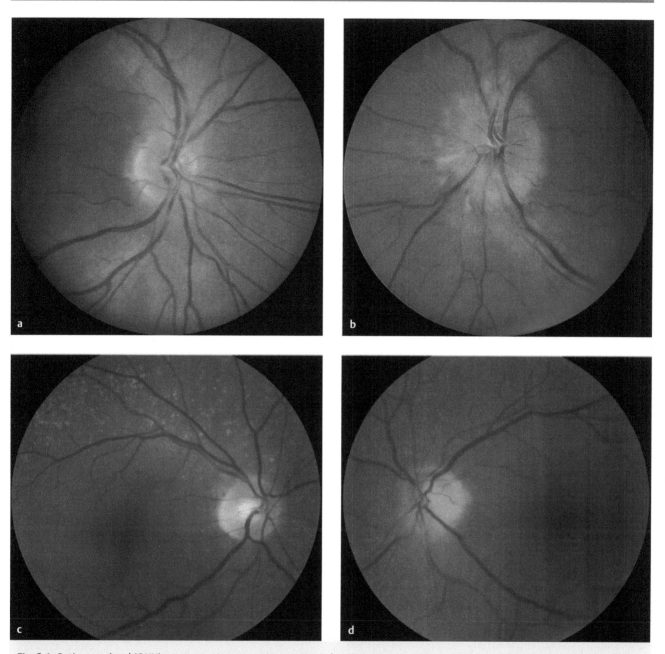

**Fig. 3.1** Optic nerve head (ONH) appearance in nonarteritic anterior ischemic optic neuropathy (NAION) and arteritic anterior ischemic optic neuropathy (AAION). **(a)** The healthy eye demonstrates a characteristic crowded appearance, which has been called "disc at risk." **(b)** ONH appearance in NAION. Edema is segmental, with mild superimposed pallor and flame hemorrhages. **(c)** The healthy eye demonstrates a normal cup-to-disc ratio. Lack of a disc at risk should suggests an AAION. **(d)** ONH appearance in AAION. Pallor is more pronounced. (Reproduced with permission from American Academy of Ophthalmology.)

## Presenting Symptoms and Signs

The most common ocular manifestation of GCA is acute unilateral painful vision loss that can initially present with episodes of transient vision loss.[5] In addition, patients with GCA may complain of jaw claudication, scalp tenderness, headache, hip and shoulder arthralgia, malaise, and fevers (see ▶ Fig. 3.2).[6]

## Clinical Considerations

### Diagnosis

The gold standard for diagnosis is a temporal artery biopsy (TAB), but note that TAB sensitivity ranges from 70 to 90%.[7] Studies also suggest the use of temporal artery ultrasound for diagnosis of

GCA, which may present with a positive "halo sign" (inflammation around the artery). Some studies have shown high specificity and moderate sensitivity, but ultrasound has not yet reached the level of replacing the TAB for the diagnosis of GCA.[89]

## Current Treatment

The current treatment of GCA remains high-dose corticosteroids.[10] Treatment courses vary but may be as long as 1 to 2 years of chronic steroids and given the need to taper steroids slowly to prevent a GCA relapse.[6] In addition, recent studies have shown the potential for tocilizumab to be therapeutic for GCA.[11] The cost of tocilizumab is $355 for a prefilled syringe of 162 mg of drugs.[12] Consultation with rheumatology

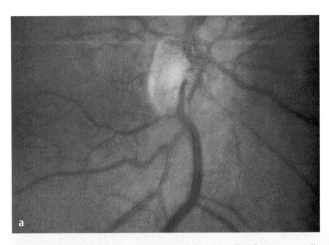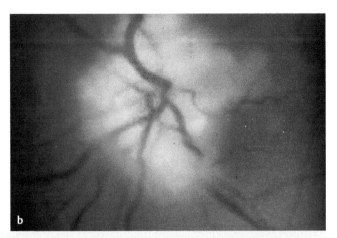

**Fig. 3.2** (a, b) The left optic disc is pallid and swollen from giant cell arteritis. Fundoscopy shows a normal right optic disc with a cup-to-disc ratio of about 0.3 and massive infarction (with a pallid white or "chalky" white appearance) of the left optic eye, with extension into the surrounding retina. (Reproduced with permission from American Academy of Ophthalmology.)

is recommended for most cases of GCA but especially for those cases requiring consideration for steroid-sparing regimens including tocilizumab.

| Cost considerations | |
| --- | --- |
| Not recommended | Lumbar puncture |
| Recommended | ESP/CRP, TAB, steroids |
| Practice option | CBC and platelet count, ultrasound, MRI, fractional anisotropy (FA) |

### 3.2.2 Posterior Ischemic Optic Neuropathy

#### Etiology and Pathophysiology

Posterior ischemic optic neuropathy (PION) is an optic nerve disorder resulting from an infarction of the retrobulbar portion of the optic nerve. This form of neuropathy is less common than anterior ischemic optic neuropathy (AION) and can be distinguished from AION by the normal-appearing optic nerve head.[8] Etiology of PION is typically divided into three groups: perioperative (surgical), arteritic (GCA), and nonarteritic (idiopathic).[9]

#### Presenting Symptoms and Signs

Patients with PION typically present with acute central or peripheral vision loss.[8] Other symptoms are based on the type of PION.

#### Clinical Considerations

##### Diagnosis

PION is a diagnosis of exclusion. It is recommended to rule out GCA, perform a thorough ophthalmologic examination, and consider a brain MRI to rule out other causes of retrobulbar optic neuropathy.[9]

##### Current Treatment

Treatment depends on the mechanism of PION. There is currently no treatment for perioperative PION and nonarteritic

PION that can significantly improve vision loss. Patients with arteritic PION may be treated with corticosteroids if GCA is suspected.[13]

| Cost considerations | |
| --- | --- |
| Not recommended | – |
| Recommended | ESP, CRP, CT, and/or MRI of the brain and orbit with and without contrast for retrobulbar optic neuropathy |
| Practice option | TAB if suspecting GCA |

### 3.2.3 Hypertensive Retinopathy

#### Etiology and Pathophysiology

Hypertensive retinopathy (HR) is a condition found in hypertensive patients characterized by retinal vascular signs.[14]

#### Presenting Symptoms and Signs

The traditional classification system of HR is known as the Keith–Wagener–Barker (KWB) scale and classifies HR as mild, moderate, or malignant depending on the extent of the disease. Malignant cases involve severe grade 4 retinopathy and papilledema.[15] Patients with hypertension may also experience NAION.

#### Clinical Considerations

##### Diagnosis

Early detection of HR is beneficial because some studies have suggested an association between retinopathy and long-term stroke risk. Fundoscopic examination and retinal photography have been recommended to determine the presence and severity of retinopathy in hypertensive patients.[16]

##### Current Treatment

HR treatment is focused around the goal of reducing systemic blood pressure.[17] Consultation with a retinal specialist may also be sought for further treatment.

## 3.2.4 Diabetic Papillitis

### Etiology and Pathophysiology

Diabetic papillitis (DP) is a rare finding in patients with type 1 or type 2 diabetes presenting with optic disc edema.[18] The pathophysiology of the disease is undetermined, but evidence does suggest that duration of diabetes is not a risk factor for DP.[19]

### Presenting Symptoms and Signs

In patients with DP, the optic nerve function is typically intact and either unilateral or bilateral hyperemic disc swelling may be present. Patients may occasionally present with decreased visual acuity but for the most part are asymptomatic.[18] In 70 to 100% of patients with DP, macular edema may be a comorbid finding. Other signs of diabetic retinopathy may be found in 35 to 90% of patients.[19]

### Clinical Considerations

### Diagnosis

DP is a diagnosis of exclusion. The current criteria listed for DP diagnosis are as follows: (1) patient must have confirmed diagnosis of either type 1 or type 2 diabetes; (2) present with optic disc edema; (3) have largely intact optic nerve function; (4) have normal intracranial pressure; and (5) be clear of inflammation, infection, and/or infiltration of the optic nerve. MRI of the brain and orbits and lumbar puncture may be performed in order to rule out other conditions.[18]

### Current Treatment

No treatment is recommended for most patients with DP since the disease usually self-resolved. Use of corticosteroids is currently debated as to whether it is effective in curbing progression of the diseases. Other treatment options such as vascular endothelial growth factor (VEGF) inhibitors to resolve swelling and improve visual acuity have been reported but require further testing to confirm their efficacy.[19]

## 3.3 Infectious

### 3.3.1 Infectious Neuroretinitis

### Etiology and Pathophysiology

Neuroretinitis may be involved in the presentation of infections. Common etiologic agents may include *Bartonella*, syphilis, and Lyme disease.

**Bartonella neuroretinitis**, also known as cat scratch disease (CSD), is the ocular manifestation of infection by *Bartonella henselae*, which is the most common infectious cause of neuroretinitis, contributing to up to 64% of all cases.[20]

**Syphilis** is a chronic, sexually transmitted infection of the spirochete *Treponema pallidum* that may affect any part of the body, including the eyes. Syphilitic infection of the eye is uncommon but can occur in later stages of the disease.[21,22]

**Lyme disease** is an *Ixodes* tick–transmitted infection caused by the spirochete *Borrelia burgdorferi*. The localized infection begins with erythema migrans "bull's eye" rash.

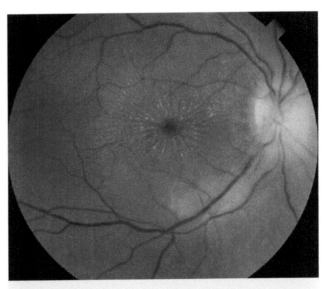

**Fig. 3.3** Disc edema and macular star in a patient with neuroretinitis due to cat-scratch disease. (Reproduced with permission from American Academy of Ophthalmology.)

After the infection becomes disseminated and in the absence of treatment, up to 15% of patients may develop neurological complications.[23]

### Presenting Symptoms and Signs

Patients may present with decreased visual acuity. Optic disc edema with a macular star figure may be noted.[20,24] Panuveitis is the most common ophthalmic finding in ocular syphilis (see ▶ Fig. 3.3).[25]

### Clinical Considerations

### Diagnosis

Diagnosis is based on history, and physical and serologic testing.

### Current Treatment

Consultation with an infectious disease specialist may be considered to assist with medical management. For bartonella neuroretinitis, data suggest use of doxycycline with rifampin for adults for 4 to 6 weeks under observation by an ophthalmologist. For children younger than 8 years, a 4- to 6-week course of rifampin and either azithromycin or trimethoprim/sulfamethoxazole can be considered.[26]

For ocular syphilis, parenteral penicillin is currently the drug of choice for treatment, typically resulting in visual improvement and management of inflammation within 1 month. Corticosteroids are typically not used, but may be considered if additional inflammatory complications, such as macular edema, arise.[25]

For treatment of early Lyme disease, oral doxycycline, amoxicillin, and cefuroxime have all demonstrated equal effectiveness. Of these antimicrobial choices, doxycycline was noted to have superior central nervous system (CNS) penetration.[27]

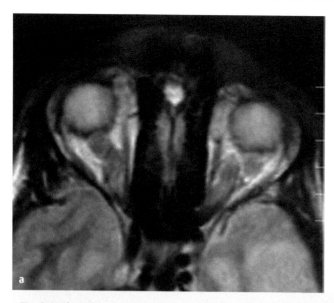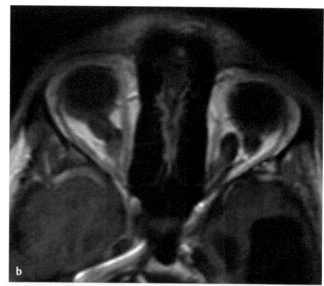

**Fig. 3.4** Bilateral optic nerve gliomas in a patient with a neurofibromatosis type 1. **(a)** Both optic nerves are expanded and hyperintense in the T2-weighted image. **(b)** They do not enhance in the postcontrast T1-weighted image. (Adapted from Forsting M, Jansen O, ed. MR Neuroimaging: Brain, Spine, Peripheral Nerves. 1st edition. New York, NY: Thieme; 2016.)

| Cost considerations | |
| --- | --- |
| Not recommended | – |
| Recommended | Serologic testing |
| Practice option | Lumbar puncture, MRI, infectious disease referral |

## 3.4 Compressive/Neoplastic

### 3.4.1 Compressive Optic Neuropathy

#### Optic Nerve Glioma

#### Etiology and Pathophysiology

Optic nerve glioma is the most common tumor of the optic nerve.[28] Benign optic nerve gliomas may present at any age, but most become symptomatic within the first two decades of life.[24] Malignant optic nerve glioma is less common, occurring predominantly in males older than 20 years.[28] Patients may also have evidence of neurofibromatosis type I (NF1).[29]

#### Presenting Symptoms and Signs

Patients with optic nerve gliomas may present with progressive decreased visual function, proptosis, optic disc swelling, and/or strabismus. Typically, ocular and orbital pains are both absent.[28]

#### Clinical Considerations

##### Diagnosis

MRI is the gold standard for imaging, but CT may be considered to visualize intratumoral calcifications (▶Fig. 3.4).[29]

## Current Treatment

Treatment and management of optic nerve glioma is patient dependent. It may be recommended that a multidisciplinary approach be undertaken, consulting an ophthalmologist, radiation oncologist, pediatric oncologist, neuroradiologist, and a neurosurgeon.[29]

| Cost considerations | |
| --- | --- |
| Not recommended | Lumbar puncture |
| Recommended | MRI |
| Practice option | Consultation with neurosurgery and/or radiation oncology |

#### Optic Nerve Sheath Meningiomas

#### Etiology and Pathophysiology

Optic nerve sheath meningiomas (ONSMs) are rare benign tumors that arise from meninges surrounding the optic nerve.[30] They are the second most common optic nerve tumor after optic nerve gliomas and account for a third of primary optic nerve tumors.[31] These tumors tend to be well defined and progress slowly, but they may still compress the anterior visual pathway leading to vision loss. Ninety-five percent of all cases are unilateral. Bilateral cases are uncommon and tend to be associated with patients with neurofibromatosis type 2.[32]

#### Presenting Symptoms and Signs

Patients may present with progressive painless visual loss over 1 to 5 years.[31] Examination via fundoscopy may reveal presence of optic disc swelling (early stage) and pallor or optociliary shunt vessels (late stage), which are retinochoroidal

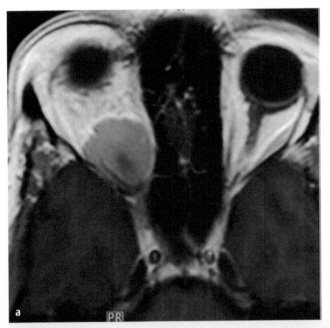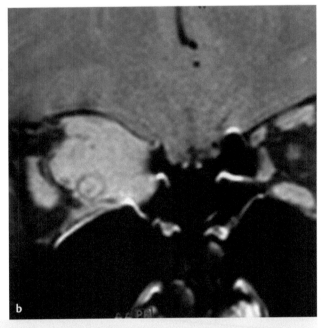

**Fig. 3.5** Optic nerve sheath meningioma. Large optic nerve sheath meningioma in a patient with a 6-year history of right-sided blindness, formerly attributed to optic neuritis. **(a)** T1-weighted (T1w) image shows a large, expansile, uniformly enhancing mass with smooth margins in the right orbital cone. The encased optic nerve is barely perceptible at the center of the mass. **(b)** Fat-saturated coronal T1w image after contrast administration more clearly demonstrates the encased optic nerve in the inferolateral quadrant of the meningioma. (Adapted from Forsting M, Jansen O, ed. MR Neuroimaging: Brain, Spine, Peripheral Nerves. 1st edition. New York, NY: Thieme; 2016.)

collaterals.[31,33] Patients may also have proptosis and extraocular motility defects depending on size of location of the tumor.

## Clinical Considerations

### Diagnosis

MRI of the brain and orbit with and without gadolinium is considered the gold standard for diagnosis of ONSM (▶Fig. 3.5).[31] CT of the head without contrast can also be useful for patients demonstrating optic canal enlargement and nerve sheath calcification, sometimes present in ONSM cases.[30]

### Current Treatment

Observation may be recommended depending on the degree of vision loss. In moderate to severe vision loss, stereotactic fractionated radiotherapy is a potential solution.[34] Surgical resection is not typically indicated for treatment of ONSM due to the position of these tumors, often resulting in permanent vision loss postoperatively.[35] A multidisciplinary approach with ophthalmology, neurosurgery, and radiation oncology may be beneficial.

| Cost considerations | |
| --- | --- |
| Not recommended | Lumbar puncture |
| Recommended | MRI of brain and orbit |
| Practice option | Head CT, consultation with neurosurgery and/or radiation oncology |

## Foster Kennedy Syndrome

### Etiology and Pathophysiology

Foster Kennedy syndrome is a rare syndrome traditionally characterized by an intracranial mass (typically a meningioma) causing ipsilateral optic nerve atrophy and anosmia with contralateral papilledema due to increased intracranial pressure.[33,36]

### Presenting Symptoms and Signs

Findings for this syndrome include progressive loss of vision in one eye due to nerve compression and concurrent papilledema in the opposite eye (possibly presenting as an enlarged blind spot).[37] Furthermore, personality changes may be noted if the frontal lobe is involved.[38]

### Clinical Considerations

### Diagnosis

The above presentation may warrant neuroimaging with MRI to confirm the diagnosis.[33]

### Current Treatment

The primary treatment involves surgical resection of the tumor. Radiation may also be considered. In some instances, however, postsurgical damage to the optic nerve may or may not be reversible.[39]

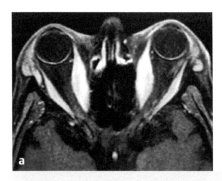 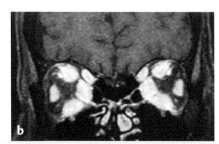 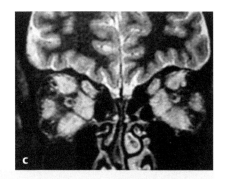

**Fig. 3.6** A 53-year-old woman with thyroid orbitopathy and bilateral proptosis. **(a)** Axial and **(b)** coronal fat-suppressed T1-weighted images show increased gadolinium contrast enhancement of asymmetrically enlarged extraocular muscles without involvement of the corresponding tendons in both orbits. **(c)** The involved muscles have fusiform shapes and have slightly high signal on coronal short tau inversion recovery (STIR). (Adapted from Meyers S, ed. Differential Diagnosis in Neuroimaging: Head and Neck. 1st ed. New York, NY: Thieme; 2016.)

| Cost considerations | |
|---|---|
| Not recommended | Lumbar puncture |
| Recommended | MRI and consultation with neurosurgery and radiation oncology |
| Practice option | – |

## Thyroid Eye Disease

### Etiology and Pathophysiology

Thyroid eye disease (TED) is an autoimmune, inflammatory, noninfectious orbitopathy associated with Grave's hyperthyroidism or Hashimoto's thyroiditis.[40,41] The etiology and pathophysiology of TED are discussed in greater detail in Chapter 4 (Cranial Nerves III, IV, VI: Ocular Motor Cranial Nerve Disorders).

### Presenting Symptoms and Signs

In some cases of TED, extraocular muscle enlargement and orbital inflammation may result in compressive optic neuropathy; optic nerve involvement has been demonstrated in 6% of TED patients.[40] Loss of color vision and peripheral vision may also be noted.[40] Other aspects of the symptoms and signs of TED, including the more common findings of eyelid retraction and exophthalmos, are discussed in greater detail in Chapter 4 (Cranial Nerves III, IV, VI: Ocular Motor Cranial Nerve Disorders).

### Clinical Considerations

#### Diagnosis

Diagnosis of TED requires thyroid hormone studies in addition to an investigation into potential thyroid autoantibodies. CT without contrast is preferred for initial imaging. For more details refer to Chapter 4 (Cranial Nerves III, IV, VI: Ocular Motor Cranial Nerve Disorders) and ▶ Fig. 3.6.

#### Current Treatment

In cases of compressive optic neuropathy, intervention may be urgent. Radiation and corticosteroids may be employed to reduce inflammation of the orbit. Furthermore, orbital

decompression surgery may be necessary in some cases.[40] Refer to Chapter 4, section 4.5.1 for a more detailed discussion of TED management.

| Cost considerations | |
|---|---|
| Not recommended | – |
| Recommended | Thyroid antibodies |
| Practice option | Orbital ultrasound, MRI, CT, steroids, radiation, decompression |

## 3.4.2 Infiltrative Optic Neuropathy

Infiltrative optic neuropathies may occur secondary to neoplasms or a variety of infectious and inflammatory etiologies. The optic nerve is most commonly infiltrated by either primary or secondary tumors. Primary tumors are significantly more prevalent. Examples of primary tumors include optic glioma (the most common), ganglioglioma, capillary hemangioma, cavernous hemangioblastoma, and melanocytomas.[36,42] Examples of secondary tumors that may infiltrate the optic nerve include metastatic carcinoma and lymphomas, leukemia, and myeloma.[36] Sarcoidosis represents the most common inflammatory and opportunistic fungi, such as *Cryptococcus*, the most common infectious etiologies.[36] Loss of visual acuity or color vision, visual scotomas, and optic disc swelling may be seen. Many cases of optic nerve infiltration, however, do not feature any signs of optic neuropathy.[36] Consider consulting with ophthalmology, oncology, or infectious disease in the treatment of these cases, depending on the underlying etiology.

## 3.5 Degenerative

### 3.5.1 Glaucoma

#### Etiology and Pathophysiology

Glaucoma is the second leading cause of blindness in the world after cataracts, defined by elevated intraocular pressure (IOP) leading to optic neuropathy. It can be divided into open-angle and closed-angle glaucoma.[43]

## Presenting Symptoms and Signs

Open-angle glaucoma is characterized by progressive peripheral vision loss prior to central visual deficits. Cupping may be a common ophthalmoscope examination finding. Patients with acute-angle closure glaucoma may present with sudden-onset, painful red eye. This represents an ophthalmologic emergency, and treatment within 24 hours to prevent irreversible blindness is recommended.[44]

## Clinical Considerations

### Diagnosis

Suspicion for glaucoma can arise if optic cup diameter is greater than 50% of the disc diameter. An IOP of greater than 20-mm $H_2O$ may warrant referral to ophthalmology.[44]

### Current Treatment

The goal of therapy is primarily to lower the IOP. The first line of therapy typically includes topical prostaglandins; multidrug therapy may be used in severe cases. The cost of generic antiglaucomatous agents is typically less than $20 per bottle. Laser therapy can also be considered before surgical intervention may be required. It may be important to consider that the use of steroids may potentially worsen glaucoma.[45]

| Cost considerations | |
| --- | --- |
| Not recommended | – |
| Recommended | IOP screening, antiglaucomatous agents |
| Practice option | Ophthalmology or glaucoma specialist |

# 3.6 Inflammatory/Autoimmune

## 3.6.1 Optic Neuritis

### Optic Neuritis Related to Multiple Sclerosis

#### Etiology and Pathophysiology

Optic neuritis, as related to multiple sclerosis (MS), is caused by demyelination of the optic nerve due to inflammation resulting in acute, monocular vision loss.[46] The condition typically develops in patients between the ages of 20 and 40 years and preferentially affects Caucasian women.[47]

#### Presenting Symptoms and Signs

Optic neuritis related to MS usually presents as monocular loss of vision.[47] Pain with eye movement and red color desaturation are also commonly seen.[47]

#### Clinical Considerations

##### Diagnosis

Diagnosis of optic neuritis related to MS is based on the newly updated 2017 McDonald criteria for MS diagnosis.[48] Patients

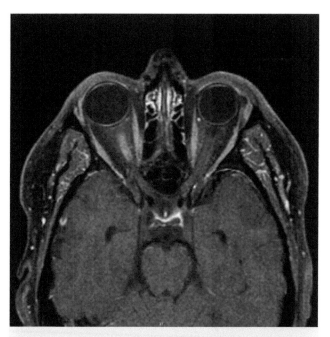

**Fig. 3.7** Acute optic neuritis. Fat-suppressed, contrast-enhanced T1-weighted TSE image angled parallel to the optic nerves demonstrates an elongated hyperintense area in the right optic nerve. (Adapted from Forsting M, Jansen O, ed. MR Neuroimaging: Brain, Spine, Peripheral Nerves. 1st ed. New York, NY: Thieme; 2016.)

suspected of having optic neuritis may undergo MRI for the brain and spinal cord with and without gadolinium.[46] If symptoms are presented in a young child (<15 y), optic neuropathy due to infection or postinfection may be considered.[49]

In cases where patients are older than 50 years, ischemic optic neuropathy such as GCA or ischemic optic neuropathy may be considered (▶ Fig. 3.7).[46]

#### Current Treatment

Treatment with intravenous methylprednisolone (IVMP) is recommended for optic neuritis.[50] More recent studies have indicated that high-dose oral corticosteroids and high-dose IV corticosteroids are bioequivalent for treatment of acute optic neuritis and may be more cost-effective and convenient for patients.[51]

| Cost considerations | |
| --- | --- |
| Not recommended | – |
| Recommended | MRI brain, orbit ± spine, neurology, steroids |
| Practice option | Lumbar puncture, neuromyelitis optica (NMO), myelin oligodendrocyte glycoprotein (MOG), IVMP or bioequivalent oral steroids |

### Optic Neuritis Related to Neuromyelitis Optica

#### Etiology and Pathophysiology

Optic neuritis related to NMO, also known as Devic's disease, is a demyelinating autoimmune disease of the CNS that selectively targets the optic nerves and the spinal cord. It is now commonly accepted that NMO is distinct from MS. The discovery of specific autoantibodies against aquaporin-4 (anti-AQP4, also known as NMO-IgG), unique to NMO and the major immunologic characteristic of the disease, has reinforced this distinction.[52]

NMO appears to be more prevalent among non-Caucasian and female populations.

## Presenting Symptoms and Signs

Patients may experience acute vision loss, either unilateral or bilateral, and may develop issues with sphincter control, paresthesias, and tetraparesis/paraparesis from transverse myelitis. A commonly affected cerebral region includes the area postrema, which may result in intractable nausea, vomiting, and hiccups.[52]

## Clinical Considerations

### Diagnosis

The most recent diagnostic criterion requires the presence of optic neuritis and acute myelitis, and the nonrequired supportive criteria include contiguous spinal cord lesion on MRI, brain MRI not meeting diagnostic criteria for MS, and anti-AQP4 seropositivity (▶Fig. 3.8).[53]

## Current Treatment

Treatment of acute attacks may include IV corticosteroids followed by plasma exchange of IVIG. Long-term immunosuppressive agents such as azathioprine, mycophenolate, and rituximab may be prescribed after the first attack. These therapies can be used alone or in tandem with oral corticosteroids for NMO maintenance treatment.[52] NMO demonstrates varying degrees of recovery within months of attack, with many patients suffering from residual disability and recurring attacks. In general, NMO has poorer prognosis and response to therapy compared to MS.[54]

| Cost considerations | |
| --- | --- |
| Not recommended | – |
| Recommended | MRI brain, orbit ± spine, NMO testing, neurology referral, steroids, immunosuppression |
| Practice option | Lumbar puncture, MOG |

## Optic Neuritis Related to NMO Spectrum Disorders

A subgroup of patients with optic neuritis have been identified as those who do not have MS and lack autoantibodies against AQP4 (present in NMO patients). These patients instead may be positive for antimyelin oligodendrocyte glycoprotein (anti-MOG) antibodies. This form of optic neuritis tends to be recurrent and is highly responsive to steroid treatment.[55] Testing for MOG antibody is currently available through the Mayo clinic.[56]

## 3.6.2 Sarcoidosis

### Etiology and Pathophysiology

Sarcoidosis is an autoimmune disorder of unknown etiology that causes an inappropriate immune system activation resulting in systemic inflammatory infiltration of tissues, granuloma formation, and fibrosis. The disorder has a higher prevalence in African Americans.[57] Among patients with neurosarcoidosis, up to one-third may have neuro-ophthalmologic manifestations.[58]

### Presenting Symptoms and Signs

Patients may present with optic neuritis, uveitis, lid inflammation, dry eyes, or other orbital diseases.[59,60]

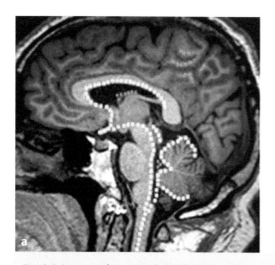
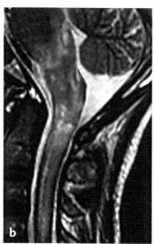
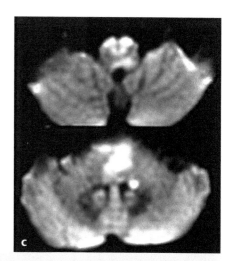

**Fig. 3.8** Neuromyelitis optica (NMO) lesions and the aquaporin-4 (AQP-4) channel distribution in the central nervous system. **(a)** Overlaid to a sagittal T1-weighted image there is a schematic view of the main distribution of AQP-4 channel protein sites in the central nervous system. There is a high concentration of AQP-4 channel protein in the central spinal cord, hypothalamus, subependymal white matter, supraoptic nuclei, optic nerve/chiasm, cerebellar cortex (*yellow spots*), ependymal cells (*blue spots*), and in the subcortical white matter (*orange spots*). **(b)** Acute NMO lesions commonly present as longitudinally extensive or transverse myelitis on sagittal T2-weighted image, commonly affecting the medulla and spinal cord junction. **(c)** Acute lesions may show restricted diffusion, with hyperintensity on diffusion-weighted imaging (axial views at the levels of medulla and pons). (Adapted from Leite C, Castillo M, ed. Diffusion Weighted and Diffusion Tensor Imaging. A Clinical Guide. 1st ed. Stuttgart: Thieme; 2015.)

## Clinical Considerations

### Diagnosis

Definitive diagnosis of sarcoidosis may require a tissue biopsy. Patients may also present with elevated serum angiotensin converting enzyme (ACE), a test that is 73% sensitive and 83% specific. Specificity of ACE testing may be increased in combination with whole-body gallium scanning.[61] ACE levels are also known to increase in the cerebrospinal fluid (CSF) but has poor sensitivity.[62]

### Current Treatment

Treatment for sarcoidosis-related optic neuropathy typically involves use of high-dose corticosteroids, either oral or IV. In the case of repeated relapses, an additional immunosuppressive agent may be added.[57] Referral to ophthalmology and rheumatology could be considered for management.

## 3.6.3 Other

Additional inflammatory diseases may have potential for involvement of the optic nerve, particularly autoimmune vasculitis. These vasculitides include but are not limited to granulomatosis with polyangiitis (GPA), eosinophilic GPA (EGPA), polyarteritis nodosa (PAN), and Behcet's disease. Serological testing may be useful for the diagnosis of vasculitis. For these conditions, consider a multidisciplinary approach with rheumatology in addition to ophthalmology.

# 3.7 Hereditary Optic Neuropathy

## 3.7.1 Dominant (Kjer) Optic Atrophy

### Etiology and Pathophysiology

Dominant optic atrophy (DOA) is the most common hereditary optic atrophy, most often caused by a mutation in the *OPA1* gene on chromosome 3.[63] The disease exhibits autosomal dominant transmission with near total penetrance and highly variable expressivity.[64]

### Presenting Symptoms and Signs

DOA is characterized by insidious onset of central vision loss and optic atrophy often occurring in early childhood.[63]

### Clinical Considerations

### Diagnosis

Diagnosis of DOA is based on clinical findings such as age and mode of onset, visual acuity changes, disc pallor, and autosomal dominant pattern of inheritance, among others.[63]

Genetic analysis of the *OPA1* gene can serve as a definitive diagnosis for DOA. If no significant mutation or deletion is found, testing for the full-length mitochondrial genome may be considered. Identification of mutation is recommended for genetic counseling.[65]

### Current Treatment

No specific treatment currently exists, but low-vision aids may be helpful in cases of severe visual acuity loss. Avoidance of tobacco, alcohol, and other drugs and medications that can interfere with mitochondrial metabolism can also be considered.[65]

| Cost considerations | |
| --- | --- |
| Not recommended | – |
| Recommended | Family history |
| Practice option | Genetic testing |

## 3.7.2 Leber Hereditary Optic Neuropathy

### Etiology and Pathophysiology

Leber hereditary optic neuropathy (LHON) is the most common mitochondrial disorder causing optic neuropathy. It is transmitted via maternal inheritance with incomplete penetrance. Environmental factors, namely, those that cause an increase in reactive oxygen species, could potentially contribute to disease development.[60]

### Presenting Symptoms and Signs

LHON typically presents in young adult males with bilateral, painless, sequential subacute vision loss.[66]

### Clinical Considerations

### Diagnosis

Diagnosis of LHON can be established together with genetic testing yielding identification of one of the three common mtDNA (mitochondrial DNA) pathogenic variants. The most common point mutation in LHON is at G11778A, followed by mutations at T14484C and G3460A, accounting for 95% of all cases.[60]

### Current Treatment

Idebenone has been shown to be beneficial in preventing further visual impairment and promotes visual recovery in some cases; however, effectiveness is potentially dose dependent.[67,68] However, this drug is currently only approved for use in Europe and not within the United States or Canada for treatment of LHON (Canadian Institutes of Health Research, https://www.drugbank.ca/drugs/DB09081). Consider cautioning patients to avoid drugs and medications that may have mitochondrial toxicity, including alcohol, tobacco, and some medications. Some suggested general mitochondrial therapies; however, there is minimal evidence that these therapies are effective in management of the disease.[69]

| Cost considerations | |
| --- | --- |
| Not recommended | – |
| Recommended | Avoidance of mitochondrial irritants |
| Practice option | Genetic testing, mitochondrial cocktail |

## 3.8 Congenital Optic Disc Abnormalities

Congenital optic disc anomalies are defined as abnormalities in the anatomy or appearance of the optic disc and retina. The optic disc is typically round and pink in color, approximately 1.5 mm in diameter with a central depression (the cup).[70] Optic disc drusen, optic disc hypoplasia, megalopapilla, tilted disc syndrome, and morning glory syndrome are among some of the congenital optic disc anomalies encountered. Ophthalmology referral and routine follow-up are often recommended (►Fig. 3.9 and ►Fig. 3.10).

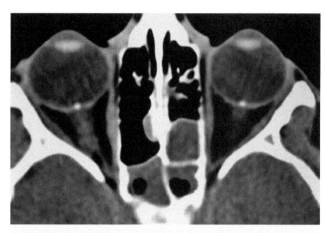

**Fig. 3.9** Axial CT shows small, focal, rounded, calcified zones at both optic disc heads representing bilateral optic nerve head drusens. (Adapted from Meyers S, ed. Differential Diagnosis in Neuroimaging: Head and Neck. 1st ed. New York, NY: Thieme; 2016.)

## 3.9 Traumatic

### 3.9.1 Traumatic Optic Neuropathy

#### Etiology and Pathophysiology

Traumatic optic neuropathy (TrON) is an uncommon cause of vision loss after blunt or penetrating injury. Direct TrON refers to a direct penetrating injury to the optic nerve. This is less common than indirect TrON, referring to injury to the optic nerve as a result of concussive force to the head causing contusion of the nerve in the optic canal.[71] The most common injury mechanisms include motor vehicle accident, assault, bike accident, and falling.[72]

#### Presenting Symptoms and Signs

Patients suffering from TrON may present with an array of ophthalmologic findings as well as neuro-ophthalmologic signs including decreased vision, decreased color vision, visual field defects, and an afferent pupillary defect.[71]

#### Clinical Considerations

##### Diagnosis

CT through the orbit and optic canal may be considered.[71]

##### Current Treatment

For direct TrON, prognosis is poor and severe visual loss is probable. For indirect TrON, there is a 40 to 60% visual recovery rate, with baseline visual acuity being an important prognostic marker.[42] While the use of "mega" dose corticosteroids was

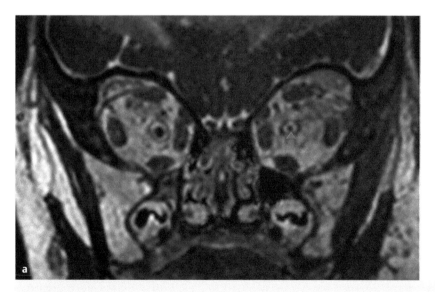
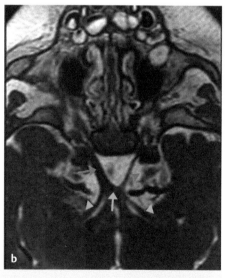

**Fig. 3.10** Optic nerve hypoplasia. **(a)** Coronal image made with fast imaging employing steady-state acquisition (FIESTA) of the head of a 1-year-old boy shows an asymmetrically decreased volume of the orbital segment of the left optic nerve (*red arrowhead*), representing optic nerve hypoplasia. **(b)** Axial oblique FIESTA image of the optic chiasm confirms a diminutive caliber of the left optic nerve (*red arrowhead*) and a normal caliber of the right optic nerve (*red arrow*). Posterior to the chiasm (*green arrow*), there is a symmetrically smaller-than-expected volume of the optic tracts (*green arrowheads*). No etiology was identified for the hypoplasia in this patient. (Adapted from Choudhri A, ed. Pediatric Neuroradiology. Clinical Practice Essentials. 1st edition. Stuttgart: Thieme; 2016.)

supported in the past for treatment of TrON, this was later disproven.[72] The 2004 CRASH trial depicted an increased mortality in patients with a Glasgow Coma Score (GCS) less than 14 who received high-dose corticosteroids.[73]

Surgical intervention in direct TrON may be beneficial for removal of the insult, but has not been shown to be beneficial for indirect TrON.[72]

| Cost considerations | |
| --- | --- |
| Not recommended | Steroids if GCS ≤ 14 |
| Recommended | CT of orbit and optic canal |
| Practice option | – |

# 3.10 Metabolic

## 3.10.1 Toxic Optic Neuropathy and Nutritional Optic Neuropathy

### Etiology and Pathophysiology

Toxic optic neuropathy (TxON) is a collection of disorders caused by damage to the optic nerve from toxins, including medications, heavy metals, organic solvents (e.g., benzene and toluene), methanol, carbon dioxide, and tobacco.[74]

The optic nerve is susceptible to damage from a variety of drugs, including amiodarone, PDE5 inhibitors, antituberculosis drugs (ethambutol and isoniazid), some antimicrobial agents (linezolid, ciprofloxacin, cimetidine, and chloramphenicol), antiepileptic drugs (vigabatrin), disulfiram, halogenated hydroquinolines (amebicidal medications), antimetabolites (e.g., methotrexate, cisplatin, carboplatin, vincristine, and cyclosporin), tamoxifen, and sildenafil.[74]

Heavy metal toxicity may also contribute to TxON.[75] Vitamin B and folate deficiencies can result in the pathogenesis of optic neuropathy, especially in the presence of toxic exposure.[74]

### Presenting Symptoms and Signs

Patients with TxON typically present with bilateral, painless, progressive decline of visual acuity. The optic nerve may be normal, swollen, or hyperemic in early stages, and optic atrophy may develop as the disease progresses.[75]

### Clinical Considerations

#### Diagnosis

Inquiring about diet, drug/toxin exposure, substance use, and occupation may be beneficial.[75] Neuroimaging is recommended to rule out alternative causes of pathology.

#### Current Treatment

In most cases of nutritional optic neuropathy, vision can be partially or fully restored with vitamin B supplements.[74] Treatment for TxON resulting from drug or chemical toxicity depends on the insulting agent in question.

| Cost considerations | |
| --- | --- |
| Not recommended | – |
| Recommended | – |
| Practice option | MRI, toxin and vitamin level testing, removal toxic agent, replacement of deficiency |

# 3.11 Idiopathic

## 3.11.1 Idiopathic Intracranial Hypertension (Pseudotumor Cerebri)

### Etiology and Pathophysiology

Idiopathic intracranial hypertension (IIH), previously known as pseudotumor cerebri (PTC), is a syndrome featuring raised intracranial pressure without intracranial ventriculomegaly, tumor, or mass.[76] CSF contents should be normal with the exception of an elevated opening pressure. IIH primarily affects obese women of childbearing age.[77]

### Presenting Symptoms and Signs

Headache is the most common presenting symptom of IIH in adults. Other common symptoms include transient visual obscurations, pulsatile tinnitus, and horizontal diplopia.[78] The most notable sign in IIH patients is bilateral papilledema, which may be present in the majority of cases.[77]

### Clinical Considerations

#### Diagnosis

MRI, MR venography (MRV), and lumbar puncture could be considered to fulfill the modified Dandy criteria (▶Fig. 3.11).

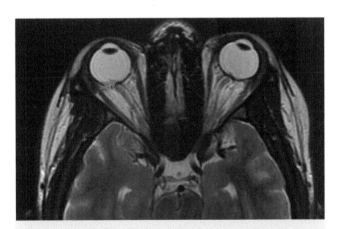

**Fig. 3.11** Papilledema. Axial T2 weighted image of the anterior head of a 16-year-old girl with severe headaches and pseudotumor cerebri shows elevation of the optic nerve head (*blue arrow*), representing the correlate on magnetic resonance imaging of elevation/papilledema of the head of the optic nerve. There is also prominence of cerebrospinal fluid within the optic nerve sheaths (*blue arrowhead*), which with papilledema is suggestive of elevated intracranial pressure. (Adapted from Choudhri A, ed. Pediatric Neuroradiology. Clinical Practice Essentials. 1st edition. Stuttgart: Thieme; 2016.)

## Current Treatment

Dietary modifications and weight loss are the first-line treatment.[77] Diuretics, particularly carbonic anhydrase inhibitors such as acetazolamide (studied in a clinical trial) or less commonly methazolamide, have been used. Topiramate possesses carbonic anhydrase-inhibiting properties and may be considered if acetazolamide fails. Furosemide is another diuretic occasionally used as a second-line treatment.[78]

Surgical intervention may be indicated for visual loss that is attributed to papilledema and occurs after failure of maximal medical therapy. Acute, fulminant IIH with visual loss may need emergent surgical intervention (e.g., optic nerve sheath fenestration [ONSF] and/or ventriculoperitoneal [VP] or lumboperitoneal [LP] shunt) Referral to neurosurgery may be suggested for a VP or LP shunt. For ONSF, referral to an oculoplastic surgeon may be considered.[78]

### Cost considerations

| | |
| --- | --- |
| Not recommended | – |
| Recommended | MRI of brain and orbit, MRV of cerebral sinus, lumbar puncture |
| Practice option | Ultrasound, ONSF, VP/LP shunt |

## 3.12 Conclusion

In general, the diagnosis of optic neuropathy requires evaluation with an ophthalmic specialist. Clinicians should be aware of the common causes of optic neuropathy, however, including ischemic, demyelinating, inflammatory, traumatic, hereditary, and infectious etiologies.

## References

[1] Tamhankar M, Nicholas J. Nonarteritic anterior ischemic optic neuropathy: Clinical features and diagnosis. Waltham, MA:UpToDate; 2016

[2] Fasler K, Traber GL, Jaggi GP, Landau K. Amiodarone-associated optic neuropathy: a clinical criteria-based diagnosis? Neuroophthalmology 2017;42(1):2–10

[3] Atkins EJ, Bruce BB, Newman NJ, Biousse V. Treatment of nonarteritic anterior ischemic optic neuropathy. Surv Ophthalmol 2010;55(1):47–63

[4] De Smit E, O'Sullivan E, Mackey DA, Hewitt AW. Giant cell arteritis: ophthalmic manifestations of a systemic disease. Graefes Arch Clin Exp Ophthalmol 2016;254(12):2291–2306

[5] Kawasaki A, Purvin V. Giant cell arteritis: an updated review. Acta Ophthalmol 2009;87(1):13–32

[6] Pineles S, Kozak A, Burkat C, Marcet M. Giant cell arteritis. EyeWiki. San Francisco, CA: American Academy of Ophthalmology; 2017

[7] Lee AW, Chen C, Cugati S. Temporal arteritis. Neurol Clin Pract 2014;4(2):106–113

[8] Hayreh SS. Posterior ischaemic optic neuropathy: clinical features, pathogenesis, and management. Eye (Lond) 2004;18(11):1188–1206

[9] Sadda SR, Nee M, Miller NR, Biousse V, Newman NJ, Kouzis A. Clinical spectrum of posterior ischemic optic neuropathy. Am J Ophthalmol 2001;132(5):743–750

[10] Bhatti MT, Tabandeh H. Giant cell arteritis: diagnosis and management. Curr Opin Ophthalmol 2001;12(6):393–399

[11] Leuchten N, Aringer M. Tocilizumab in the treatment of giant cell arteritis. Immunotherapy 2018;10(6):465–472

[12] Tocilizumab (Actemra): Adult patients with moderately to severely active rheumatoid arthritis [Internet]. Ottawa (ON): Canadian agency for drugs and technologies in health; 2015 Aug. Available from: https://www.ncbi.nlm.nih.gov/books/NBK349521/

[13] Tamhankar M, Nicholas JV. Posterior Ischemic Optic Neuropathy. UpToDate. Waltham, MA: UpToDate; 2017

[14] Karaca M, Coban E, Ozdem S, Unal M, Salim O, Yucel O. The association between endothelial dysfunction and hypertensive retinopathy in essential hypertension. Med Sci Monit 2014;20:78–82

[15] Aissopou EK, Papathanassiou M, Nasothimiou EG, et al. The Keith-Wagener-Barker and Mitchell-Wong grading systems for hypertensive retinopathy: association with target organ damage in individuals below 55 years. J Hypertens 2015;33(11):2303–2309

[16] Ong YT, Wong TY, Klein R, et al. Hypertensive retinopathy and risk of stroke. Hypertension 2013;62(4):706–711

[17] Harjasouliha A, Raiji V, Garcia Gonzalez JM. Review of hypertensive retinopathy. Dis Mon 2017;63(3):63–69

[18] Slagle WS, Musick AN, Eckermann DR. Diabetic papillopathy and its relation to optic nerve ischemia. Optom Vis Sci 2009;86(4):e395–e403

[19] Tamhankar M, Nicholas J. Diabetic papillopathy. In: Wilterdink J, ed. UpToDate. Waltham, MA: UpToDate; 2016

[20] Spach D, Kaplan S. Microbiology, epidemiology, clinical manifestations, and diagnosis of cat scratch disease. In: Mitty J, ed. UpToDate. Waltham, MA: UpToDate; 2017

[21] Moradi A, Salek S, Daniel E, et al. Clinical features and incidence rates of ocular complications in patients with ocular syphilis. Am J Ophthalmol 2015;159(2):334–343

[22] Lee SY, Cheng V, Rodger D, Rao N. Clinical and laboratory characteristics of ocular syphilis: a new face in the era of HIV co-infection. J Ophthalmic Inflamm Infect 2015;5(1):56

[23] Lozano A, Rodriguez-Garcia A, Feldman B. Lyme disease. EyeWiki. San Francisco, CA: American Academy of Ophthalmology

[24] Rush JA, Younge BR, Campbell RJ, MacCarty CS. Optic glioma. Long-term follow-up of 85 histopathologically verified cases. Ophthalmology 1982;89(11):1213–1219

[25] Davis JL. Ocular syphilis. Curr Opin Ophthalmol 2014;25(6):513–518

[26] Spach D, Kaplan S. Treatment of cat scratch disease. In: Mitty J, ed. UpToDate. Waltham, MA: UpToDate; 2018

[27] Hu L. Treatment of Lyme disease. In: Mitty J, ed. UpToDate. Waltham, MA: UpToDate; 2017

[28] Miller NR. Primary tumours of the optic nerve and its sheath. Eye (Lond) 2004;18(11):1026–1037

[29] Recht L. Optic pathway glioma. In: Eichler A, ed. UpToDate. Waltham, MA: UpToDate; 2017

[30] O'Brien J, Pineles S. Optic Nerve Sheath Meningioma. In: O'Brien J, ed. EyeWiki. San Francisco, CA: American Academy of Ophthalmology; 2015

[31] Shapey J, Sabin HI, Danesh-Meyer HV, Kaye AH. Diagnosis and management of optic nerve sheath meningiomas. J Clin Neurosci 2013;20(8):1045–1056

[32] Najem K, Margolin E. Meningioma, Optic Nerve Sheath. Treasure Island, FL: StatPearls; 2018

[33] Lai AT, Chiu SL, Lin IC, Sanders M. Foster Kennedy syndrome: now and then. J Neuroophthalmol 2014;34(1):92–94

[34] Eddleman CS, Liu JK. Optic nerve sheath meningioma: current diagnosis and treatment. Neurosurg Focus 2007;23(5):E4

[35] Schick U, Dott U, Hassler W. Surgical management of meningiomas involving the optic nerve sheath. J Neurosurg 2004;101(6):951–959

[36] Hoyt Wa. Compressive and infiltrative optic neuropathies In: Miller N, Newman N, Biousse V, Kerrison J, eds. Walsh & Hoyt's Clinical Neuro-Ophthalmology. Philadelphia, PA: Lippincott Williams & Wilkins; 2005

[37] Pastora-Salvador N, Peralta-Calvo J. Foster Kennedy syndrome: papilledema in one eye with optic atrophy in the other eye. CMAJ 2011;183(18):2135

[38] Lotfipour S, Chiles K, Kahn JA, Bey T, Rudkin S. An unusual presentation of subfrontal meningioma: a case report and literature review for Foster Kennedy syndrome. Intern Emerg Med 2011;6(3):267–269

[39] Parafita-Fernández A, Sampil M, Cores C, Cores FJ, Viso E. Foster Kennedy syndrome: an atypical presentation. Optom Vis Sci 2015;92(12):e425–e430

[40] Durairaj VD. Clinical perspectives of thyroid eye disease. Am J Med 2006;119(12):1027–1028

[41] Kumari R, Chandra Saha B. Advances in the management of thyroid eye diseases: an overview. Int Ophthalmol 2017

[42] Yu-Wai-Man P. Traumatic optic neuropathy: clinical features and management issues. Taiwan J Ophthalmol 2015;5(1):3–8

[43] Kingman S. Glaucoma is second leading cause of blindness globally. Bull World Health Organ 2004;82(11):887–888

[44] Jacobs D. Open-angle glaucoma: epidemiology, clinical presentation, and diagnosis. In: Sullivan D, ed. UpToDate. Waltham, MA: UpToDate; 2018

[45] Jacobs D. Open-angle glaucoma: treatment. In: Sullivan D, ed. UpToDate. Waltham, MA: UpToDate; 2018

[46] Osborne B, Balcer LJ. Optic neuritis: pathophysiology, clinical features, and diagnosis. In: Wilterdink J, ed. Waltham, MA: UpToDate; 2016

[47] Optic Neuritis Study Group. The clinical profile of optic neuritis. Experience of the optic neuritis treatment trial. Arch Ophthalmol 1991;109(12): 1673–1678

[48] Thompson AJ, Banwell BL, Barkhof F, et al. Diagnosis of multiple sclerosis: 2017 revisions of the McDonald criteria. Lancet Neurol 2018;17(2):162–173

[49] Boomer JA, Siatkowski RM. Optic neuritis in adults and children. Semin Ophthalmol 2003;18(4):174–180

[50] Osborne B, Balcer LJ. Optic neuritis: prognosis and treatment. In: Wilterdink J, ed. UpToDate. Waltham, MA: UpToDate;. 2018

[51] Morrow SA, Fraser JA, Day C, et al. Effect of treating acute optic neuritis with bioequivalent oral vs intravenous corticosteroids: a randomized clinical trial. JAMA Neurol 2018;75(6):690–696

[52] Pereira WL, Reiche EM, Kallaur AP, Kaimen-Maciel DR. Epidemiological, clinical, and immunological characteristics of neuromyelitis optica: a review. J Neurol Sci 2015;355(1–2):7–17

[53] National Multiple Sclerosis Society. Symptoms and Diagnosis of NMO. New York, NY: National Multiple Sclerosis Society; 2018

[54] Drori T, Chapman J. Diagnosis and classification of neuromyelitis optica (Devic's syndrome). Autoimmun Rev 2014;13(4–5):531–533

[55] Chalmoukou K, Alexopoulos H, Akrivou S, Stathopoulos P, Reindl M, Dalakas MC. Anti-MOG antibodies are frequently associated with steroid-sensitive recurrent optic neuritis. Neurol Neuroimmunol Neuroinflamm 2015;2(4):e131

[56] Mayo Clinic Mayo Medical Laboratories. Myelin Oligodendrocyte Glycoprotein (MOGIgG1) Fluorescence-Activated Cell Sorting (FACS) Assay, Serum. Rochester, MN: Mayo Clinic Mayo Medical Laboratories; 2018

[57] Kidd DP, Burton BJ, Graham EM, Plant GT. Optic neuropathy associated with systemic sarcoidosis. Neurol Neuroimmunol Neuroinflamm 2016;3(5):e270

[58] Baughman RP, Weiss KL, Golnik KC. Neuro-ophthalmic sarcoidosis. Eye Brain 2012;4:13–25

[59] Rosenbaum J. Uveitis: etiology, clinical manifestations, and diagnosis. In: Trobe J, Romain P, eds. UpToDate. Waltham, MA: UpToDate; 2017

[60] Rasool N, Lessell S, Cestari DM. Leber hereditary optic neuropathy: bringing the lab to the clinic. Semin Ophthalmol 2016;31(1–2):107–116

[61] Pillai P, Hossain K. Sarcoid uveitis. EyeWiki. San Francisco, CA: American Academy of Ophthalmology; 2019

[62] Khoury J, Wellik KE, Demaerschalk BM, Wingerchuk DM. Cerebrospinal fluid angiotensin-converting enzyme for diagnosis of central nervous system sarcoidosis. Neurologist 2009;15(2):108–111

[63] Kjer B, Eiberg H, Kjer P, Rosenberg T. Dominant optic atrophy mapped to chromosome 3q region. II. Clinical and epidemiological aspects. Acta Ophthalmol Scand 1996;74(1):3–7

[64] Eiberg H, Kjer B, Kjer P, Rosenberg T. Dominant optic atrophy (OPA1) mapped to chromosome 3q region. I. Linkage analysis. Hum Mol Genet 1994;3(6):977–980

[65] Lenaers G, Hamel C, Delettre C, et al. Dominant optic atrophy. Orphanet J Rare Dis 2012;7:46

[66] Yu-Wai-Man P, Chinnery PF. Leber hereditary optic neuropathy. In: Adam MP, Ardinger HH, Pagon RA, et al, eds. GeneReviews((R)). Seattle, WA: University of Washington; 1993

[67] Lyseng-Williamson KA. Idebenone: a review in Leber's hereditary optic neuropathy. Drugs 2016;76(7):805–813

[68] Chen J, Ren M, Du Y. Ineffectiveness of low-dosage Idebenone on Chinese patients with Leber's hereditary optic neuropathy: report of two cases. Kuwait Med J 2018;50(1):95–99

[69] Newman NJ. Treatment of Leber hereditary optic neuropathy. Brain 2011;134(Pt 9):2447–2450

[70] Golnik KC. Congenital anomalies and acquired abnormalities of the optic nerve. In: Paysse E, Armsby C, eds. UpToDate. Waltham, MA: UpToDate; 2017

[71] Gardiner M. Overview of eye injuries in the emergency department. In: Torrey S, Wiley J, eds. UpToDate. Waltham, MA: UpToDate; 2017

[72] Levin LA, Beck RW, Joseph MP, Seiff S, Kraker R. The treatment of traumatic optic neuropathy: the International Optic Nerve Trauma Study. Ophthalmology 1999;106(7):1268–1277

[73] Roberts I, Yates D, Sandercock P, et al; CRASH trial collaborators. Effect of intravenous corticosteroids on death within 14 days in 10008 adults with clinically significant head injury (MRC CRASH trial): randomised placebo-controlled trial. Lancet 2004;364(9442):1321–1328

[74] Grzybowski A, Zülsdorff M, Wilhelm H, Tonagel F. Toxic optic neuropathies: an updated review. Acta Ophthalmol 2015;93(5):402–410

[75] Altiparmak UE. Toxic optic neuropathies. Curr Opin Ophthalmol 2013; 24(6):534–539

[76] McGeeney BE, Friedman DI. Pseudotumor cerebri pathophysiology. Headache 2014;54(3):445–458

[77] Spennato P, Ruggiero C, Parlato RS, et al. Pseudotumor cerebri. Childs Nerv Syst 2011;27(2):215–235

[78] Friedman DI. The pseudotumor cerebri syndrome. Neurol Clin 2014; 32(2):363–396

# 4 Cranial Nerves III, IV, VI: Ocular Motor Cranial Nerve Disorders

*Michael Duan, Junru Yan, Aroucha Vickers, Claudia M. Prospero Ponce, and Andrew G. Lee*

**Abstract**

This chapter discusses ocular motor cranial nerve disorders (i.e., cranial nerves [CN] III, IV, and VI). Special attention will be given to pertinent patient presentations, suggestions regarding diagnosis and referral, and details regarding overall cost considerations. The evaluation of diplopia in general, however, is beyond the scope of this chapter. The initial evaluation for an ocular motor cranial neuropathy begins with a complete history and physical examination. Patients with a neurologically nonisolated ocular motor cranial neuropathy (e.g., systemic or constitutional symptoms or signs or localizing neurologic signs) should undergo directed laboratory and imaging evaluations. Patients with neurologically isolated ocular motor cranial neuropathy may require directed neuroimaging (e.g., preferably magnetic resonance imaging [MRI] of the brain and orbit with and without gadolinium), but other imaging modalities may be necessary (e.g., computed tomography [CT] scans or orbital ultrasound) for patients who cannot undergo MRI or for whom specific indications exist for alternative imaging (e.g., thyroid eye disease, sinus disease). Other screening laboratory studies or additional diagnostic modalities (e.g., positron emission tomography [PET] scan or CT of other areas of the body, e.g., chest, abdomen, and pelvis) may be necessary to look for alternative diagnoses (e.g., sarcoid, lymphoma) or sources for potential diagnostic biopsy. The estimated costs for some of these diagnostic tests and procedures are described in the text.

*Keywords:* diplopia, strabismus, phoria, oscillopsia, ophthalmoplegia, cranial neuropathy, oculomotor nerve, trochlear nerve, abducens nerve

## 4.1 General Considerations

### 4.1.1 Diplopia

Diplopia, defined as double vision or the simultaneous perception of two relatively displaced images, is one of the most common symptoms for which patients may seek ophthalmic care. Diplopia can be monocular or binocular: binocular diplopia disappears with the occlusion of one eye, while monocular diplopia persists. Monocular diplopia typically stems from optical and ocular causes such as glasses, contact lenses, cataracts, and corneal disease, while binocular diplopia is more often associated with brain, nerve, or muscle pathologies.[1] In general, the evaluation of monocular diplopia is limited to optical corrections and does not require additional laboratory testing or neuroimaging.

It is important to distinguish paretic etiologies of diplopia, which can be neurogenic in nature, from restrictive etiologies of diplopia involving some mechanical obstruction of the extraocular muscles (EOMs). This chapter is primarily concerned with ocular motor dysfunction resulting from neurogenic (i.e., ocular motor cranial neuropathy) paresis, although some important restrictive etiologies are also discussed.

Oculomotor disorders may be broadly categorized as conditions of the supranuclear, nuclear, or infranuclear regions.

Supranuclear disorders involve any structure upstream of the cranial nerve nucleus (CNN), including the cerebral cortex and subcortex. Nuclear disorders are the result of lesions to the CNN in the brainstem. Infranuclear disorders include diseases of the peripheral cranial nerves (CNs) themselves, in addition to disease affecting the neuromuscular junction or muscles. This chapter is primarily concerned with nuclear and infranuclear disorders.

### 4.1.2 Cranial Nerve III, IV, and VI Palsy

The classical presentation of each CN palsy in isolation will be reviewed. In a CN III (oculomotor nerve) palsy, the affected eye can be deviated downward (hypotropia) and outward (exotropia); this can be accompanied by partial or complete ptosis and possibly pupillary dilation (anisocoria). In a CN IV (trochlear nerve) palsy, the affected eye may be extorted with a small-angle ipsilateral hypertropia (HT). Patients with CN IV palsy will classically develop a worsening HT in contralateral gaze and ipsilateral head tilt. The patient may tilt their head away from the affected side so as to correct this misalignment. In a CN VI (abducens nerve) palsy, the affected eye may be deviated inward (esotropia) and can demonstrate a partial or complete abduction deficit (▶Fig. 4.1, ▶Fig. 4.2 and ▶Fig. 4.3).[1] The most common etiologies of these neurologically isolated ocular motor cranial neuropathies are ischemic small vessel infarcts. Compressive lesions including intracranial aneurysm (predominantly posterior communicating artery aneurysm producing a pupil-involved CN III palsy), trauma (predominantly CN IV but also CN VI), and neoplasm (one or more CNs may be involved) can produce ocular motor CN-related diplopia. Even in the post-neuroimaging era, over a quarter of isolated ocular motor cranial neuropathies remain "idiopathic" in origin.[1] The most common etiologies for ocular motor cranial neuropathy will be discussed in more detail later. Also, please refer to section 3.1, Initial Evaluation and General Considerations. ▶Table 4.1. summarizes estimated costs for some diagnostic tests and procedures that may be indicated in the workup of ocular motor cranial palsy.

**Table 4.1** Medicare allowables (2018) of some common and possible procedures in testing for ocular motor disorders

| Test (CPT code) | Cost: Medicare allowables ($) |
| --- | --- |
| Brain MRI (70553) | 400 |
| Head MRA with and without dye (70546) | 510 |
| Head CT with and without contrast (70470) | 201 |
| CT cerebral angiography (73706) | 375 |
| MRI orbit with and without contrast (70543) | 460 |
| Orbital ultrasound (76510) | 150 per eye |
| Lumbar puncture (62270) | 180 |
| Cerebral angiography (36224) | 2,200 |

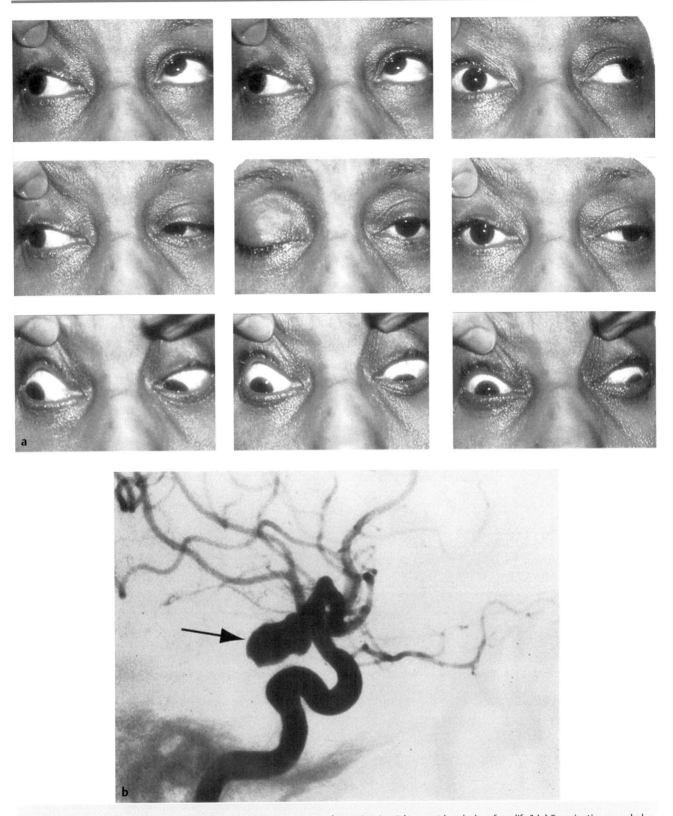

**Fig. 4.1** Complete third nerve palsy. This 62-year-old woman reported experiencing "the worst headache of my life." (**a**) Examination revealed complete ptosis on the right; a nonreactive, dilated pupil; and severely limited extraocular movement except for abduction. (**b**) Lateral view of a cerebral angiogram demonstrated a posterior communicating artery aneurysm (*arrow*). (Reproduced with permission from American Academy of Ophthalmology.)

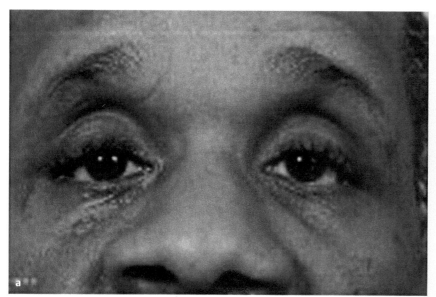

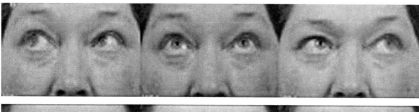

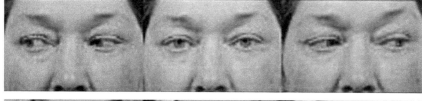

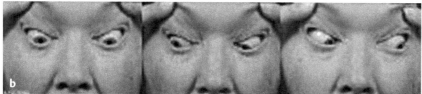

**Fig. 4.2** CN IV palsy. **(a)** Traumatic left fourth nerve palsy showing left hypertropia in primary gaze. **(b)** Patient with left fourth nerve palsy. Note the left eye hypertropia and the limitation of the left eye to look down compared with the right eye. (Adapted from Sekhar L, Fessler R, ed. Atlas of Neurosurgical Techniques: Brain. Vol. 2. 2nd ed. New York, NY: Thieme; 2015.)

## 4.2 Vascular

### 4.2.1 Stroke

#### Etiology and Pathophysiology

Stroke is an acute injury to the brain caused by either ischemia or hemorrhage. Ischemic strokes can be further divided by etiology into thrombosis, embolism, thromboembolism, and systemic hypoperfusion.[2] Depending on the location of the stroke, patients may present with very specific CN findings as described below.[1]

#### Presenting Symptoms and Signs

The presenting symptoms and signs of a stroke largely depend on the location of the pathology, which may include the cortex, the brainstem, or the peripheral nerve:

- **Cortical stroke** affecting the frontal eye field regions may result in gaze palsies causing the eye to deviate toward the source of the lesion.[3]

- **Brainstem lesions** affecting the midbrain may lead CN III or CN IV nuclear or fascicular palsy, while pontine lesions may present with CN VI palsy. Concurrent neurological deficits based on the location of the lesions may occur.
- **Peripheral ocular motor cranial mononeuropathies** are commonly accepted to be caused by microvascular ischemia. Specific clinical symptoms depend on the nerve affected. Some of the common etiologies, such as diabetic neuropathy, are discussed in greater detail in the following sections.[4]

#### Clinical Decisions

#### Diagnosis

Diagnosis of an acute cortical or brainstem stroke includes stabilization of vital signs, especially blood pressure, breathing, and body temperature. A noncontrast CT is typically ordered, which is highly sensitive for hemorrhage detection. If a subarachnoid hemorrhage (SAH) is suspected but not present on

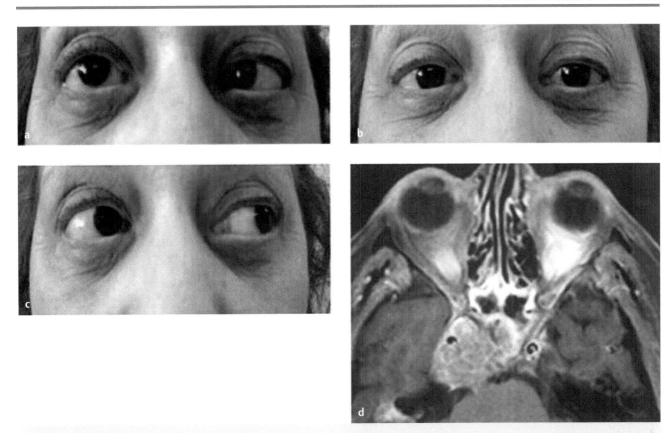

**Fig. 4.3** **(a–c)** Example of sixth nerve examination. Note the palsy of the right abducens nerve. **(d)** Magnetic resonance imaging demonstrates tumor involving the right cavernous sinus. (Adapted from Stamm A, ed. Transnasal Endoscopic Skull Base and Brain Surgery: Tips and Pearls. 1st ed. New York, NY: Thieme; 2011.)

CT, a lumbar puncture (LP) may be ordered. MRI with and without contrast can also be considered. Consultation with neurology is often requested to assist with the diagnosis.[5]

### Current Treatment

Although an eyepatch may be worn for symptomatic relief of diplopia, the main concern is differentiating small vessel ischemic, neurologically isolated CN palsy from brainstem infarct. The brainstem stroke is typically defined by other neurologic symptoms and signs that localize to the brainstem (i.e., "the company it keeps"). Typically, diplopia caused by small vessel ischemic strokes is expected to improve over time. Brainstem infarction, however, has a variable prognosis depending on severity and etiology (e.g., hemorrhage). Treatment for the different types of stroke depends on the etiology of the stroke. In general, admission to the hospital and emergent consultation with neurologists, neurosurgeons, interventionalists, and intensivists are often considered based on time of symptoms onset of a brainstem infarct.

| Cost considerations for evaluation of non-isolated or non-vasculopathic isolated ocular motor cranial neuropathy | |
| --- | --- |
| Recommended | Initial head CT followed by MRI with and without contrast and CTA/ MR angiography (MRA), and hospital admission and stroke consultation in acute brainstem strokes |
| Practice option | Conventional catheter angiography may be necessary in some cases (especially pupil involved third nerve palsy) |

## 4.2.2 Aneurysm

### Etiology and Pathophysiology

One of the most common causes of an acute, neurologically isolated CN III palsy is due to compression by an expanding aneurysm, typically of the posterior communicating artery.[6] These aneurysms are at risk of rupturing, resulting in SAH within hours or days of initial onset of symptoms.[7]

### Presenting Symptoms and Signs

Patients with SAH may present with the worst headache of their life, ptosis, and ophthalmoplegia. The pupil of the affected eye may be dilated.[6]

### Clinical Decisions

### Diagnosis

In general, patients with an acute, painful, CN III palsy with or without pupil involvement should undergo a CT head without contrast emergently. A contrast CTA should be performed in the acute setting in cases where aneurysm is suspected. In patients with an unexplained nonaneurysmal CN III palsy, cranial MRI and MRA may still be necessary despite negative CT/CTA to exclude nonaneurysmal causes of CN III palsy. Patients with a high suspicion for aneurysm, despite a negative CT/CTA and MRI/MRA, may still require standard catheter angiography.[6]

## Current Treatment

Patients with acute symptomatic aneurysms causing a CN III palsy should be admitted to the hospital. Surgical clipping and endovascular coiling are commonly used techniques for treatment of aneurysms.[8] Diplopia and ptosis may variably recover over time after treatment. If diplopia or ptosis are persistent, prisms or strabismus surgery and/or ptosis repair may be employed.[7]

| Cost considerations | |
| --- | --- |
| Not recommended | Pupil-involved, painful CN III palsy do not require evaluation for myasthenia gravis |
| Recommended | CT head without contrast initially followed by contrast CTA in the acute setting. MRI and MRA with and without contrast should be considered for nonaneurysmal causes of CN III palsy. Standard catheter angiogram may still be required if the clinical suspicion for aneurysm remains high despite negative non-catheter-based neuroimaging (e.g., CT/MRI). Evaluation for myasthenia gravis and other etiologies for CN III palsy presentation should be performed especially in isolated, pupil-spared, and painless CN III palsy |
| Practice option | LP may be necessary if neuroimaging is negative. Neurology, interventionalist, or neurosurgery consultations may be required depending on findings |

## 4.2.3 Cavernous Sinus Fistula

### Etiology and Pathophysiology

Carotid-cavernous fistula (CCF) occurs when an abnormal connection is formed between the arteries (e.g., internal or external carotid artery) and the cavernous sinus (refer to ▶ Fig. 4.4 for anatomy of the cavernous sinus). These connections can appear spontaneously (typically low-flow dural CCF) or may result from head trauma (typically high-flow direct CCF).[9]

### Presenting Symptoms and Signs

CCF may present with a multitude of symptoms such as vision loss (optic neuropathy, retinal vein occlusion, ocular ischemic syndrome, or glaucoma), exophthalmos, conjunctival congestion and chemosis, and ophthalmoplegia (from CN or EOM dysfunction). CCF can also produce intracranial bleeding.[9] Other findings may include subjective bruit, diplopia, tearing, red eye, ptosis, sensation of ocular foreign body, blurred vision, and headache (▶ Fig. 4.5).[10]

### Clinical Decisions

#### Diagnosis

Both CT/CTA and MR/MRA have modest sensitivities and specificities for CCF.[10] Imaging of the orbit may show an enlarged

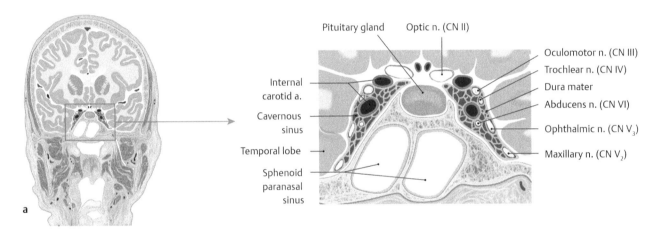

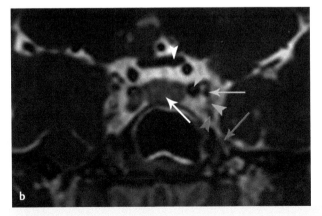

**Fig. 4.4** Cavernous sinus. **(a)** Artist's rendering of the cavernous sinus, with **(b)** a companion coronal fast imaging employing steady-state acquisition after contrast administration image showing the cavernous sinus lateral to the pituitary gland (*white arrow*). Within the cavernous sinus is the internal carotid artery (*blue arrowhead*) and the abducens nerve (CN VI). Along the lateral margin are CN III (*green arrow*), CN IV (*green arrowhead*), CN V1 (*red arrowhead*), and CN V2 (*red arrow*). For reference, the optic chiasm is marked (*white arrowhead*); however, the optic nerve does not course within the cavernous sinus. (a: Adapted from Gilroy et al., Atlas of Anatomy. 3rd ed. 2017. Based on: Schuenke M, Schulte E, Schumacher U. THIEME Atlas of Anatomy. Head and Neuroanatomy. Illustrations by Voll M and Wesker K. 2nd ed. New York: Thieme Medical Publishers; 2016.)

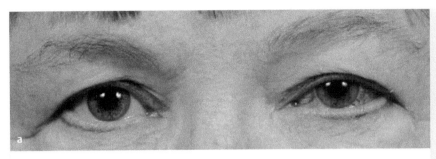

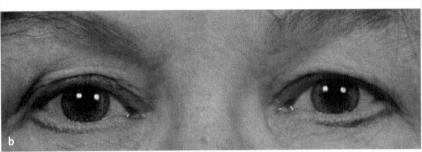

**Fig. 4.5** Orbital appearance. **(a)** Two weeks before and **(b)** 3 months after transvenous coil embolization of a carotid-cavernous fistula. Note the chemosis and mild ptosis of the left eye before intervention. (Adapted from Sekhar L, Fessler R, ed. Atlas of Neurosurgical Techniques: Brain. Vol. 1. 2nd ed. New York, NY: Thieme; 2015.)

superior ophthalmic vein. However, standard catheter angiogram is typically required both for diagnosis and for treatment (endovascular) of CCF.

## Current Treatment

Options for dural CCF treatment include observation for spontaneous improvement (in low-flow CCF) and symptomatic treatment with intraocular pressure-lowering agents and endovascular intervention with closure of the CCF.[10] Observation may be the preferred approach to treatment of low-risk, low-flow CCF cases, as up to 70% of dural CCFs will spontaneously close.[10] Endovascular interventional techniques have replaced open surgical procedures as the preferred treatment for direct CCFs, offering a 90 to 100% cure rate with some rare complications.

| Cost considerations | |
| --- | --- |
| Not recommended | Laboratory testing and LP are not typically necessary in the evaluation of CCF |
| Recommended | CT/MRI and CTA/MRA; most cases require standard catheter angiogram for diagnosis |
| Practice option | Consultation with endovascular interventionalist |

# 4.3 Infectious

## 4.3.1 Herpes Zoster, Syphilis, Lyme Disease, and HIV

### Etiology and Pathophysiology

Although relatively uncommon, infectious etiologic agents can cause diplopia from ocular motor cranial neuropathy. These include herpes zoster ophthalmicus (HZO), Lyme disease, neurosyphilis, and human immunodeficiency virus (HIV)/acquired immunodeficiency syndrome (AIDS).

**Herpes zoster** is caused by the reactivation of varicella zoster infection from childhood. In 20% of cases, the disease manifests

in CN V along the ophthalmic division and is called HZO.[11] The nerve most commonly affected is CN III, followed by CN VI and then CN IV. Typically the elderly tend to be more affected and the disease is typically self-limiting when immunocompetent.[12] The etiology is usually obvious because of the presence of the cutaneous V1 distribution vesicular rash, but some cases have no rash (herpes zoster sine herpete) or may have vesicles in the distribution of CN VII in the posterior auricular area or palate (Ramsay–Hunt syndrome).

**Lyme disease** is an infectious disease caused by the spirochete *Borrelia burgdorferi* resulting in systemic inflammation. Neuropathy of the CNs may be present in the second stage of the disease most commonly affecting CN V but also affecting CN III to CN VI, CN VII, and CN VIII.[13] The diagnosis is usually suggested by seasonal exposure or travel to an endemic area for Lyme disease and a tick bite, the presence of a rash (e.g., target lesion of erythema chronicum migrans), and other symptoms or signs of Lyme disease.

**Neurosyphilis** is caused by infection by the spirochete *Treponema pallidum* and can present with central nervous system (CNS) involvement with CN involvement and ocular findings.[14] CN II, CN VI, CN VII, and CN VIII can be commonly affected.[15]

**HIV/AIDS** is caused by the HIV ribonucleic acid (RNA) retrovirus and may result in neuro-ophthalmic side effects either by direct effect of the virus or by indirect effects of opportunistic infections and malignancies as the immune state of the patient declines. Between 50 and 75% of patients with HIV will present with ocular findings. The abducens nerve is most frequently affected, but CN III and CN IV can also be affected. Infections and malignancies most likely to result in neuro-ophthalmic pathologies include syphilis, cryptococcosis, and lymphoma.[16]

### Presenting Symptoms and Signs

Vertical, horizontal, or oblique diplopia may occur depending on the affected nerve(s) as well as headaches and meningismus among other symptoms.[15,17] Patients with HZO may present with Hutchinson's sign (involvement of the tip of the nose from

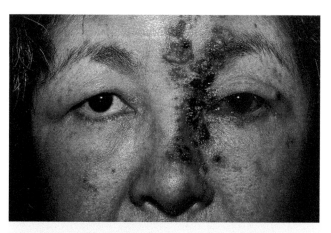

**Fig. 4.6** Reactivation of the herpes zoster virus, or shingles, in the fifth cranial nerve can lead to herpes zoster ophthalmicus. In this condition, dendrite keratopathy along with uveitis can lead to marked pain and visual loss. Involvement of the skin at the tip of the nose, supplied by the nasociliary nerve, is often associated with ocular involvement. Treatment with oral acyclovir or its derivatives often can reduce symptoms and shorten the course of the disease. If ophthalmic involvement is suspected, the patient should be evaluated by an ophthalmologist. The recent introduction of a vaccine to prevent herpes zoster in patients older than 60 years may have an impact on the incidence of herpes zoster ophthalmicus in the future. (Reproduced with permission from American Academy of Ophthalmology.)

nasociliary nerve) and unilateral vesicular dermatitis in the ophthalmic division of the trigeminal nerve prior to the development of ophthalmoplegia (▶Fig. 4.6).[11]

## Clinical Decisions

### Diagnosis

Serologic testing for the above culprits may be considered. MRI of the brain with and without contrast may help rule out other causes of CN palsies.[11,17,18] LP may be considered to test for both opening pressure etiologic agents.[17]

### Current Treatment

Any patient who is immunocompromised or pregnant with a single or multiple cranial neuropathies due to infection should be considered for admission to the hospital.

Treatment for typical HZO usually consists of oral acyclovir with or without corticosteroids; however, when HZO involves any CNs, intravenous (IV) acyclovir and IV corticosteroids are often recommended.[11,19] Treatment for Lyme disease with neurological involvement typically includes IV antibiotics such as ceftriaxone.[17] Treatment for neurosyphilis is IV penicillin G.[18] Treatment for HIV-induced ophthalmoplegia is highly variable depending on the cause. Aside from antiviral therapy given for HIV, it may be beneficial to consult infectious disease, neurology, in addition to ophthalmology to optimize management.[16]

| Cost considerations | |
| --- | --- |
| Not recommended | – |
| Recommended | Infectious disease serology and polymerase chain reaction (PCR) in the cerebrospinal fluid (CSF) |
| Practice option | MRI, LP, and infectious disease consultation |

# 4.4 Neoplastic

## 4.4.1 Leptomeningeal Carcinomatous

### Etiology and Pathophysiology

Leptomeningeal carcinomatosis is an uncommon complication of cancer that occurs when the disease metastasizes to the leptomeninges. The terminal condition typically has poor prognosis, with overall survival of approximately 6 to 8 weeks without treatment.[20] It may be present in 5 to 15% of patients with lymphomas or leukemia and in 1 to 5% of solid tumor patients, where most cases are associated with adenocarcinoma. Breast cancer represents the most common primary tumor source of leptomeningeal carcinomatosis, followed by lung carcinoma and melanoma.[21]

### Presenting Symptoms and Signs

Because leptomeningeal carcinomatosis may involve any level of the CNS, it can exhibit a wide range of presenting symptoms including multiple unilateral or bilateral CN palsies.[22,23]

### Clinical Decisions

### Diagnosis

MRI of brain with contrast is typically indicated and may show meningeal enhancement in 75 to 90% of patients with positive CSF findings (▶Fig. 4.7).[23] CSF cytology may be positive in about 70 to 90% of cases.[21] Nonspecific CSF markers may include elevated opening pressure, lymphocytic pleocytosis, and elevated CSF protein.

### Current Treatment

Therapy for leptomeningeal carcinomatosis is generally palliative in nature. Three modalities that have been explored include radiation therapy, systemic therapy, and intrathecal therapy, each possessing significant drawback.[23] Recent studies have demonstrated promise for the combination of small molecular weight target inhibitors and intrathecal chemotherapeutic agents in prolonging survival.[20]

| Cost considerations | |
| --- | --- |
| Not recommended | – |
| Recommended | MRI head and spine with and without contrast |
| Practice option | LP and oncology |

## 4.4.2 Other Tumors

### Etiology and Pathophysiology

Neoplastic processes in the orbit, superior orbital fissure, orbital apex, and cavernous sinus may result in ophthalmoplegia.[24] Lesions producing an ipsilateral optic neuropathy in addition to ocular motor cranial neuropathy are often due to an underlying orbital apex syndrome (OAS).[25] Primary parasellar tumors that may invade the orbital apex or cavernous sinus include pituitary adenoma, meningioma, craniopharyngioma, and chordoma. Metastatic malignancies from nasopharyngeal

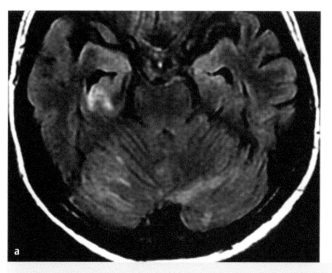 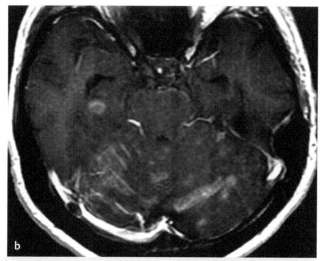

**Fig. 4.7** Leptomeningeal carcinomatosis in a patient with metastatic breast cancer. **(a)** Axial T2-weighted (T2w) fluid-attenuated inversion recovery (FLAIR) image demonstrates abnormal hyperintensity focally along the medial right temporal lobe and along the bilateral cerebellar folia. **(b)** Axial T1W postcontrast image demonstrates marked smooth, predominantly linear enhancement in regions of FLAIR signal abnormality confirming the presence of leptomeningeal disease. (Adapted from: Tsiouris A, Sanelli P, Comunale J, ed. Case-Based Brain Imaging. 2nd ed. New York, NY: Thieme; 2013.)

tumors, lymphoma, squamous cell carcinoma, or distant solid organ tumors (breast, lung, melanoma, and prostate) may also invade the orbital system.[24]

## Presenting Symptoms and Signs

Diplopia, ophthalmoplegia, proptosis, and visual loss are the predominant symptoms in OAS.[25]

## Clinical Decisions

### Diagnosis

High-resolution MRI of the brain and orbit with contrast and fat suppression sequences is indicated for diagnosis of lesions in the orbit and contiguous anatomical locations. Surgical biopsy is typically a requisite for confirmation of the diagnosis.[25]

### Current Treatment

Symptoms in neoplastic OAS may initially respond to corticosteroids.[25] Management of the underlying neoplastic process is of central concern in these cases; consider consulting with neurosurgery and oncology.

| Cost considerations | |
| --- | --- |
| Not recommended | – |
| Recommended | MRI brain and orbit |
| Practice option | Biopsy, steroids, neurosurgery, and oncology |

# 4.5 Inflammatory/Autoimmune
## 4.5.1 Thyroid Eye Disease

### Etiology and Pathophysiology

Although thyroid eye disease (TED) causes a restrictive extraocular myopathy and not an ocular motor cranial neuropathy, it can mimic CN palsy. TED is the most common cause of orbital disease in adults, most commonly occurring in patients with Grave's disease but also in those with Hashimoto's thyroiditis or even euthyroid state. It is an autoimmune, inflammatory, noninfectious orbitopathy that is six times more likely to affect women than men.[26]

## Presenting Symptoms and Signs

TED may produce an ophthalmoplegia that mimics a third, fourth, or sixth CN palsy. Enlargement of EOMs and adipose tissue hypertrophy are responsible for many of the clinical signs and symptoms of TED. EOM involvement typically occurs in the following order: inferior rectus, medial rectus, superior rectus, lateral rectus, and finally the obliques.[27] Eyelid retraction and proptosis commonly occur along with dry eyes, pain, cornea irritation, or ulceration (▶Fig. 4.8).[28]

## Clinical Decisions

### Diagnosis

Thyroid laboratory screening may be a useful diagnostic tool; free T4, free or total T3, and thyroid-stimulating hormone (TSH) may be targeted for initial screening.[27] However, TED may present in euthyroid patients who harbor thyroid autoantibodies. These autoantibodies include those against thyrotropin receptor (TRAb), thyroglobulin (TgAb), thyroid peroxidase (TPOAb), TSH (TSHAb), and thyrotropin-binding inhibitory immunoglobulins (TBII).[29]

CT without contrast is preferred in order to visualize the EOMs and orbital content.[27] Imaging modalities such as MRI, and ultrasound, may also be useful to confirm the TED diagnosis while excluding others in the differential.

### Current Treatment

Consider referral to endocrinology to assist in medical management. Corticosteroids may be considered; selenium

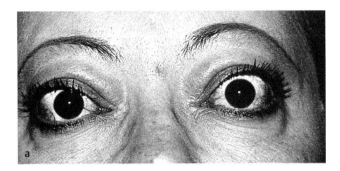

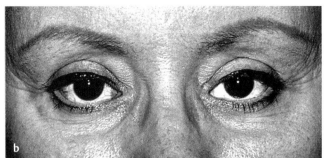

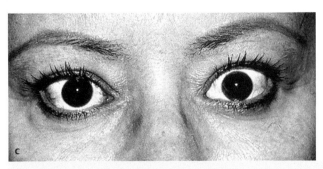

**Fig. 4.8** (a-c) Thyroid-related orbitopathy. (Reproduced with permission from American Academy of Ophthalmology.)

supplementation has also improved symptoms in some studies, although further research is needed. In refractory cases, orbital radiation or surgical rehabilitation may be considered.[27] Radioactive iodine and thyroidectomy may also be considered in cases necessitating long-term hyperthyroidism control.[28] Procedures to consider include eyelid surgery to correct eyelid retraction, eye muscle surgery to correct diplopia and dysfunction of EOMs, and orbital decompression surgery to relieve orbital pressure especially if vision is compromised.[26] Consider referral to an oculoplastic surgeon.

| Cost considerations | |
| --- | --- |
| Not recommended | Iodinated contrast CT scan may worsen uncontrolled systemic thyroid disease |
| Recommended | Thyroid function studies and thyroid antibodies |
| Practice option | Orbital CT/MRI/ultrasound and endocrinology |

## 4.5.2 Myasthenia Gravis

### Etiology and Pathophysiology

Myasthenia gravis (MG) is the most common neuromuscular disease in which antibodies target acetylcholine receptor (AChR) in the neuromuscular junction. It is an acquired autoimmune condition that typically presents in the 20 to 30s for females and late 60s to 80s for males. Approximately 50% of ocular MG patients are seropositive for the AChR or may be seronegative. Seronegative cases of MG (especially with bulbar involvement) might be positive for other antibodies for MG including muscle-specific receptor tyrosine kinase (MuSK). Ten to 15% of MG cases may coincide with an underlying thymoma.[30] MG may be exacerbated by a variety of medications, including antibiotics, calcium channel blockers, beta blockers, and sedatives, among others.[31]

### Presenting Symptoms and Signs

The symptoms of MG may include fatigability and variability.[30] Patients typically experience fluctuating muscle weakness worsening throughout the day. Fatigable ptosis and external ophthalmoplegia may be seen, mimicking CN III, CN IV, and/or CN VI palsies. Pupillary reactions are never compromised in MG.[31] Other ocular signs may include Cogan's lid twitch and orbicularis oculi weakness. Bulbar involvement, such as dysarthria, dysphagia, and dyspnea should be considered. Systemic symptoms may develop including proximal muscle weakness and respiratory muscle fatigability.

### Clinical Decisions

#### Diagnosis

Classically, the ice pack test and IV edrophonium have been used to aid in the diagnosis; however, they are associated with false-positive and false-negative results. Therefore, it may be recommended that physicians obtain serological testing against antibodies for AChR, and in seronegative cases, additional testing may be needed (e.g., MuSK). Electrophysiologic studies may also be recommended for confirmation, via either repeat repetitive nerve stimulation (RNS) studies or single-fiber electromyography (SFEMG). A chest CT or MRI is also recommended to rule out a thymoma in patients suspected of having MG.[32]

#### Current Treatment

The first line of treatment recommended is acetylcholinesterase blockers, among which pyridostigmine is commonly used for symptomatic relief. Further immunotherapy may be prescribed such as glucocorticoids (slowly tapering upward to avoid adverse events) or other long-term immunosuppressants such as azathioprine or mycophenolate. Plasmapheresis and IV immunoglobulin (IVIG) are fast- but short-acting solutions that are also sometimes used. Thymectomy may be recommended for some patients; therefore, consultation with thoracic surgery is recommended.[33]

| Cost considerations | |
|---|---|
| Not recommended | – |
| Recommended | MG antibody panel and CT chest |
| Practice option | RNS, SFEMG, immunosuppression, thymectomy, and neurology |

### 4.5.3 Miller Fisher's Syndrome

#### Etiology and Pathophysiology

Miller Fisher's syndrome (MFS) is considered a variant of the Guillain–Barré syndrome (GBS). The disease is an autoimmune antibody-mediated peripheral neuropathy.[34] MFS often develops after upper respiratory infection or, less commonly, after gastrointestinal disorders. Asians and males tend to have a higher risk for developing MFS.[35]

#### Presenting Symptoms and Signs

MFS is characterized by the classic triad symptoms of external ophthalmoplegia, ataxia, and areflexia.[36] MFS can mimic one or more, unilateral or bilateral CN palsies.

#### Clinical Decisions

#### Diagnosis

Testing for anti-GQ1b antibodies may help narrow the differential, since antibody titers are thought to correlate with the severity of MFS. CSF studies may show high protein with normal white blood cell count (albuminocytologic dissociation), which is a nonspecific finding.[35]

#### Current Treatment

MFS may often be self-resolving with overall good prognosis and low recurrence and mortality rates. Supportive therapy is generally sufficient so long as respiratory function is spared. Medical therapies exist, but unlike GBS, randomized controlled trials have not been conducted. Preliminary data show that treatments like IVIG and plasmapheresis used for GBS treatment are minimally effective for MFS.[35]

| Cost considerations | |
|---|---|
| Not recommended | – |
| Recommended | Ganglioside serology<br>MRI brain and orbit |
| Practice option | LP for albuminocytologic dissociation |

### 4.5.4 Tolosa–Hunt Syndrome

#### Etiology and Pathophysiology

The Tolosa–Hunt syndrome (THS) is an idiopathic granulomatous inflammation of the cavernous sinus that can affect CN III, CN IV, and CN VI, and produce a steroid-responsive, painful ophthalmoplegia. THS, however, should be considered a diagnosis of exclusion.[22]

#### Presenting Symptoms and Signs

THS is a painful ophthalmoplegia that presents with recurrent unilateral orbital pain and ipsilateral oculomotor paralysis.[24]

#### Clinical Decisions

#### Diagnosis

MRI is the most useful imaging modality for diagnosis of THS, as it provides better resolution of the cavernous sinus soft tissue than CT (▶Fig. 4.9). Diagnostic criteria for THS include prompt response (within 72 h) of the paresis and pain to corticosteroid treatment.[22]

#### Current Treatment

THS typically resolves quickly and completely with corticosteroid treatment. If steroid-induced complications arise or in the case of recurrent attacks, focal radiotherapy may be effective.[24]

| Cost considerations | |
|---|---|
| Not recommended | CT alone |
| Recommended | MRI brain and orbit, and steroids |
| Practice option | LP and laboratory testing |

### 4.5.5 Demyelinating Disease: MS-Related INO

#### Etiology and Pathophysiology

Multiple sclerosis (MS) is a disease that causes inflammation, demyelination, and degeneration of axons, with an unknown etiology.[37] One of the most common ophthalmic presentations of MS is internuclear ophthalmoplegia (INO), a finding present in 17 to 41% of MS patients resulting from a lesion in the medial longitudinal fasciculus (MLF).[38] The INO can be mistaken for a "partial third nerve palsy," especially in the setting of concomitant skew deviation.

#### Presenting Symptoms and Signs

Patients with MS-induced INO may often complain of horizontal diplopia on lateral gaze (▶Fig. 4.10).[38] For other potential ophthalmic signs of MS, refer to Chapter 3, section 3.6.1.

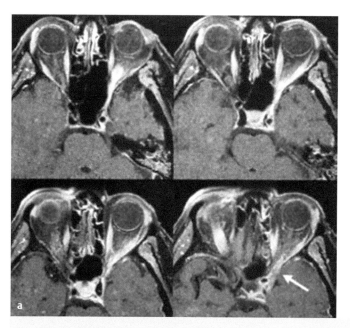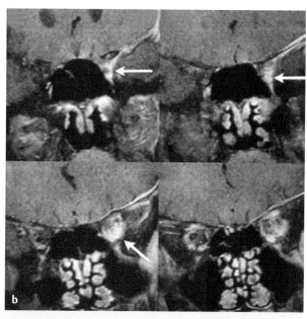

**Fig. 4.9** Tolosa–Hunt syndrome. **(a)** Axial and **(b)** coronal fat-suppressed T1-weighted images show poorly defined gadolinium contrast enhancement in the left orbital apex extending posteriorly into the left superior orbital fissure and left cavernous sinus (*arrows*). (Adapted from Meyers S, ed. Differential Diagnosis in Neuroimaging: Head and Neck. 1st ed. New York, NY: Thieme; 2016.)

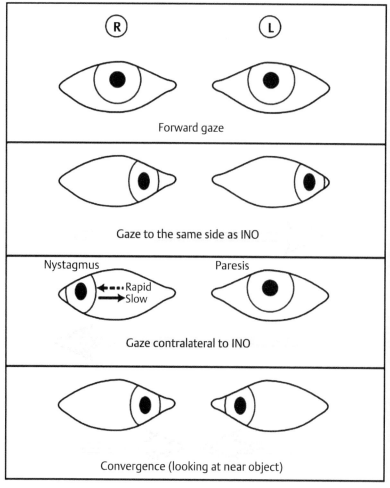

**Fig. 4.10** Illustration of gaze findings with a left internuclear ophthalmoplegia. Convergence may be intact (lower panel) if the lesion producing the INO is in the pons rather than the midbrain. INO, internuclear ophthalmoplegia. (Adapted from Greenberg M, ed. Handbook of Neurosurgery. 8th ed. New York, NY: Thieme; 2016.)

## Clinical Decisions

### Diagnosis

MRI with and without contrast in the MLF region of the brainstem is recommended for confirmation of diagnosis, but many cases have negative imaging.[38] For other diagnostic criteria of MS, refer to Chapter 3. Evaluation for a pseudo-INO (e.g., myasthenia gravis) should also be performed, especially with a negative cranial MRI.

### Current Treatment

INO typically resolves on its own over a period of several weeks to months, during which an eye patch may be worn to aid with diplopia.[38] Steroids may be employed.

| Cost considerations | |
|---|---|
| Not recommended | – |
| Recommended | MRI and neurology |
| Practice option | Eye patch, steroids, and MG evaluation for pseudo-INO |

## 4.5.6 Vasculitides

Autoimmune vasculitides, many of which were mentioned in Chapter 3, may produce an oculomotor disorder. The most important of these to consider is giant cell arteritis (GCA; also known as temporal arteritis), a systemic vasculitis affecting medium- to large-caliber arteries that presents in patients older than 50 years.[39] While visual loss is overwhelmingly the most common ophthalmic manifestation of GCA (appearing in 98% of patients), diplopia may also occur in approximately 6 to 21% of patients. Diplopia may precede visual loss in some cases and serve as the only ophthalmic manifestation of GCA in others.[40] Refer to Chapter 3 (Cranial Nerve II: Visual Disorders) for a more detailed discussion of diagnostic and management considerations in GCA.

# 4.6 Congenital

## 4.6.1 Congenital Fourth Nerve Palsy

### Etiology and Pathophysiology

Congenital palsy of CN IV is the most common CN palsy, as well as the most common pediatric cause of ocular torticollis (head tilt). The most typical variety of this congenital palsy involves complete absence of the trochlear nerve, leading to a congenital cranial dysinnervation disorder (CCDD).[41] Congenital CN IV palsies, in some cases, may be hereditary.[42]

### Presenting Symptoms and Signs

Patients with CN IV palsy may present with head tilt, diplopia, HT, and diminished binocular vision.[41] There may be evidence of a long-standing head tilt when looking at old photographs of the patient.[43]

## Clinical Decisions

### Diagnosis

Clinical diagnosis of a CN IV palsy is most frequently done using the Parks–Bielschowsky three-step test; the sensitivity of this clinical three-step test is 70%.[41]

### Current Treatment

Any symptom of congenital CN IV palsy, particularly a significant head tilt, may serve as an indication for surgery. If the head tilt is severe, surgery becomes a more pressing consideration because unresolved torticollis may result in progressive asymmetry of the face. Surgical intervention carries the risk of inducing a secondary acquired Brown syndrome.[41]

| Cost considerations | |
|---|---|
| Not recommended | – |
| Recommended | Old photographs and strabismus specialist |
| Practice option | Surgical intervention |

## 4.6.2 Brown Syndrome

### Etiology and Pathophysiology

Brown syndrome is a disorder characterized by impaired elevation of the eye that is most apparent in adduction. It can be attributed to abnormalities in the superior oblique muscle or tendon, either congenital or acquired via trauma, surgery, or an inflammatory etiology.[43]

### Presenting Symptoms and Signs

Limited elevation of the eye, particularly during adduction, is the most important clinical sign of Brown syndrome. Other findings may include exotropia in up-gaze, hypotropia in primary gaze, and palpebral fissure widening on adduction (▶ Fig. 4.11).[43,44]

## Clinical Decisions

### Diagnosis

Diagnosis of Brown syndrome is a clinical diagnosis based on the above signs. All three criteria in the three-step test used for congenital CN IV palsy should be negative in Brown syndrome.[45]

### Current Treatment

While Brown syndrome may spontaneously resolve in some cases, surgical intervention may be considered.[45]

| Cost considerations | |
|---|---|
| Not recommended | – |
| Recommended | Strabismus specialist |
| Practice option | – |

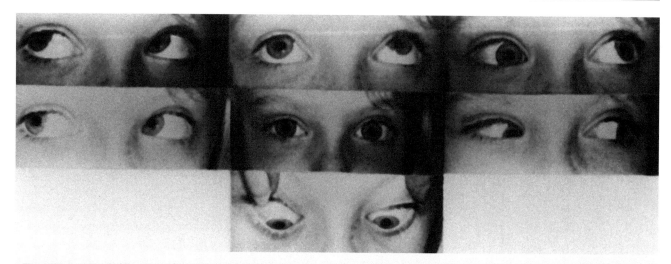

**Fig. 4.11** A congenital Brown syndrome, showing the eyes in various gazing positions. Note the markedly limited elevation of the right eye in the upward midline position (top middle), which is even more pronounced on adduction of the right eye (top right). (Adapted from Valvassori G, Mafee M, Becker M, ed. Imaging of the Head and Neck. 2nd ed. New York, NY: Thieme; 2004.)

### 4.6.3 CPEO and KSS

#### Etiology and Pathophysiology

Chronic progressive external ophthalmoplegia (CPEO) is a mitochondrial disease that involves ophthalmoplegia and progressive, bilateral ptosis. Kearns–Sayre syndrome (KSS) is a related disorder involving multiple systems, featuring progressive external ophthalmoplegia (PEO) alongside cardiac block and pigmentary retinopathy.[46]

#### Presenting Symptoms and Signs

Patients with CPEO may present with blurred vision, increasing difficulty in opening both eyes, and possible weakness of the proximal limbs. As symptoms worsen, patients may become unstable and ultimately become unable to walk.[46] Dysarthria and dysphagia are other symptoms that may afflict patients with CPEO.[46,47]

#### Clinical Decisions

#### Diagnosis

Diagnostic modalities to consider include MRI to look for CNS atrophy, muscle biopsy, histological analysis, and genetic testing for mitochondrial mutations. Mutation screening may also help elucidate whether the CPEO phenotype is heritable or sporadic.[46]

#### Current Treatment

There are currently no treatments for CPEO that have demonstrated widespread effectiveness in patients. Proposed treatments, albeit with little to no supportive evidence, include CoQ10, vitamin cocktails, dichloroacetate, carnitine, and creatine.[46]

| Cost considerations | |
| --- | --- |
| Not recommended | – |
| Recommended | – |
| Practice option | MRI, muscle biopsy, genetic testing, and mitochondrial cocktail |

## 4.7 Trauma

### 4.7.1 Trauma-Induced Palsies

#### Etiology and Pathophysiology

Head trauma is a major cause of isolated or combined palsies of CN III, CN IV, and CN VI.[1]

**Traumatic CN IV palsy** is the most common nonidiopathic etiology of CN IV palsy, owing to its unique dorsal exit from the brainstem.[48] **Traumatic CN VI palsy** and, less frequently, **traumatic CN III palsy** may also occur.

#### Presenting Symptoms and Signs

The classical presentations for isolated ocular motility CN palsies are discussed in the "Abstract".

#### Clinical Decisions

#### Diagnosis

Consider that any combination of cranial neuropathies may be present in cases of head or facial trauma. CT of the head and orbit may be considered in the acute setting. High-resolution MRI may be considered for conclusive diagnosis and potential localization of traumatic cranial neuropathies.

## Current Treatment

Traumatic ocular motor neuropathies may first be managed with such temporary measures as observation, occlusion, or prisms, with spontaneous recovery being the hoped-for result.[48] In accordance with the CRASH trial, steroids may be employed if the Glasgow Coma Scale is not ≤14.[49] In refractory cases, typically after 6 months of injury, surgery may be considered.[50]

| Cost considerations | |
| --- | --- |
| Not recommended | – |
| Recommended | CT |
| Practice option | MRI, observation, occlusion, prism, and surgery |

# 4.8 Metabolic/Toxic

## 4.8.1 Diabetes

### Etiology and Pathophysiology

Diabetes-induced cranial neuropathy typically occurs in older patients with long-standing diabetes. The pathophysiology is likely due to microvascular ischemia-induced focal demyelination of the nerves.[51] The involvement of CN VI is most prevalent, followed by CN III and lastly CN IV.[52]

### Presenting Symptoms and Signs

Patients with CN VI palsy typically present with abrupt, painless diplopia.[53] CN III palsy typically presents with ipsilateral pain in addition to acute-onset ptosis and diplopia. Pupils are generally spared.[51]

### Clinical Decisions

### Diagnosis

Diagnosis is based on the previously mentioned clinical symptoms and signs. However, neuroimaging may be recommended if aneurysm-induced CN III palsy is suspected.[53]

### Current Treatment

No specific treatment is indicated for diabetic cranial neuropathy. Prismatic help may be indicated for diplopia and patients should maintain optimal glycemic levels to lower risk factors for further ischemic events. Recovery typically occurs over a span of 3 to 6 months.[51,53]

| Cost considerations | |
| --- | --- |
| Not recommended | |
| Recommended | CT/CTA, followed by MR/MRA for CN III palsy |
| Practice option | Prism and eye patch |

## 4.8.2 Wernicke Encephalopathy

### Etiology and Pathophysiology

Wernicke encephalopathy is a neurological disorder caused by thiamine, or vitamin B1, deficiency; it is the most common encephalopathy resulting from a single deficient vitamin. It is traditionally associated with alcoholism, although nonalcoholic cases involving excessive vomiting or postbariatric surgery have been reported.[54] Korsakoff's syndrome represents the chronic irreversible sequelae of Wernicke encephalopathy.

### Presenting Symptoms and Signs

Wernicke encephalopathy features a classic triad of symptoms including ophthalmoplegia, ataxia, and altered mental status.[55] Other diseases may manifest as a result of thiamine deficiency, including wet or dry beriberi and Marchiafava–Bignami syndrome.[54]

### Clinical Decisions

### Diagnosis

Total blood thiamine and transketolase (may not be universally available) may be obtained, but high-dose thiamine treatment should be initiated without waiting for these test results.[54] MRI is the standard for radioimaging in patients with suspected Wernicke encephalopathy, as it may reveal characteristic features, but the MRI may be normal. These features may include hyperintensity in the mammillary bodies, medial thalami, periaqueductal gray, and tectum (▶Fig. 4.12). The sensitivity of CT was found to be low. The final diagnosis of Wernicke encephalopathy may also be confirmed by neurological response after treatment with thiamine supplementation.[55]

### Current Treatment

Urgent, high-dose, parenteral thiamine supplementation forms the crux of therapy for acute Wernicke encephalopathy. Thiamine has demonstrated good overall safety via any administration route and should be administered as quickly as possible in suspected cases. In countries or populations at risk of thiamine deficiency, prophylactic supplementation of food with thiamine may be considered.[54] Concomitant magnesium replacement may also be helpful.

| Cost considerations | |
| --- | --- |
| Not recommended | CT alone |
| Recommended | Urgent, high-dose, parenteral thiamine supplementation |
| Practice option | Thiamine level and MRI |

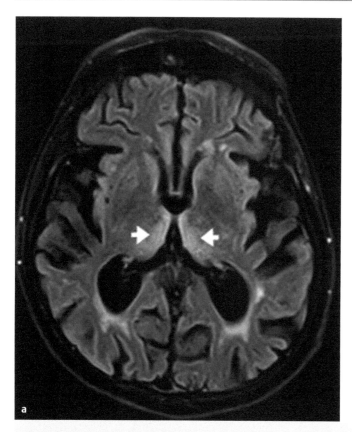 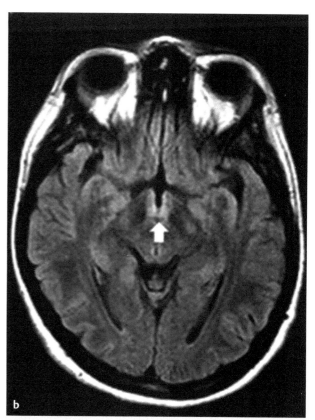

**Fig. 4.12** Wernicke encephalopathy. **(a, b)** Axial fluid-attenuated inversion recovery (FLAIR) images show bilateral symmetric hyperintensity in the medial aspect of the thalami (*arrows*; **a**). Edema and hyperintensity are also seen in the mammillary bodies (*fat arrow*; **b**). (Adapted from Kanekar S, ed. Imaging of Neurodegenerative Disorders. 1st ed. New York, NY: Thieme; 2015.)

### 4.8.3 Medication, Toxin, Vitamin Deficiency–Induced Ophthalmoparesis

A variety of medication-induced, toxin-induced, and vitamin deficiency–related etiologies exist for patients with ophthalmoplegia. High concentrations of the antiepileptic drug phenytoin have been associated with ophthalmoplegia.[56] Other drugs found to be associated with ophthalmoplegia in larger doses include phenobarbital, carbamazepine, primidone, and amitriptyline.[57] Anti–tumor necrosis factor-α (anti-TNF-α) drugs (such as adalimumab),[58] in addition to Tiratricol or dexfenfluramine (anti-obesity drugs),[59] have been reported as causes of INO. Ophthalmoplegia may be a presenting sign of botulism[60] or heavy metal poisoning, and rarely due to snake-bite injuries.[61] Many other drugs or toxins are possible etiologies of ocular motility disorders, as this list is not exhaustive. Vitamin E[62] and, in rare cases, Vitamin B12 deficiency[63] can also result in ophthalmoplegia. Giving special attention to diet, drug/toxin exposure, and social history during history taking can help elucidate a toxic- or metabolite-induced etiology of ophthalmoplegia. Management for toxic- or medication-induced ocular motility disorders is dependent on the offending substance, whereas vitamin supplementation can be considered in etiologies of vitamin deficiency.

## 4.9 Idiopathic

### 4.9.1 Idiopathic Intracranial Hypertension

#### Etiology and Pathophysiology

The etiology and pathophysiology of idiopathic intracranial hypertension (IIH) have been discussed in Chapter 3 (Cranial Nerve II: Visual Disorders).

#### Presenting Symptoms and Signs

Abducens nerve palsy may occur in around 20% of IIH cases as a nonlocalizing sign of increased intracranial pressure. Palsies of CNs other than the abducens nerve (including CN III and CN IV) are considered atypical findings that may be more common in pediatric cases or suggest secondary etiologies of the disease.[64]

Other presenting symptoms and signs of IIH, including headache, pulsatile tinnitus, and vision loss, are discussed in Chapter 3 (Cranial Nerve II: Visual Disorders).

## Clinical Decisions

### Diagnosis

Diagnosis of IIH may involve MRI, MR venography (MRV), and lumbar puncture to fulfill the modified Dandy criteria.

### Current Treatment

Weight loss and diuretics (particularly carbonic anhydrase inhibitors such as acetazolamide) form the first-line treatment for IIH. Surgical intervention with optic nerve sheath fenestration (ONSF) or VP shunt may be considered in cases of IIH refractory to medical management or involving vision loss. For more details, refer to Chapter 3, section 3.11.1.

## 4.10 Conclusion

A number of various etiologies of ocular motility disorders due to ocular motor cranial neuropathies or CN palsy mimics (e.g., giant cell arteritis, TED, MG, MFS, Wernicke encephalopathy) have been explored over the course of this chapter. The differential diagnosis of diplopia and ophthalmoplegia is wide, and clinical evaluation is made difficult by the presentation of CN palsies not always in isolation but often in combination. Consultation with a number of different specialties may often be required for management of these diseases. Referral suggestions, recommendations for preferred diagnostic modalities or tests, presentations of management options, and indications to pursue invasive interventions found in the chapter may be used to guide cost-effective patient care.

## References

[1] McGee S. Nerves of the eye muscles (III, IV, and VI): approach to diplopia. Evidence-Based Physical Diagnosis. Amsterdam: Elsevier Health Sciences; 2016

[2] Caplan L. Etiology, classification, and epidemiology of stroke. In: Kasner S, Dashe J, eds. UpToDate. Waltham, MA: UpToDate; 2017

[3] Tanaka H, Arai M, Kubo J, Hirata K. Conjugate eye deviation with head version due to a cortical infarction of the frontal eye field. Stroke 2002;33(2):642–643

[4] Evliyaoglu F, Karadag R, Burakgazi AZ. Ocular neuropathy in peripheral neuropathies. Muscle Nerve 2012;46(5):681–686

[5] Caplan L. Overview of the evaluation of stroke. In: Kasner S, Dashe J, eds. UpToDate. Waltham, MA: UpToDate; 2018

[6] Lee TY, Ting CY, Tsai MJ, Tsai MJ. Third nerve palsy and internal carotid aneurysm. QJM 2016;109(11):755–756

[7] Lee AG. Third cranial nerve (oculomotor nerve) palsy in adults. In: Brazis PW, Wilterdink J, eds. UpToDate. Waltham, MA: UpToDate; 2017

[8] Singer R, Ogilvy C, Rordorf G. Treatment of cerebral aneurysm. In: Biller J, Wilterdink J, eds. UpToDate. Waltham, MA: UpToDate; 2013

[9] Maciej W, Tadeusz P, Pawel B, et al. Posttraumatic bilateral carotid-cavernous fistula. J Int Adv Otol 2013;9(3):417–422

[10] Henderson AD, Miller NR. Carotid-cavernous fistula: current concepts in aetiology, investigation, and management. Eye (Lond) 2018;32(2):164–172

[11] Harthan JS, Borgman CJ. Herpes zoster ophthalmicus-induced oculomotor nerve palsy. J Optom 2012;6:60–65

[12] Park KC, Yoon SS, Yoon JE, Rhee HY. A case of herpes zoster ophthalmicus with isolated trochlear nerve involvement. J Clin Neurol 2011;7(1):47–49

[13] Savas R, Sommer A, Gueckel F, Georgi M. Isolated oculomotor nerve paralysis in Lyme disease: MRI. Neuroradiology 1997;39(2):139–141

[14] Çoban E, Aldan M, Gez S, et al. A case of neurosyphilis presenting with multiple cranial neuropathy. Turkish J Neurol. 2016;22:127–129

[15] Berger JR, Dean D. Neurosyphilis. Handb Clin Neurol 2014;121:1461–1472

[16] Rajasekhar P, Manjula B, Kumari S, Deepthi D. A clinical study of multiple ocular motor nerve palsies in people living with HIV/AIDS in a tertiary eye care hospital. J Dental Med Sci. 2015;14(5):35–38

[17] Bababeygy SR, Quiros PA. Isolated trochlear palsy secondary to Lyme neuroborreliosis. Int Ophthalmol 2011;31(6):493–495

[18] Seeley WW, Venna N. Neurosyphilis presenting with gummatous oculomotor nerve palsy. J Neurol Neurosurg Psychiatry 2004;75(5):789

[19] Chaker N, Bouladi M, Chebil A, Jemmeli M, Mghaieth F, El Matri L. Herpes zoster ophthalmicus associated with abducens palsy. J Neurosci Rural Pract 2014;5(2):180–182

[20] Gwak HS, Lee SH, Park WS, Shin SH, Yoo H, Lee SH. Recent advancements of treatment for leptomeningeal carcinomatosis. J Korean Neurosurg Soc 2015;58(1):1–8

[21] Nuvoli S, Contu S, Pung BLJ, Solinas P, Madeddu G, Spanu A. Intracranial leptomeningeal carcinomatosis: a diagnostic study with 18F-fluorodeoxyglucose positron emission tomography/computed tomography. Case Rep Neurol 2018;10(1):45–53

[22] La Mantia L, Curone M, Rapoport AM, Bussone G; International Headache Society. Tolosa-Hunt syndrome: critical literature review based on IHS 2004 criteria. Cephalalgia 2006;26(7):772–781

[23] Kak M, Nanda R, Ramsdale EE, Lukas RV. Treatment of leptomeningeal carcinomatosis: current challenges and future opportunities. J Clin Neurosci 2015;22(4):632–637

[24] Gladstone JP. An approach to the patient with painful ophthalmoplegia, with a focus on Tolosa-Hunt syndrome. Curr Pain Headache Rep 2007;11(4):317–325

[25] Yeh S, Foroozan R. Orbital apex syndrome. Curr Opin Ophthalmol 2004;15(6):490–498

[26] Durairaj VD. Clinical perspectives of thyroid eye disease. Am J Med 2006;119(12):1027–1028

[27] Weiler DL. Thyroid eye disease: a review. Clin Exp Optom 2017;100(1):20–25

[28] Yang DD, Gonzalez MO, Durairaj VD. Medical management of thyroid eye disease. Saudi J Ophthalmol 2011;25(1):3–13

[29] Kumari R, Chandra Saha B. Advances in the management of thyroid eye diseases: an overview. Int Ophthalmol 2017

[30] Bird S. Clinical manifestation of myasthenia gravis. In: Shefner J, Targoff I, Eichler A, eds. UpToDate. Waltham, MA: UpToDate; 2017

[31] Noel M, Burkat C, Jirawuthiworavong G, Marcet M. Myasthenia gravis. In: Burkat C, Jirawuthiworavong G, eds. EyeWiki. San Francisco, CA: American Academy of Ophthalmology; 2017

[32] Bird S. Diagnosis of myasthenia gravis. In: Shefner J, Targoff I, Eichler A, eds. UpToDate. Waltham, MA: UpToDate; 2017

[33] Bird S. Treatment of myasthenia gravis. In: Shefner J, Targoff I, Eichler A, eds. UpToDate. Waltham, MA: UpToDate; 2017

[34] Vriesendorp F. Guillain-Barré syndrome in adults: clinical features and diagnosis. In: Shefner J, Targoff I, Eichler A, eds. UpToDate. Waltham, MA: UpToDate; 2017

[35] Rezaei S, Ponce CP, Vickers A, Lee AG. Miller Fisher variant of Guillain–Barre syndrome. In: Lee A, Ponce C, eds. EyeWiki. San Francisco, CA: American Academy of Ophthalmology; 2017

[36] Mori M, Kuwabara S, Yuki N. Fisher syndrome: clinical features, immuno-pathogenesis and management. Expert Rev Neurother 2012;12(1):39–51

[37] Olek MJ, Mowry EM. Pathogenesis and epidemiology of multiple sclerosis. In: González-Scarano F, Dasche JF, eds. UpToDate. Waltham, MA: UpToDate; 2018

[38] Frohman TC, Frohman EM. Intranuclear ophthalmoparesis. In: Brazis PW, Wilterdink J, eds. UpToDate. Waltham, MA: UpToDate; 2017

[39] Bhatti MT, Tabandeh H. Giant cell arteritis: diagnosis and management. Curr Opin Ophthalmol 2001;12(6):393–399

[40] Kawasaki A, Purvin V. Giant cell arteritis: an updated review. Acta Ophthalmol 2009;87(1):13–32

[41] Engel JM. Treatment and diagnosis of congenital fourth nerve palsies: an update. Curr Opin Ophthalmol 2015;26(5):353–356

[42] Bale JF Jr, Scott WE, Yuh W, Sato Y, Menezes A. Congenital fourth nerve palsy and occult cranium bifidum. Pediatr Neurol 1988;4(5):320–321

[43] Kaeser PF, Brodsky MC. Fourth cranial nerve palsy and Brown syndrome: two interrelated congenital cranial dysinnervation disorders? Curr Neurol Neurosci Rep 2013;13(6):352

[44] Wang Y, McCulley TJ, Doyle JJ, Chang J, Lee MS, McClelland CM. Brown syndrome following upper eyelid ptosis repair. Neuroophthalmology 2017;42(1):49–51

[45] Manley DR, Alvi RA. Brown's syndrome. Curr Opin Ophthalmol 2011; 22(5):432–440

[46] Lv ZY, Xu XM, Cao XF, et al. Mitochondrial mutations in 12S rRNA and 16S rRNA presenting as chronic progressive external ophthalmoplegia (CPEO) plus: a case report. Medicine (Baltimore) 2017;96(48):e8869

[47] Hedermann G, Løkken N, Dahlqvist JR, Vissing J. Dysphagia is prevalent in patients with CPEO and single, large-scale deletions in mtDNA. Mitochondrion 2017;32:27–30

[48] Prosst RL, Majetschak M. Traumatic unilateral trochlear nerve palsy. J Trauma 2007;62(6):E1–E3

[49] Roberts I, Yates D, Sandercock P, et al; CRASH trial collaborators. Effect of intravenous corticosteroids on death within 14 days in 10008 adults with clinically significant head injury (MRC CRASH trial): randomised placebo-controlled trial. Lancet 2004;364(9442):1321–1328

[50] Asproudis I, Vourda E, Zafeiropoulos P, Katsanos A, Tzoufi M. Isolated abducens nerve palsy after closed head injury in a child. Oman J Ophthalmol 2015;8(3):179–180

[51] Boulton AJ, Malik RA, Arezzo JC, Sosenko JM. Diabetic somatic neuropathies. Diabetes Care 2004;27(6):1458–1486

[52] Tracy JA, Dyck PJ. The spectrum of diabetic neuropathies. Phys Med Rehabil Clin N Am 2008;19(1):1–26, v

[53] Llewelyn JG. The diabetic neuropathies: types, diagnosis and management. J Neurol Neurosurg Psychiatry 2003;74(Suppl 2):ii15–ii19

[54] Galvin R, Bråthen G, Ivashynka A, Hillbom M, Tanasescu R, Leone MA; EFNS. EFNS guidelines for diagnosis, therapy and prevention of Wernicke encephalopathy. Eur J Neurol 2010;17(12):1408–1418

[55] Kim TE, Lee EJ, Young JB, Shin DJ, Kim JH. Wernicke encephalopathy and ethanol-related syndromes. Semin Ultrasound CT MR 2014;35(2):85–96

[56] Perucca P, Mula M. Antiepileptic drug effects on mood and behavior: molecular targets. Epilepsy Behav 2013;26(3):440–449

[57] Puri V, Chaudhry N. Total external ophthalmoplegia induced by phenytoin: a case report and review of literature. Neurol India 2004;52(3):386–387

[58] Drury J, Hickman SJ. Internuclear ophthalmoplegia associated with anti-TNFα medication. Strabismus 2015;23(1):30–32

[59] Lledo Carreres M, Lajo Garrido JL, Gonzalez Rico M, Navarro Polo JN, Escobar Cava P, Aznar Saliente T. Toxic internuclear ophthalmoplegia related to antiobesity treatment. Ann Pharmacother 1992;26(11):1457–1458

[60] Ehrenreich H, Garner CG, Witt TN. Complete bilateral internal ophthalmoplegia as sole clinical sign of botulism: confirmation of diagnosis by single fibre electromyography. J Neurol 1989;236(4):243–245

[61] Praveen Kumar KV, Praveen Kumar S, Kasturi N, Ahuja S. Ocular manifestations of venomous snake bite over a one-year period in a tertiary care hospital. Korean J Ophthalmol 2015;29(4):256–262

[62] Dhawan PS, Goodman BP. Neurologic manifestations of nutritional disorders. Aminoff's Neurology and General Medicine. Amsterdam: Elsevier Inc.; 2014

[63] Akdal G, Yener GG, Ada E, Halmagyi GM. Eye movement disorders in vitamin B12 deficiency: two new cases and a review of the literature. Eur J Neurol 2007;14(10):1170–1172

[64] Spennato P, Ruggiero C, Parlato RS, et al. Pseudotumor cerebri. Childs Nerv Syst 2011;27(2):215–235

# 5 Cranial Nerve V: Trigeminal Nerve

*Wissam Elfallal and Jeff Jacob*

## Abstract

Trigeminal neuralgia is the most common pathology of cranial nerve V encountered in clinical practice. It is a clinical diagnosis characterized by severe, paroxysmal stabbing facial pains. It was given the name "tic douloureux," which translates as "painful tic," due to the characteristic painful facial spasms that occur during attacks. This disease entity can be devastating to patients, causing severe debilitation of daily activities and earning it the label the "suicide disease." Trigeminal neuralgia tends to peak in the 50s to 60s, with a female-to-male ratio of 2:1. The overall prevalence is 10 to 300/100,000 worldwide. The relatively high prevalence of trigeminal neuralgia contributes to high costs of care on the medical system. The diagnosis and evaluation of trigeminal neuralgia is based on clinical features and history. Imaging may be obtained to rule out other etiologies or in cases of atypical facial pain and is considered a level C recommendation by the American Academy of Neurology. The treatment and surgical management accounts for the majority of the health care cost for trigeminal neuralgia. For instance, many patients with trigeminal neuralgia are referred to dental offices for root canals and dental extraction from inaccurate diagnosis, leading to unnecessary treatment and costs. There are many modalities in the treatment of trigeminal neuralgia including pharmacologic, interventional procedures, such as percutaneous radiofrequency, Gamma Knife stereotactic surgery, and microvascular decompression. Careful, individualized care of each patient can allow for cost-effective options along with providing good clinical outcomes and high patient satisfaction.

*Keywords:* trigeminal neuralgia, facial pain syndrome, suicide disease, tic douloureux

## 5.1 Introduction

The trigeminal nerve has two primary physiologic functions, the first being sensation to the face, anterior two-thirds of tongue, and to the dura of the anterior and middle cranial fossa. Sensory modalities include light touch, pain/temperature perception, and proprioception. The second component of the nerve is motor innervation to the muscles of mastication, that is, the masseter, temporalis, medial/lateral pterygoids, mylohyoid, and anterior belly of the digastric.[1] A multitude of disease pathologies can affect the trigeminal nerve including basilar skull fractures, dental trauma, metastatic tumors, aneurysms, lupus, scleroderma, sarcoidosis, and arterial ectasia. These pathologies affect the peripheral component of cranial nerve V after it has left the brainstem. The gasserian ganglion may be also affected by herpes zoster, as well as by primary and metastatic tumors.[1] Like trigeminal neuralgia, all these conditions generally present with facial pain, which can be unilateral, paroxysmal, and stabbing in nature. However, unlike classic trigeminal neuralgia, neurologic deficits such as loss of sensation of varying degrees may be present.

The pathophysiology of trigeminal neuralgia is complex and not fully understood. Trigeminal neuralgia may be due to injury or compression of the afferent fibers at the nerve root or due to injury of the trigeminal ganglion in Meckel's cave. Injury to the trigeminal nerve can lead to over-activation and a low threshold for nerve root firing. The touch sensation A-beta fibers lie in close proximity to the pain C-fibers, leading to cross-activation of these fibers.[2]

Overall, a low stimulus is needed to activate the nerve, which may explain why relatively light stimuli can be a trigger for significant facial pain.

## 5.2 Anatomy

The trigeminal nerve begins in the upper pons, exiting the brainstem as the portio major sensory branch and portio minor motor branch. As the nerve exits the brainstem and travels into the prepontine cistern, it transitions from central myelination by oligodendrocytes to peripheral myelination by Schwann cells, an area of change known as the "transition zone."[3] Once in the prepontine cistern, the nerve courses toward the skull base into Meckel's cave, where it forms the gasserian ganglion. At the gasserian ganglion, the nerve diverges into its three peripheral segments: ophthalmic (V1), maxillary (V2), and mandibular (V3) branches. The upper segment V1 exits out of the orbit via the superior orbital fissure, the maxillary or V2 segment exits out of the foramen rotundum after leaving the pterygopalatine fossa, and the mandibular segment V3 exits the cranium via the foramen ovale. The various sensory afferents and the motor efferent of cranial nerve V are carried in separate tracts, with a total of three sensory and one motor nuclei. The nucleus of the spinal trigeminal tract contains three parts known as the pars oralis, pars caudalis, and pars interpolaris. These subnuclei transmit pain and temperature sensation. The principal sensory nucleus integrates tactile sensation and light touch. The final sensory nucleus is the mesencephalic, which transmits proprioception of the face. These nuclei all project to the ventral posteromedial nucleus of the thalamus where they synapse, and project to the primary somatosensory nucleus of the parietal lobe. The motor nuclei innervate muscles of the first brachial arch, which includes muscles of mastication as previously described.[1,3,4,5] Critical understanding of trigeminal anatomy is key in localization of the lesion and initiating the appropriate management.

## 5.3 Clinical Evaluation

Trigeminal neuralgia is a disease entity characterized by sudden, unilateral, severe episodes of stabbing pain in the trigeminal nerve distribution, involving one or more of the peripheral nerve segments, as defined by the International Association for the Study of Pain.[6] The initial approach to trigeminal neuralgia begins with a proper history to assure an accurate clinical diagnosis. In order to properly evaluate trigeminal neuralgia, history should include inquiring about pain patterns, location, the presence of triggers, the duration of symptoms, and looking for possible causalgia. Many people suffering from trigeminal neuralgia may become aware of specific triggers that elicit their pain such as light sensation to face, cold air, brushing of teeth, drinking from a straw, stroking the hair on their face, shaving, stress, fatigue, smiling, laughing, or even kissing. It is also important to ask about the conditions that have an increased prevalence and association in developing trigeminal neuralgia, such as multiple sclerosis, stroke, hypertension, and Charcot–Marie–Tooth disease. These conditions may initially present like trigeminal neuralgia or be the causative agent.[2,4] Physical examination must include a full neurologic examination, with special attention to the head and neck, with high suspicion for secondary etiologies including mass lesions or orofacial conditions.

Classification of trigeminal neuralgia can be made on the basis of history and physical examination and, if needed, using advanced imaging such as MRI. ▶Table 5.1 lists seven different types of trigeminal neuralgia and their distinct features as well as complex grading scheme that is useful in standardizing the diagnosis into specific categories.[7] However, a more simplified categorization that can be used by primary care physicians is to organize trigeminal neuralgia into one of two groups: classic trigeminal neuralgia (CTN) and symptomatic trigeminal neuralgia (STN). CTN refers to a typical presentation of paroxysmal pain described as intense, sharp, or stabbing in nature with an associated trigger, lasting no more than a few seconds to 2 minutes. CTN does not involve neurologic deficits on physical examination and may be idiopathic or due to vascular compression with no other underlying etiology.[2,6,7] A clinical picture suggestive of CTN does not require further neuroimaging for confirmation of the disease, but an MRI is still important to obtain to rule out other pathologies. STN, on the other hand, is trigeminal neuralgia secondary to an underlying pathology other than vascular compression that may be causing injury or mass effect on the trigeminal nerve.[6,8] Atypical presentation includes those with bilateral symptoms, neurologic deficit on examination, or pain lasting more than 2 minutes, all of which should prompt suspicion of STN. A comprehensive medical history and physical examination, along with neuroimaging, can help categorize and diagnose other underlying disease pathologies.

## 5.4 Differential Diagnosis

The differential diagnosis is broad and involves a multitude of disorders arising from the head and neck. Part of the differential includes headache disorders such as cluster headache and trigeminal autonomic cephalalgias; dental pain such as tooth fracture, tooth infection, and temporomandibular joint disorders (TMJ); sinusitis; and cerebellopontine angle (CPA) tumors such as a schwannoma and meningioma.[8] Other neuralgias with features that may mimic trigeminal neuralgia include occipital neuralgia, glossopharyngeal neuralgia, postherpetic neuralgia, and atypical facial pain.[7] After clinical diagnosis is established, health care providers may classify trigeminal neuralgia and other facial pain–related syndromes.

**Table 5.1** Classification scheme for trigeminal neuralgia (TN) and distinctions

| | |
|---|---|
| TN 1 | Idiopathic spontaneous facial pain episodic in nature |
| TN 2 | Similar to type 1 but pain is constant |
| TN 3 | TN pain but secondary to unintended trauma or surgery to the trigeminal nerve |
| TN 4 | Deafferentation pain after peripheral nerve ablation in treatment of TN or facial pain |
| TN 5 | TN due to multiple sclerosis |
| TN 6 | Postherpetic neuralgia manifesting as TN |
| TN 7 | Atypical facial pain, due to somatoform manifestation from psychiatric illness |

## 5.5 Diagnostic Evaluation and Challenges

Diagnostic modalities are limited to a few useful studies. Workup may initially involve basic laboratory studies including a complete blood count (CBC) with differential and a basic metabolic profile. If there is high suspicion of an underlying condition, one may consider obtaining a lumbar puncture, angiotensin-converting enzyme (ACE) levels, and/ or erythrocyte sedimentation rate (ESR)/C-reactive protein (CRP). These laboratory investigations are generally not productive in eliciting a diagnosis in the workup of trigeminal nerve pathology. Further workup may include electromyographic (EMG) testing for trigeminal nerve reflexes, specifically the blink reflex. EMG of the blink reflex evaluates the latency and amplitude of facial muscle activation after stimulation of the first division of the trigeminal nerve. Multiple studies have shown that EMG blink reflex tests were useful in differentiating CTN from STN; the diagnostic accuracy of identifying STN with an abnormal blink reflex test had a pooled sensitivity of 94% and a pooled specificity of 87%.[2,6,8] Neuroimaging in the form of CT and MRI may identify secondary causes of trigeminal neuralgia including multiple sclerosis or mass lesions. In patients initially presenting with clinically painful trigeminal neuralgia with normal neurologic examinations, neuroimaging may still identify abnormalities in up to 10 to 18% of patients. A pooled analysis found that the overall yield of imaging is 15% in patients presenting as CTN; this was supported by class III studies.[2,6,8,9] The majority of these patients tend to present to primary care providers for initial evaluation and care. In this setting, even without neurologic deficit, it is reasonable to begin with a brain MRI. This imaging modality is the preferred study to rule out other causes and guide patients early on to the appropriate specialist such as a neurologist or a neurosurgeon if an abnormality is found. ▶Fig. 5.1 demonstrates an MRI with the normal course of the trigeminal nerve exiting the brainstem entering into Meckel's cave. Other imaging modalities such ultrasound, fluorodeoxyglucose positron emission tomography (FDG-PET)/CT, diffusion tensor imaging, fractional anisotropy, and virtual endoscopy have been investigated but generally not used for the evaluation of cranial nerve V disorders. MR and CT scan imaging have become essential for advanced practitioners and necessary due to the advent of radiosurgery therapy and for preoperative surgical planning. However, repeat imaging is not routinely performed

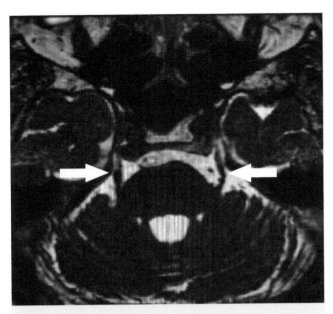

**Fig. 5.1** MRI axial brain constructive interference in steady state imaging demonstrating the trigeminal nerve exiting the pons and entering into Meckel's cave, as indicated by the right and left *arrows*.

or recommended unless a new neurologic deficit is found or a significant change in the disease is encountered. In general, MR imaging without contrast is the best initial diagnostic test, due to its high imaging quality, lack of radiation exposure, and excellent detection of soft-tissue lesions.[6] If an abnormality is found, further imaging may be obtained such as contrasted MRI studies, constructive interference in steady state (CISS), and/or CT scan to delineate seen pathology. However, to maintain a cost-effective workup, these studies are unnecessary in the primary care setting and it is advised to refer to a specialist to decide the best imaging needed and for surgical planning if needed. In this paradigm, unnecessary tests are not ordered and cost-effective efficient care is provided by a highly specialized team.

## 5.6 Medical Management

A multitude of pharmacological treatments have been used in the management of trigeminal neuralgia. The initial group of drugs used are anticonvulsants. It is recommended to begin with oral monotherapy. The most effective medication recognized in the treatment of CTN is carbamazepine, which is supported by multiple class I and II studies.[6] Other treatment options used in the management of CTN include oxcarbazepine, which is supported by class II studies.[6] Other effective but less commonly used modalities include baclofen, lamotrigine, and pimozide as oral agents.[6] Topical anesthetics on the other hand have been found to be ineffective toward pain relief or prevention of attacks. In STN, some studies have shown better pain relief using medications such as lamotrigine, gabapentin, topiramate, and misoprostol.[6] First-line treatment with carbamazepine starts with 200 to 1,200 mg/d split into two doses generally starting with 100 mg twice a day, and dose may be escalated by a 100 mg every other day until symptoms are relieved or side effects are intolerable.[10] It is reasonable to begin with oxcarbazepine as it is generally

better tolerated with less side effects, but it is generally less effective. The cost of each medication can vary year by year and from different companies. Generic carbamazepine is covered by most Medicare and insurance plans. The price may vary from $27.50 to an average retail price of $65.63 for 60 200-mg tablets (GoodRx. https://www.goodrx.com/). In comparison, oxcarbazepine's lowest price was found to be $9.00 with an average retail cost of $112.88 for 60 300-mg tablets. These costs can vary year by year and are dependent on insurance coverage. Though these medications are efficacious in over 80% of patients, dose escalation is required over time due to medication autoinduction and reduced plasma dose with only 50% efficacy rate.[10] Second-line agents such as lamotrigine, baclofen, and pimozide may be added alongside or as solo agents if patients are unable to tolerate first-line medications. Failure rates vary; for instance, baclofen followed over a 1- to 5-year period was found to be only effective in 30% of patients.[6,10] Individual circumstances, side effects, changing costs over time, and most importantly patient response will help guide cost-effective treatment. Medical management is considered a failure when patient symptomatology is no longer controlled by medications, side effects are intolerable, or patients may request surgery in fear of pain returning despite control with medications. In these situations, three primary treatments exist, which can be broken up into two categories, either ablative in the form of percutaneous procedures and stereotactic radiosurgery or nonablative microvascular decompression for CTN. If patients suffer from STN caused by a secondary process such as multiple sclerosis or tumor, then treatment would be targeted at the underlying cause. In certain situations, however, STN may be managed with the above-mentioned treatments.

## 5.7 Surgical Management

It is estimated that annually over 8,000 patients undergo surgical intervention for trigeminal neuralgia, Annually, this cost amounts to over $100 million in health care costs.[9] In the current climate of health care, medical costs and utilization are under great scrutiny. Along with implementation of the Affordable Care Act, many clinicians have become very mindful of treatment costs and burden on the system. There has been a great push for cost-effective methods for treatment of diseases. After failure of pharmacologic therapy, three primary treatment modalities are used. Microvascular decompression (MVD) is nonablative and has the longest lasting effect but has the highest cost and risk of all treatment modalities. An MVD is completed by a neurosurgeon, in which a craniotomy, or opening into the skull, allows the surgeon to explore and expose the fifth nerve throughout its entire course from the brainstem to Meckel's cave. This is a delicate procedure requiring endotracheal anesthesia and microsurgical techniques. Postoperatively, the patient is admitted in the intensive care unit but usually discharged on the second or third day after surgery.[11] Ablative procedures that are less invasive include percutaneous stereotactic rhizotomy (PSR) and stereotactic radiosurgery (SRS). Both have lower overall costs and morbidity associated with treatment, but pain does reoccur more often.[12] PSR is a less invasive procedure in which a microelectrode is inserted through the cheek entering the skull through foramen ovale to access the trigeminal nerve. Then, using an electric current to heat the electrode, a portion of the nerve is destroyed by thermal injury, in order to alleviate pain. This procedure can be done in an outpatient setting with discharge the same day without admission into the hospital.[9] SRS is an outpatient procedure where a frame is fixated to the head with pins by a neurosurgeon, assisted by a radiation oncologist, and highly focused radiation is used to destroy trigeminal nerve fibers to alleviate pain, requiring no inpatient stay.[13]

An investigation by Mazur et al took a unique approach by evaluating the quality-adjusted life-year known as the QALY calculation. This score reviewed pain relief over a 10-year period comparing the aforementioned treatment modalities. Retrospective analysis of data was obtained from Medicare claims. Overall, it was found that MVD was the number one utilized treatment modality of the three in over 51% of cases reviewed. In addition, it had the most satisfactory outcome, but it did have the highest cost. MVD QALY score was 8.22, with the total cost of the procedure being $40,435. PSR was used in 7% of cases, with a QALY score of 6.53 and overall cost of $3,911, and finally SRS therapy was used 42% of the time with a QALY score of 4.92 and a cost of $38,062. Interestingly, it was found that PSR is 11.5 time more cost-effective than MVD and SRS.[12,14] Although it was found that PSR was the most cost-effective treatment strategy, this only evaluated the direct cost of the procedure. The study did not include outpatient and in-patient services, medication use and status, need for additional procedures, out-of-pocket costs, and days lost of working. No specific study has evaluated these individual factors and the overall cost of each treatment modality. Even though PSR is the most cost appealing, it did have the highest retreatment rate, which is an important factor when considering long-term management. In the long term, MVD in fact may be the best option in carefully selected patients, taking into account durability of treatment, less need for retreatment, and overall patient satisfaction, with minimal morbidity when done by an experienced team in high-volume centers.

Treatment modalities had great variability due to age, patient's ability to tolerate certain treatments, and symptomatology making a prospective study difficult to perform. MVD was most likely to be performed on younger and healthier patients and was of highest cost, but did have the longest lasting effect, which is preferable for patients who can tolerate surgery. SRS was utilized on more elderly patients. Tarricone et al found that pain recurrence of SRS-treated patients was similar to that of MVD patients.[12] This retrospective study was completed between 2003 and 2013 reviewing 89 patients. Overall, looking at both fee and outcome, radiofrequency ablation was considered the most practical, then microvascular decompression, followed by SRS.[12,15,16] Advanced age is not considered a contraindication to surgery, but is a factor in decision making. Pollock et al evaluated the cost per quality-adjusted pain-free year and found that PSR was $6,342, MVD was $8,174, and SRS was $8269.[9] This study reinforced the usefulness of SRS for elderly patients, but MVD was projected to be more cost-effective in the long term and is recommended as the ideal treatment if surgical risk is satisfactory. A case-by-case scenario of each patient's presenting symptoms, severity, age, prior treatments, and expectations is needed to help guide the best treatment options in a cost-effective manner.

## 5.8 Outcomes

CTN consisting of sharp short-lived lancinating painful episodes in the trigeminal nerve distribution tends to respond better to surgical treatment. Patients with STN tend to have atypical symptoms and present with constant aching pain or bilateral symptoms and may have some features of CTN, leading to a mixed clinical presentation. Patients with CTN have a good clinical response, but patients with atypical features tend to have poorer response and the benefit of surgical treatment in this group is unclear. It was found that patients who suffered from atypical trigeminal neuralgia had a 91.8% relief following MVD and those with CTN had a 93% relief in pain during the immediate postoperative period. However, the recurrence rate of symptoms was 60.3% in atypical versus 19.9% in CTN patients.[11] Clinical features are very key in helping decide which patients are best suited for MVD. In our clinical practice, we generally offer MVD in CTN and in a select few scenarios for patients with atypical features.

Gamma Knife radiosurgery is also a reasonable treatment modality. The success rate reported varies, but therapy is known to delay pain relief response. Patients treated with SRS found pain relief 80.5% of time after treatment, but the average time to relief was 1.6 months. Karam et al treated patients with median radiation dose of 45 Gy with a single 4-mm isocenter. At 3 years, only 67% of patients were pain free, but 75% still reported good, satisfactory outcomes. At 69 months, only 32% were pain free and 63% were free from severe discomfort. Patients older than 70 years appeared to have a better propensity of response to SRS therapy.[13] Trigeminal neuralgia is also known as the "suicide disease" and takes a great toll on an individual's life and mental health. Kotecha et al reviewed the quality of life (QOL) and depression rates after treatment of SRS. In this study, 92% of patients were found to be pain free at 12 months. The average time to improvement of QOL score was noted at 9 months. Lower rates of depression in these groups were also noted.[17] It is of utmost importance to have thorough dialogue of patient expectations to each surgical treatment and associated costs. In addition, discussion regarding acceptable complications, such as facial numbness, as well as the need for possible retreatment must occur.

## 5.9 Conclusion

Trigeminal neuralgia is a painful neuropathic facial pain syndrome with debilitating symptoms leaving patients in a great deal of suffering. The gold standard of diagnosis is clinical diagnosis along with history to determine whether symptoms fit a CTN pattern versus STN from other causes. MRI is used to determine secondary causes including possible vascular ectasia causing trigeminal nerve compression. Secondary tests such as EMG can help differentiate CTN from STN, but they are generally not used in primary evaluation. First-line treatment is pharmacologic oral therapy. Failure of symptom control or inability to tolerate medication regimen generally requires surgical intervention. Surgical treatments include percutaneous procedures, SRS, and microvascular decompression. Each treatment has different risks, costs, benefits, and outcomes. Overall, PSR is the most cost-effective measurement, but not the most durable. MVD has the highest upfront cost, but it provides the best long-term pain relief. No specific time line of when surgical intervention should be implemented is recommended, but two class IV studies found that patients who completed surgery in retrospect would have preferred to have had surgery earlier.

# References

[1] Walker HK. Cranial nerve V: the trigeminal nerve. In: Walker HK, Hall WD, Hurst JW, eds. Clinical Methods: The History, Physical, and Laboratory Examinations. 3rd ed. Boston, MA: Butterworths; 1990

[2] Zakrzewska JM, Relton C, Krovvidi H. Trigeminal neuralgia. Neurosurg Clin N Am 2016;27(3):353–363

[3] Hughes MA, Frederickson AM, Branstetter BF, Zhu X, Sekula RF Jr. MRI of the trigeminal nerve in patients with trigeminal neuralgia secondary to vascular compression. AJR Am J Roentgenol 2016;206(3):595–600

[4] Bathla G, Hegde AN. The trigeminal nerve: an illustrated review of its imaging anatomy and pathology. Clin Radiol 2013;68(2):203–213

[5] Krafft RM. Trigeminal neuralgia. Am Fam Physician 2008;77(9):1291–1296

[6] Gronseth G, Cruccu G, Alksne J, et al. Practice parameter: the diagnostic evaluation and treatment of trigeminal neuralgia (an evidence-based review): report of the Quality Standards Subcommittee of the American Academy of Neurology and the European Federation of Neurological Societies. Neurology 2008;71(15):1183–1190

[7] Eller JL, Raslan AM, Burchiel KJ. Trigeminal neuralgia: definition and classification. Neurosurg Focus 2005;18(5):E3

[8] Lambert M. AAN and EFNS guideline on diagnosing and treating trigeminal neuralgia. Am Fam Physician 2009;79(11):1001–1002

[9] Pollock BE, Ecker RD. A prospective cost-effectiveness study of trigeminal neuralgia surgery. Clin J Pain 2005;21(4):317–322

[10] Obermann M. Treatment options in trigeminal neuralgia. Ther Adv Neurol Disorder 2010;3(2):107–115

[11] Wu A, Doshi T, Hung A, et al. Immediate and long-term outcomes of microvascular decompression for mixed trigeminal neuralgia. World Neurosurg 2018;117:e300–e307

[12] Tarricone R, Aguzzi G, Musi F, Fariselli L, Casasco A. Cost-effectiveness analysis for trigeminal neuralgia: cyberknife vs microvascular decompression. Neuropsychiatr Dis Treat 2008;4(3):647–652

[13] Karam SD, Tai A, Wooster M, et al. Trigeminal neuralgia treatment outcomes following Gamma Knife radiosurgery with a minimum 3-year follow-up. J Radiat Oncol 2014;3(2):125–130

[14] Mazur MD, Ravindra VM. Journal club: surgical management of trigeminal neuralgia: use and cost-effectiveness from an analysis of the Medicare claims database. Neurosurgery 2015;77(5):832–834

[15] Holland M, Noeller J, Buatti J, He W, Shivapour ET, Hitchon PW. The cost-effectiveness of surgery for trigeminal neuralgia in surgically naïve patients: a retrospective study. Clin Neurol Neurosurg 2015;137:34–37

[16] Sivakanthan S, Van Gompel JJ, Alikhani P, van Loveren H, Chen R, Agazzi S. Surgical management of trigeminal neuralgia: use and cost-effectiveness from an analysis of the Medicare Claims Database. Neurosurgery 2014;75(3):220–226, discussion 225–226

[17] Kotecha R, Miller JA, Modugula S, et al. Stereotactic radiosurgery for trigeminal neuralgia improves patient-reported quality of life and reduces depression. Int J Radiat Oncol Biol Phys 2017;98(5):1078–1086

# 6 Cranial Nerve VII: Facial Nerve Disorders

*Matthew Kircher, Abigail Thomas, and John Leonetti*

**Abstract**

A cost-effective approach to facial nerve disorders starts with a complete history and physical examination. The routine use of imaging, laboratory, and/or electrophysiologic studies is typically not warranted in the most common case of facial paralysis, Bell's palsy. The cost of addressing Bell's palsy can be significant, and the routine use of ancillary testing in a situation where the result is unlikely to alter diagnosis or treatment is not cost-effective. However, other causes of facial paralysis need consideration, and this analysis begins once again with the history and physical examination. Selective testing is therefore warranted on an individual basis with sufficient clinical suspicion.

*Keywords:* Bell's palsy, facial paralysis, facial paresis

## 6.1 Introduction

The facial nerve is responsible for a myriad of head and neck functions: innervating motor fibers to the muscles of facial expression and middle ear, taste receptors from the anterior two-thirds of the tongue, parasympathetic fibers to salivary glands, and somatic afferents from the external auditory canal and pinna. This nerve takes a long anatomic course through the cerebellopontine angle, temporal bone, and parotid gland, and may be at risk of injury due to inflammatory, infectious, neoplastic, traumatic, and congenital disorders. Facial nerve disorders result in life-changing functional and social deficits for many patients. About one-half of 22,594 patients surveyed at the Edinburgh facial palsy clinic demonstrated a considerable degree of psychological distress and restriction in social activities as a consequence of their facial palsy.[1] The workup of this disorder requires an in-depth understanding of anatomy and pathophysiology in order to provide efficient, cost-effective diagnoses and treatment.

## 6.2 Anatomy

The facial nerve exits the pontomedullary junction as a motor root and a mixed visceral root known as the nervus intermedius. The nerve traverses the cerebellopontine angle and enters the internal auditory canal along with the branches of the vestibulocochlear nerve before traversing the meatal foramen. The fallopian canal extends from the meatal foramen down to the stylomastoid foramen and consists of the labyrinthine segment, geniculate ganglion, horizontal tympanic segment, second genu, and vertical mastoid segment of the facial nerve. The meatal foramen is the narrowest segment of the fallopian canal with an average diameter of 0.68 mm, and it is in this region that the nerve can become compressed and dysfunction as a result of inflammation and/or trauma.

The greater petrosal nerve branches off the facial nerve at the geniculate ganglion and travels along the middle cranial fossa floor before exiting through the foramen lacerum toward the pterygopalatine ganglion to supply lacrimal and palatine glands. The nerve to the stapedius muscle branches at a point just distal to the second genu. The chorda tympani, carrying secretomotor fibers to salivary glands and taste fibers from the tongue, branches from the mastoid segment, passes under the tympanic membrane, and continues anterior to join the lingual nerve. The remaining facial nerve fibers emerge at the stylomastoid foramen to supply motor function to the muscles of facial expression (▶ Fig. 6.1).[2]

## 6.3 Clinical Assessment

History and physical examination are the most important step in evaluating facial paralysis. Timing of onset, degree of weakness (partial vs. complete), duration, and associated signs and symptoms should dictate the diagnostic workup. Patients will commonly present to an emergency department (ED) or primary care physician. The cost-effective evaluation of these patients begins with these front-line care providers to assess the patient and exclude identifiable causes of facial paresis or paralysis.

Comprehensive history and physical examination are the most readily available, informative, and cost-effective method of determining etiology of facial nerve disorder. This includes a complete head and neck examination with special attention to regional facial movement, facial resting tone, and parotid palpation. The patient may complain of dry eye secondary to incomplete eye closure (lagophthalmos) and decreased tearing ability due to loss of parasympathetic innervation of lacrimal gland by the greater superficial petrosal nerve. The efferent aspect of the corneal reflex may be absent or reduced if the motor branches to the orbicularis oculi are involved. Associated facial or auricular congenital or traumatic defects should also be noted. Sensation in the posterior auricular region can be painful or diminished, and patients may complain of hyperacusis due to stapedius muscle involvement and taste disturbance due to chorda tympani involvement. An otologic examination should document any periauricular vesicle eruption or middle ear lesions, and a neurologic examination should also be performed. The House–Brackmann (HB) scale (▶ Table 6.1) may be used to classify and communicate the degree of facial paralysis.

## 6.4 Peripheral versus Central Lesions

An upper motor neuron lesion causing facial nerve weakness will spare the forehead muscles and leave the corneal reflex intact on the affected side because of bilateral innervation to this area. Patients presenting with isolated lower facial weakness with or without other focal neurologic findings require acute evaluation for an intracranial event. However, not all isolated lower facial weakness is due to an upper motor neuron lesion. An intraparotid lesion involving the lower division of

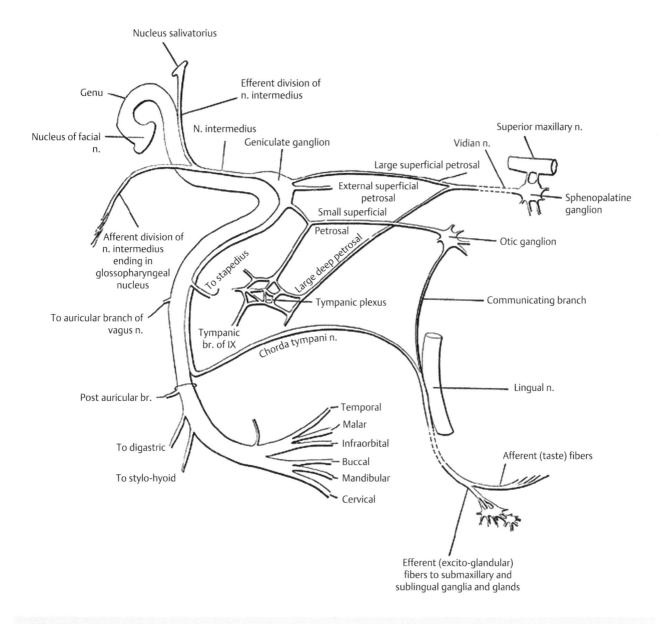

**Fig. 6.1** Facial nerve anatomy (Adapted from Carter HV, Gray H. Anatomy of the Human Body; 1918. Bartleby.com: Gray's Anatomy, Plate 788.)

the facial nerve and sparing the superior division can present in a similar manner. A peripheral or lower motor neuron lesion involves disruption of the nerve at any point from the facial nucleus to the parotid gland and will cause upper and lower face paresis or paralysis of the ipsilateral affected side with an impaired corneal reflex.

## 6.5 Diagnostic Studies

Diagnostic studies available to evaluate facial paralysis include computed tomography (CT), magnetic resonance imaging (MRI), electrophysiology, and lab studies. The fallopian canal is well defined on high-resolution CT, making this test useful in cases of suspected temporal bone pathology such as

cholesteatoma, trauma, and neoplasm. MRI can be useful in patients with suspected retrocochlear pathology or parotid gland lesions. Electrophysiologic studies such as electroneuronography (ENoG) and electromyography (EMG) may have a role in selected cases of facial nerve injury offering prognostic information in patients with complete facial paralysis. Lab studies including Lyme titers and lumbar puncture can also be considered in cases of suspected infectious or inflammatory processes.

## 6.6 Differential Diagnosis

▶Table 6.2 provides a list of potential causes for facial paralysis. This chapter will focus on a cost-effective approach to some of the more common presenting facial nerve disorders.

**Table 6.1** House–Brackmann scale

| Grade | | Function |
|---|---|---|
| I | Normal | Normal facial function in all areas. |
| II | Mild dysfunction | Slight weakness noticeable on close inspection.<br>At rest: normal symmetry of forehead; able to completely close eye with minimal effort.<br>No to slight synkinesis. |
| III[a] | Moderate dysfunction | Obvious, but not disfiguring difference between sides; noticeable but not severe synkinesis, contracture, and/or hemifacial spasm.<br>At rest: normal symmetry and tone.<br>Motion: slight to no forehead movement, able to completely close eye with maximal effort and obvious asymmetry, and able to move corners of mouth with maximal effort and obvious asymmetry. |
| IV[b] | Moderately severe dysfunction | Obvious weakness and/or disfiguring asymmetry.<br>At rest: normal symmetry and tone.<br>Motion: no forehead movement; incomplete eye closure with maximal effort. |
| V | Severe dysfunction | Only barely perceptible motion.<br>At rest: asymmetry.<br>Motion: no forehead movement; incomplete eye closure and only slight lid movement with maximal effort; slight corner of mouth movement.<br>Synkinesis, contracture, and hemifacial spasm usually absent. |
| VI | Total paralysis | Loss of tone; asymmetry; no motion; no synkinesis, contracture, or hemifacial spasm. |

[a]Obvious but no disfiguring synkinesis, contracture, and/or hemifacial spasm are grade III regardless of motor ability.
[b]Patients with synkinesis, mass action, and/or hemifacial spasm severe enough to interfere with function are grade IV regardless of motor ability.

**Table 6.2** Differential diagnosis of facial paralysis

| Acute paralysis | Chronic or progressive paralysis |
|---|---|
| Polyneuritis<br>• Bell' s palsy<br>• Herpes zoster<br>• Guillain–Barre syndrome<br>• Autoimmune disease<br>• Lyme disease<br>• Human immunodeficiency virus infection<br>• Kawasaki's disease<br><br>Trauma<br>• Temporal bone fracture<br>• Barotauma<br>• Birth trauma<br><br>Otitis media<br>• Acute bacterial<br>• Chronic bacterial<br>• Cholesteatoma<br><br>Sarcoidosis<br>• Melkersson-Rosenthal syndrome<br>• Neurologic disorders<br>• Human immunodeficiency virus infection<br>• Cerebrovascular disorder–central or peripheral | Malignancies<br>• Primary parotid tumor<br>• Metastatic tumor<br>Benign tumor<br>• Schwannoma<br>• Glomus tumor Cholesteatoma |

*Source:* Reproduced with permission from Mattox D. Clinical disorders of the facial nerve. In: Flint PW, Haughey BH, Lund VJ, et al. Cummings Otolaryngology–Head and Neck Surgery. Philadelphia, PA: Elsevier; 2010:2391–2402.

# 6.7 Bell's Palsy

The most common form of facial nerve disorder is Bell's palsy.[3] The condition is named for Sir Charles Bell, a 19th-century Scottish surgeon. Facial paralysis is acute in onset, may be partial or complete, is usually unilateral, and without another identified inciting event. Bell's palsy is by definition idiopathic; however, evidence suggests that herpes simplex virus (HSV) activation and inflammation plays a role.[4] The viral hypothesis posits that HSV reactivation leads to inflammation, edema, and subsequent nerve compression. Nerve compression at the meatal foramen and labyrinthine segment of the peripheral facial nerve leads to ischemia and nerve dysfunction. While HSV is implicated in the onset of Bell's palsy, there is no direct association. Studies of specimens in unaffected control and Bell's palsy patients have shown the presence of HSV-1 in facial nerve ganglia in both populations.[5]

Risk factors for developing Bell's palsy include diabetes, pregnancy, preeclampsia, obesity, and hypertension. The prognosis for return of function is very good with 70% of patients achieving complete resolution even without treatment.[6]

## 6.7.1 Clinical Features

The presentation of a patient with Bell's palsy includes sudden-onset unilateral facial paresis or paralysis. Decreased tearing, hyperacusis, and/or change in taste may also be evident. Bell's palsy is a diagnosis of exclusion requiring the careful elimination of other causes of facial paresis or paralysis with weakness. Presence of other focal neurological deficits is a strong indicator of intracranial event and should exclude Bell's palsy. Bilateral symptoms would also indicate alternate etiologies, such as Lyme disease or Guillain–Barré syndrome. Bell's palsy onset occurs rapidly over 1 to 2 days and reaches maximal clinical weakness within 3 weeks. Recovery of some degree of function within 6 months is expected with diagnosis of Bell's palsy in doubt if some degree of function has not returned within 3 months.[7,8] Risk factors for incomplete recovery include diabetes, pregnancy, development of postauricular pain, and age older than 60 years.

## 6.7.2 Electrodiagnostic Studies

Electrophysiologic testing may be considered to provide prognostic information on return of function only in patients with complete paralysis and has no role in partial paralysis. Electroneurography (ENOG) is an evoked compound muscle action potential derived from the muscles of facial expression. EMG measures action potentials during voluntary muscle contraction with fibrillation potentials indicative of denervated muscle and polyphasic potentials indicative of recovery.[9]

These tests are performed only on patients with complete paralysis to provide prognostic information on functional recovery. ENOG degeneration greater than 90% has been shown to predict poor recovery,[10] and EMG has been found to be up to 92% accurate in predicting recovery and up to 80% accurate in predicting poor outcomes.[11] Downsides to the test include patient discomfort from facial needle electrode placement/stimulation and cost. Per the 2017 and 2018 Medicare Fee schedules, ENOG and EMG costs range from $100 to $140, respectively.[12]

## 6.7.3 Medical Treatment

The mainstay of treatment for Bell's palsy is oral corticosteroid within 72 hours of onset. Several double-blind, placebo-controlled, randomized trials have looked at the efficacy of various steroid-dosing regimens and found no evidence to support one regimen over another.[13,14,15,16,17,18] Our practice involves administration of a 12-day oral prednisone taper of 60 mg for 4 days, 40 mg for 4 days, and 20 mg for 4 days.

Eye protection should be implemented in those with impaired eye closure. Eye protection is inexpensive, imperative to the prevention of long-term deficits, and includes the use of Lacri-Lube, artificial tear drops, taping eyes closed at night, and/or use of goggles for protection.

Antivirals may be added to the regimen, although there is mixed evidence for their use. Two large clinical trials by Sullivan et al and Engström et al found no significant differences in recovery between antivirals and placebo or between steroids only and steroids and antivirals.[16,17] However, both of these studies included patients with all degrees of facial weakness, so there is the question of whether beneficial antiviral response in patients with severe or complete paralysis was masked by those patients with mild paresis that would have recovered without any treatment.

## 6.7.4 Surgical Decompression

Despite medical therapy, some patients may still achieve poor functional recovery. Gantz et al demonstrated that patients with poor prognosis for recovery on electrophysiologic testing can benefit from middle fossa facial nerve decompression in the acute setting.[10] In this study, ENOG and EMG were performed within 2 weeks' onset of Bell's palsy with complete paralysis. All patients with less than 90% ENOG degeneration ($n = 54$) returned to HB I to II. Those patients with greater than 90% degeneration on ENOG and no EMG recovery potentials were offered middle fossa facial nerve decompression versus medical treatment alone. Thirty-four patients elected surgery and 36 elected medical treatment alone. In the medical treatment group, 42% achieved HB I to II and 58% achieved HB III to IV. In the surgical group, 91% achieved HB I to II and 9% achieved HB III to IV. In this study, surgical decompression significantly improved facial function.

## 6.7.5 Bell's Palsy Clinical Guidelines

In 2013, the American Academy of Otolaryngology–Head and Neck Surgery released clinical practice guidelines for Bell's palsy based on best available evidence (▶Table 6.3).[19] The expert panel made strong recommendations that clinicians should perform history and physical examination to exclude identifiable causes of facial paresis or paralysis, start oral steroids within 72 hours of symptom onset, and implement dry eye precautions in patients with impaired eye closure. These recommendations also happen to be a cost-effective approach.

The panel also made recommendations that routine laboratory testing and diagnostic imaging should not be obtained.

**Table 6.3** AAO clinical practice guidelines: Bell's palsy

| Strong recommendation | Recommendation | Option | No recommendation |
|---|---|---|---|
| Assess patient using history and physical examination (AEQ: Grade C; Confidence: high) | AGAINST obtaining routine lab testing (AEQ: Grade C; Confidence: high) | Offer antiviral therapy in addition to oral steroids within 72 h of symptom onset (AEC: Grade B; Confidence: medium) | Surgical decompression (AEC: Grade D; Confidence: low) |
| Prescribe oral steroids within 72 h of symptom onset for patients ≥ 16 y (AEC: Grade A; Confidence: high) | AGAINST routinely performing diagnostic imaging (AEC: Grade C; Confidence: high) | Offer electrodiagnostic testing to patients with complete facial paralysis (AEC: Grade C; Confidence: medium) | Acupuncture (AEC: Grade B; Confidence: low) |
| AGAINST prescribing oral antiviral therapy alone (AEC: Grade A; Confidence: high) | AGAINST performing electrodiagnostic testing in patients with incomplete paralysis (AEC: Grade C; Confidence: high) | | Physical therapy (AEC: Grade D; Confidence: low) |
| Implement eye protection for patients with impaired eye closure (AEC: Grade X; Confidence: high) | Reassess/refer to facial nerve specialist patients with: new/worsening neuro finding, ocular symptoms, incomplete recovery 3 mo after initial onset (AEC: Grade C; Confidence: high) | | |

*Abbreviations:* AEQ: aggregate evidence quality (based on evidence, benefit vs. harm and diagnosis); Confidence: level of confidence in evidence.

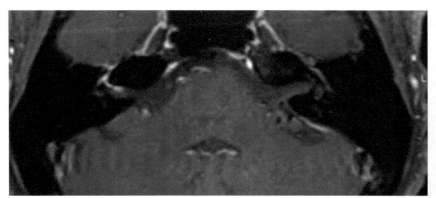

**Fig. 6.2** MRI with facial nerve enhancement.

Routine diagnostic imaging was discouraged, as history and physical examination have been shown to be the most informative investigation, and acute facial paresis/paralysis in the absence of explanatory history or physical findings is idiopathic in the vast majority of cases.[20,21] CT of the temporal bone is not indicated in cases of suspected Bell's palsy, and MRI studies may show enhancement along the involved facial nerve (►Fig. 6.2); however, this finding often does not influence the course of therapy and may in fact be mistaken for a primary facial nerve neoplasm.[22] Imaging may be indicated in the event of suggestive history or physical findings, such as temporal bone trauma, paralysis of isolated facial nerve branches, recurrent or progressive paralysis, concern for neoplasm, and no sign of recovery after 3 months (►Fig. 6.3). In addition, the panel made no recommendation regarding the role of surgical decompression in Bell's palsy, citing low-quality, nonrandomized trials and equilibrium of benefit and harm. Additional panel recommendations, options, or no recommendations statements are detailed in ►Table 6.3.

## 6.8 Herpes Zoster Oticus

Herpes zoster oticus or Ramsey–Hunt syndrome is the second most common viral infection associated with facial palsy. In a large series of 1,701 cases of acute peripheral facial nerve palsy, 116 had herpes zoster.[6] These patients present with acute facial paralysis coinciding with the herpetiform periauricular vesicles of a shingles outbreak and often vestibulocochlear dysfunction (see ►Fig. 6.1). The vesicles cause severe pain involving the external auditory canal and pinna, and can be evident prior to facial paralysis, serving as a herald sign. Patients ailed with Ramsey–Hunt syndrome can exhibit concurrent vertigo and balance issues. Prognosis for return of function is not as favorable as Bell's palsy, with only about half of patients with HB grade V to VI function returning to HB grade I to II.[23]

Diagnostic imaging is rarely indicated with classic presentation of herpes zoster oticus. Should MRI be acquired, high signal enhancement of the nerve will show up on contrast-enhanced scans. Audiologic and/or vestibular testing may be pursued in those cases with complaint. Treatment includes steroids, analgesics, anticonvulsants, and antiviral agents.

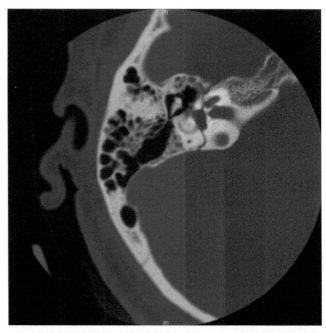

**Fig. 6.3** CT scan of temporal bone fracture involving fallopian canal.

## 6.9 Trauma

Obvious trauma or basal skull fracture would indicate traumatic facial nerve palsy ►Fig. 6.4. Timing of facial paralysis after trauma can give clue to mechanism of injury, with delayed paralysis suggesting nerve edema, while immediate paralysis is indicative of complete nerve disruption. Delayed-onset paralysis after temporal bone fracture should be treated with steroids with good prognosis for recovery expected and surgery rarely indicated. Immediate-onset paralysis often warrants facial nerve exploration, decompression, and repair, as described in ►Fig. 6.5.

## 6.10 Acute Otitis Media

Acute otitis media is a rare cause of facial paralysis due to the introduction of antibiotics. Prior to the antibiotic era, infection

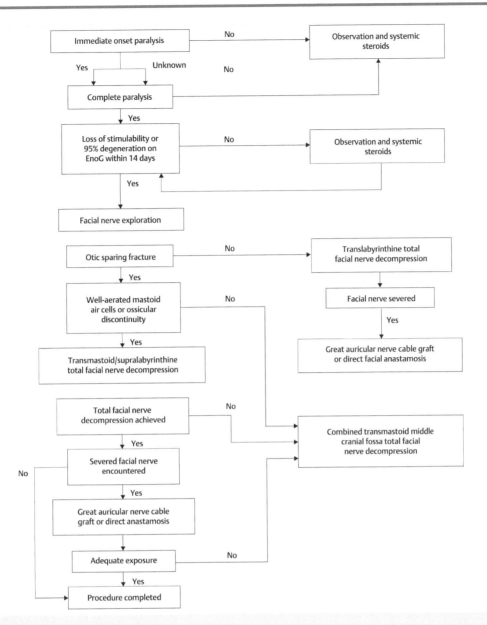

**Fig. 6.4** Management of temporal bone trauma (Reproduced with permission from Brodie H. Management of facial nerve trauma, In: Flint PW, Haughey BH, Lund VJ, et al. Cummings Otolaryngology–Head and Neck Surgery. Philadelphia, PA: Elsevier; 2010:2036–2048.)

extension into the nerve sheath caused an incidence in up to 0.5% of cases.[2] Imaging is usually unnecessary, as obvious signs of infection are evident in the initial workup, except in rare cases of intracranial complication. Most cases are managed effectively with systemic antibiotics with or without myringotomy and tube insertion (▶Fig. 6.5).

## 6.11 Chronic Otitis Media

Chronic otitis media with or without cholesteatoma can put patients at risk for facial paralysis secondary to facial nerve compression, chronic inflammation, and/or erosion. Audiometry, CT temporal bone imaging, and surgery would be indicated in this scenario.

## 6.12 Lyme Disease

Indications of Lyme disease include recent tick bites or travel to endemic areas, along with the classic bull's eye rash, fatigue, and joint pain and swelling. Facial paralysis can occur in 6 to 11% of patients and can be unilateral or bilateral. Symptoms often appear in the early disseminated phase of illness.[2] Diagnosis is often clinical but can be supported by Lyme disease serology.

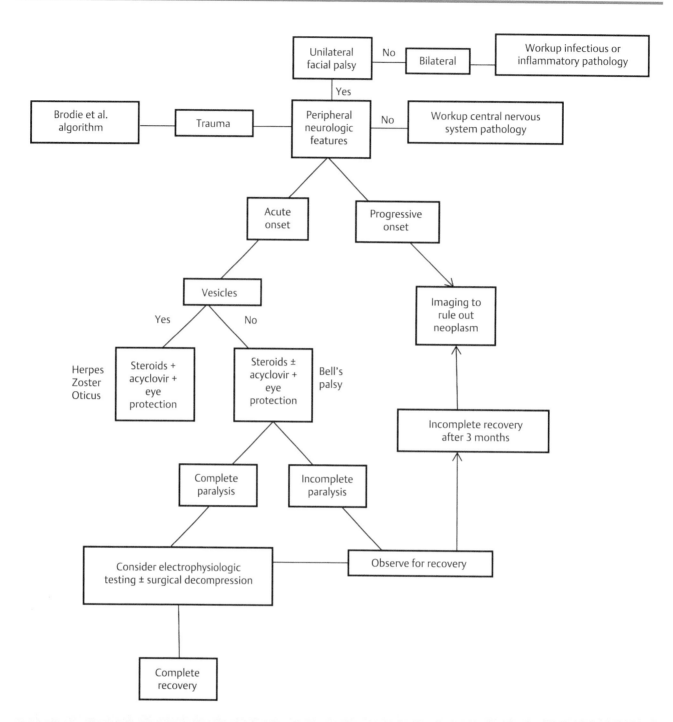

**Fig. 6.5** Cost-effective treatment algorithm for unilateral facial palsy.

## 6.13 Facial Nerve Tumors or Neoplasm

Slow, progressive onset of facial paralysis is a red flag for neoplastic activity. Symptoms lasting beyond 3 weeks and/or no return of function by 3 months would indicate further workup and imaging. Patients presenting with facial weakness, pain, and associated lymphadenopathy should be considered for malignancy and worked up accordingly.

## 6.14 Cost Discussion

Costs associated with the evaluation of facial paralysis can be attributed to visits to the emergency room, urgent care, primary care, specialists, and diagnostic testing as previously discussed. The cost of addressing Bell's palsy is no doubt significant with 35,000 to 100,000 cases annually in the United States.[19] In California EDs between 2005 and 2011, there were 43,979 total patients discharged with a diagnosis of Bell's palsy. A total of 6,224 (14.2%) underwent neuroimaging as part of their ED evaluation; 5,763 (13.2%) had CT alone, 238 (0.6%) had MRI alone, and 223 (0.5%) had both. On 90-day follow-up, 356 patients (0.8%) received an alternative diagnosis such as stroke, intracranial hemorrhage, subarachnoid hemorrhage, brain tumor, central nervous system infection, Guillain–Barré syndrome, Lyme disease, otitis media/mastoiditis, and herpes zoster.[24] This study demonstrates the rare occurrence of alternative diagnoses when Bell's palsy is suspected and argues for a complete history and physical examination and against routine diagnostic testing. Selective testing is warranted when alternative pathology is considered and should be directed with clinical suspicion and cost considerations in mind.

## 6.14.1 Cost-Effective Treatment Algorithm

The cost-effective treatment algorithm is shown in detail in ▶ Fig. 6.5.

# 6.15 Long-Term Sequelae of Facial Paralysis

Some patients suffering a facial nerve injury will develop permanent dysfunction and may benefit from a variety of static and dynamic facial reanimation procedures. Depending on the type and degree of injury, facial nerve recovery can range from mild facial asymmetry to complete paralysis. In those patients with partial recovery, synkinesis may be evident and routine outpatient Botox facial chemodenervation can be used in relaxing synkinesis and improving facial symmetry. Protection of the cornea from drying is paramount in these patients and so eyelid weight placement with or without lid-tightening procedures is often employed. Improvement in lower facial tone and movement may include static sling procedures, nerve grafting, and regional and free muscle tissue transfer.

# References

[1] Weir A, Pentland B, Crosswaite A, Murray J, Mountain R. Bell's palsy: the effect on self-image, mood state and social activity. Clin Rehabil 1995;9(2):121–125

[2] Kumar A, Mafee MF, Mason T. Value of imaging in disorders of the facial nerve. Top Magn Reson Imaging 2000;11(1):38–51

[3] Gilden DH. Clinical practice. Bell's palsy. N Engl J Med 2004;351(13):1323–1331

[4] Musani MA, Farooqui AN, Usman A, et al. Association of herpes simplex virus infection and Bell's palsy. J Pak Med Assoc 2009;59(12):823–825

[5] Linder T, Bossart W, Bodmer D. Bell's palsy and Herpes simplex virus: fact or mystery? Otol Neurotol 2005;26(1):109–113

[6] Peitersen E. Bell's palsy: the spontaneous course of 2,500 peripheral facial nerve palsies of different etiologies. Acta Otolaryngol Suppl 2002(549):4–30

[7] Hashisaki GT. Medical management of Bell's palsy. Compr Ther 1997; 23(11):715–718

[8] Selesnick SH, Patwardhan A. Acute facial paralysis: evaluation and early management. Am J Otolaryngol 1994;15(6):387–408

[9] Gordin E, Lee TS, Ducic Y, Arnaoutakis D. Facial nerve trauma: evaluation and considerations in management. Craniomaxillofac Trauma Reconstr 2015;8(1):1–13

[10] Gantz BJ, Rubinstein JT, Gidley P, Woodworth GG. Surgical management of Bell's palsy. Laryngoscope 1999;109(8):1177–1188

[11] Sittel C, Stennert E. Prognostic value of electromyography in acute peripheral facial nerve palsy. Otol Neurotol 2001;22(1):100–104

[12] American Speech-Language-Hearing Association. 2017 Medicare Fee Schedule for Audiologists. http://www.asha.org/uploadedFiles/2017-Medicare-Physician-Fee-Schedule-Audiology.pdf. Published 2017. Accessed July 25, 2018

[13] Adour KK, Ruboyianes JM, Von Doersten PG, et al. Bell's palsy treatment with acyclovir and prednisone compared with prednisone alone: a double-blind, randomized, controlled trial. Ann Otol Rhinol Laryngol 1996;105(5):371–378

[14] Hato N, Yamada H, Kohno H, et al. Valacyclovir and prednisolone treatment for Bell's palsy: a multicenter, randomized, placebo-controlled study. Otol Neurotol 2007;28(3):408–413

[15] Kawaguchi K, Inamura H, Abe Y, et al. Reactivation of herpes simplex virus type 1 and varicella-zoster virus and therapeutic effects of combination therapy with prednisolone and valacyclovir in patients with Bell's palsy. Laryngoscope 2007;117(1):147–156

[16] Sullivan FM, Swan IR, Donnan PT, et al. Early treatment with prednisolone or acyclovir in Bell's palsy. N Engl J Med 2007;357(16):1598–1607

[17] Engström M, Berg T, Stjernquist-Desatnik A, et al. Prednisolone and valaciclovir in Bell's palsy: a randomised, double-blind, placebo-controlled, multicentre trial. Lancet Neurol 2008;7(11):993–1000

[18] Yeo SG, Lee YC, Park DC, Cha CI. Acyclovir plus steroid vs steroid alone in the treatment of Bell's palsy. Am J Otolaryngol 2008;29(3):163–166

[19] Baugh RF, Basura GJ, Ishii LE, et al. Clinical practice guideline: Bell's palsy. Otolaryngol Head Neck Surg 2013;149(3, Suppl):S1–S27

[20] Holland NJ, Weiner GM. Recent developments in Bell's palsy. BMJ 2004;329(7465):553–557

[21] Holland J. Bell's palsy. BMJ Clin Evid 2008;2008:1204

[22] Kinoshita T, Ishii K, Okitsu T, Okudera T, Ogawa T. Facial nerve palsy: evaluation by contrast-enhanced MR imaging. Clin Radiol 2001;56(11):926–932

[23] Monsanto RD, Bittencourt AG, Bobato Neto NJ, Beilke SC, Lorenzetti FT, Salomone R. Treatment and prognosis of facial palsy on Ramsay Hunt syndrome: results based on a review of the literature. Int Arch Otorhinolaryngol 2016;20(4):394–400

[24] Fahimi J, Navi BB, Kamel H. Potential misdiagnoses of Bell's palsy in the emergency department. Ann Emerg Med 2014;63(4):428–434

# 7 Cranial Nerve VIII: Hearing Disorders

*Eric N. Appelbaum and Daniel H. Coelho*

**Abstract**

Cost-effective evaluation of audiovestibular disorders relies on a detailed and directed history and physical examination. Audiologic evaluation is the primary ancillary examination for auditory and vestibular disorders. Laboratory testing and imaging of the inner ear and brain should be guided by specific findings on history, physical examination, and audiological evaluation. Hearing loss is common, especially in patients older than 60 years. Patients with a complaint of hearing loss should undergo audiological evaluation. Patients with asymmetric sensorineural hearing loss (SNHL) noted on audiogram, including sudden SNHL (SSNHL), should undergo MRI to evaluate for retrocochlear pathology (most commonly vestibular schwannoma). Patients with conductive hearing loss (other than cerumen impaction that can be resolved by the primary care physician) should be referred to an otolaryngologist for further evaluation. Treatment options for conductive hearing loss include observation, hearing aid, and surgery. SNHL is common in older adults but can occur at any age. Treatment options for SNHL include observation, hearing aids, and cochlear implants. All newborns should be screened for hearing loss. Newborns with abnormalities on hearing screening should be further evaluated until hearing loss is definitively ruled in or out. Loss of follow-up is a major concern in this population. Stepwise, algorithmic evaluation of congenital hearing loss is critical to perform a thorough evaluation in a cost-effective manner.

*Keywords:* audiovestibular disorders, hearing loss, presbycusis, dizziness, vertigo, otosclerosis, vestibular schwannoma, Meniere's disease, vestibular neuritis, superior canal dehiscence syndrome

## 7.1 Introduction

Hearing and vestibular sensation are functions of the ears. While there are disorders that affect both hearing and vestibular function (Meniere's disease, vestibular schwannoma [VS] tumors, labyrinthitis), most disorders affect only one system. Therefore, hearing and balance disorders will be addressed separately. Most of the content applies to patients of all ages. There are, however, special sections dedicated to newborn hearing evaluation and cochlear implantation. These are divided into separate sections in this chapter.

## 7.2 Hearing Loss

### 7.2.1 Auditory Anatomy and Physiology

The ear can be thought of comprising three components: the outer ear (pinna and external auditory canal), the middle ear (from the tympanic membrane [TM] to the stapes footplate), and the inner ear (the cochlea and the semicircular canals). In a healthy ear, sound first arrives at the outer ear, transmitted as air vibrations. Sound then travels past the pinna through the external auditory canal (ear canal) to the TM. Air vibrations are transformed into mechanical vibrations, first of the TM and then of the ossicular chain (malleus, incus, stapes bones) in the middle ear. The energy of the oscillating stapes is transferred through the oval window of the cochlea. Within the cochlea, the sound energy is transmitted as inner ear fluid waves. These waves cause the movement of hair cells within the cochlea. Hair cell movement leads to excitation of the cochlear nerve. The signal from the cochlear nerve travels through the internal auditory canal (IAC) to the cochlear nucleus in the brainstem (retrocochlear pathway). The central auditory pathway then carries the neural input onto appropriate regions of the brain.

### 7.2.2 Epidemiology and Economic Impact of Hearing Loss

Hearing loss is one of the most common and debilitating cranial neuropathies worldwide. In the United States alone, it is estimated that 68% of adults older than 70 years experience hearing loss but that only approximately 20% seek treatment.[1,2] The economic burden related to hearing loss is enormous in the billions of dollars in the United States.[3] Medical expenses alone related hearing loss are estimated to be $12.8 billion.[4] This figure includes indirectly related medical expenses as individuals with hearing loss are at increased risk for falls, hospitalizations, and cognitive decline.[5,6,7]

In addition to simply not being able to hear the surrounding environment, hearing loss can lead to a reduction in overall quality of life (QOL) and reduced ability to engage with others and can predispose to development of depression.[8] A study of individuals with severe hearing loss prior to cochlear implantation showed an average health utility index (HUI; a measure of disability with 1 being perfect health and 0 being dead) score of 0.49 to 0.54, similar to stroke survivors or those with end-stage renal disease.[9]

Beyond the direct and indirect medical costs are estimated losses in productivity. Kochkin estimated that the amount of lost income attributable to hearing loss in the United States may be as high as $176 billion with an additional $26 billion of unrealized federal taxes.[10] Treatment of hearing loss is of paramount importance and potentially will prevent billions of dollars' worth of disability and, more importantly, restore a fundamental ability to interact with one's environment.

### 7.2.3 Clinical Approach of Hearing Loss

Hearing loss can be conductive, sensorineural, or mixed. Conductive hearing loss (CHL) is caused by a problem with transference of sound energy from the air to the cochlea. CHL generally relates to a problem of the external or middle ear. Sensorineural hearing loss (SNHL) is caused by a problem within the cochlea (inner ear), the cochlear nerve, or the auditory pathway (the latter two of which comprise the retrocochlear pathway). There can be simultaneous conductive and SNHL, which is considered a mixed hearing loss.

Hearing loss can be caused by a myriad of conditions. Some causes are easily diagnosed and treated such as cerumen impaction, a mechanical obstruction of the external auditory canal by wax build-up. Other pathologies, such as VS, are rare causes of hearing loss that present diagnostic challenges to the physician. In order to choose appropriate ancillary tests and to arrive at an accurate diagnosis of the underlying etiology of hearing loss, a pertinent history and physical examination must be performed. In addition, an audiological evaluation is an essential tool for the evaluation of hearing loss.

## 7.2.4 History

Essential elements of a history for a patient with hearing loss include description of hearing loss onset (sudden vs. gradual), duration, severity, unilateral versus bilateral, progressive versus stable, and stable versus fluctuating. Additionally, the patient should be asked about otalgia, tinnitus, drainage from the ear canals (otorrhea), aural fullness, and dizziness. History related to head trauma, barotrauma, noise exposure, exposure to ototoxic medications, previous ear infections, previous otologic surgery, and family history of otologic problems should also be ascertained. A full history including current medications, past medical and surgical history, social background, and family history should be performed.

## 7.2.5 Physical Examination

A complete head and neck examination should be performed on patients complaining of hearing loss, including an examination of the cranial nerves, face, scalp, eyes, nose, oral cavity, neck, pinna, external auditory canals, and TMs. Examination of the external auditory canals and TMs should be performed with a microscope as opposed to a handheld otoscope whenever possible. Pneumatic otoscopy should be performed to test for TM mobility. A tuning fork examination should be performed, typically with a 512-Hz tuning fork. In the Weber test, the tuning fork is placed on the center of the forehead. The sound of the tuning fork lateralizes away from the side with a SNHL and toward the side with a CHL. In the Rinne test, the sound intensity is compared between air conduction and bone conduction by placing the tuning fork in front of the ear and directly onto the mastoid bone behind the ear to see which is subjectively louder to the patient. If the air conduction condition is considered louder, the result is positive. If the bone conduction condition is considered louder, the result is negative and typically reflects at least a 25-dB CHL on that side.

## 7.2.6 Audiological Evaluation

An audiological evaluation should routinely be performed for those complaining of hearing loss, except in the case where the hearing loss can be resolved by removing cerumen from the external auditory canals.[11] Audiometric evaluation includes pure-tone audiometry, tympanometry, and speech audiometry.

## 7.2.7 Pure-Tone Audiometry

Pure-tone audiometry is a behavioral test in which the patient responds to pure-tone stimuli. Pure-tone audiometry allows for determination of the type of hearing loss (SNHL, CHL, or mixed), the pattern, and the severity of the hearing loss. In pure-tone audiometry, thresholds are obtained from the patient at a sequence of pure-tone frequencies. Thresholds are typically assessed at 250, 500, 1,000, 2,000, 4,000, and 8,000 Hz. A threshold is defined as the lowest intensity at which the patient is able to respond to the pure-tone stimulus at least 50% of the time. Pure-tone thresholds are obtained for both air conduction (through earphones or ear inserts) and bone conduction (through vibration of the mastoid bone). Pure-tone average (PTA) is a measure of hearing loss and is defined as the average of the 500-, 1,000-, and 2,000-Hz thresholds.

## 7.2.8 Speech Audiometry

Speech reception threshold (SRT) is the quietest level at which the patient can correctly recognize two-syllable words at least 50% of the time. Word recognition score (WRS) is the percentage of words correctly identified by the patient from a standard phonetically balanced word list presented about 40 dB above the PTA. WRS is routinely tested on the Central Institute for the Deaf (CID) Auditory Test W-22. WRSs are considered excellent (90–100%), good (80–90%), fair (70–80%), or poor (<70%). WRSs are expected to increase to a maximum accuracy as the intensity level that they are presented at increase from the PTA with the exception for patients with eighth cranial nerve pathology (such as a VS), where increasing the sound intensity above a certain point can lead to a decrease in WRS (also known as rollover).

## 7.2.9 Acoustic Immittance Testing

Acoustic immittance testing is generally composed of tympanometry and acoustic reflex testing.

### Tympanometry

Tympanometry is a test by which energy is transmitted through the ear canal and the reflection of the energy back to the probe is measured. Tympanometry provides information about middle ear function by giving an estimate of admittance, which can be thought of as the compliance of the TM as well as an estimate of the ear canal volume. Low compliance (e.g., flat tympanogram) with a large estimated ear canal volume can be seen in a TM perforation. Low compliance with a normal ear canal volume can be seen in patients with middle ear effusion.

### Acoustic Reflex Testing

The acoustic reflex, also known as the stapedial reflex, is the contraction of the stapedius muscle in response to high-intensity sound. The acoustic reflex is triggered bilaterally when high-intensity sound is presented to either ear. The reflex can be detected by a change in compliance of the TM. The acoustic reflex threshold is the lowest intensity level at which a change in TM compliance can be measured. In a patient with bilateral CHL, acoustic reflexes are generally absent bilaterally.

In a patient with unilateral CHL, stimulation of the unaffected ear will result in an ipsilateral acoustic reflex, while stimulation of the affected ear may or may not lead to an acoustic reflex depending on the severity of the CHL. In a patient with sensory (cochlear) hearing loss greater than 80 dB, acoustic reflexes are generally absent. In a patient with sensory hearing loss less than 80 dB, acoustic reflexes are generally present at higher intensity thresholds. Acoustic reflexes will be diminished or absent in patients with facial nerve disorders proximal to the branch of the nerve to the stapedius muscle.

## 7.2.10 Otoacoustic Emissions

Cochlear outer hair cell movements generate sounds called otoacoustic emissions (OAEs). The presence of OAEs therefore gives objective evidence to the presence of outer hair cells in the cochlea. OAEs can be measured by placing a microphone in the ear canal. Transient-evoked otoacoustic emissions (TEOAEs) are evoked by use of a broadband click. TEOAEs are generally used for newborn hearing screening (▶ Fig. 7.1). TEOAEs are present in most normal hearing ears. The presence of TEOAEs suggests hearing thresholds of at least 20-dB hearing level. Distortion product otoacoustic emissions (DPOAEs) are evoked by simultaneous application of two pure-tone frequencies. DPOAEs are able to assess higher frequencies than TEOAEs. DPOAEs are used for hearing screening for patients with concern for ototoxicity and noise-induced hearing loss.

## 7.2.11 Auditory Evoked Potentials

Auditory evoked potentials are neuroelectrical events that can be measured in response to auditory stimulus that reflects transmission of signal in the auditory system. Both electrocochleography (ECochG) and auditory brainstem response (ABR) are tests that rely on auditory evoked potentials.

### Electrocochleography

During the first 2 to 3 milliseconds after an auditory stimulus is delivered to the ear canal, it will result in the ECOG response that can be measured with electrodes placed onto or near the TM. The summating potential (SP) and the compound action potential (AP) are measured. An elevated SP/AP ratio greater than 0.45 is generally considered abnormal and suggests increased labyrinthine pressure, although institutions may have a higher or lower limit of normal. This can be used to aid in the diagnosis and monitoring of Meniere's disease and superior semicircular canal dehiscence syndrome.

### Auditory Brainstem Response

Auditory stimulus delivered to the ear canal will result in an ABR during the first 10 milliseconds after delivery of the stimulus. The response is measured by multiple electrodes placed on the scalp. The response is characterized by five waves approximating different locations along the auditory pathway: (1) wave I corresponds to the distal portion of CN VIII; (2) wave II to the proximal portion of CN VIII; (3) wave to III the cochlear nucleus, (4) wave IV to the superior olivary complex, and (5) wave V the inferior colliculus. ABR can be used for hearing screening and pure-tone threshold estimation in all ages (including newborns) by determining the lowest threshold at which wave V of the ABR is present. ABR can also be used to monitor hearing during neurotologic procedures (e.g., middle cranial fossa VS resection).

## 7.2.12 Imaging

### Computed Tomography Scan of the Temporal Bone

High-resolution computed tomography (HRCT) of the temporal bones without intravenous contrast provides excellent structural detail of the bony anatomy of the auditory pathway.

### Magnetic Resonance Imaging

Magnetic resonance imaging (MRI) with attention to the IACs with and without intravenous contrast such as gadolinium provides detailed soft-tissue evaluation of the auditory pathway.

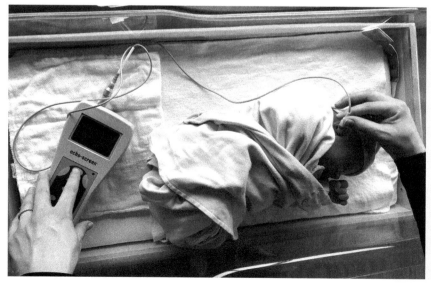

**Fig. 7.1** A newborn undergoing otoacoustic emission (OAE) for hearing screening on the second day of life prior to discharge home.

# 7.3 Cost-Effective Clinical Approach to Specific Hearing Loss Disorders

## 7.3.1 Presbycusis

Progressive hearing loss with age is common, affecting greater than 50% of individuals older than 60 years.[3,12] The majority of cases are thought to be caused by degeneration of hair cells within the cochlea due to age and cumulative noise exposure. While there is limited evidence to support the cost-effectiveness of routine audiometric hearing screen in adults older than 50 years, any older adult who complains of hearing loss should be referred for audiometric evaluation.[4,13] Patients who are found to have symmetric down-sloping SNHL should be referred to an otolaryngologist for evaluation (▶Fig. 7.2). Further workup including imaging is not needed in cases of gradual, symmetric down-sloping hearing loss in older adults as this is the pattern associated with age-related hearing loss. However, a sudden decline in hearing bilaterally should be investigated as this is not typical of aging. Treatment options include observation, hearing aid amplification, and cochlear implants in bilateral severe hearing loss.

## Hearing Aids

For those who are suffering from mild to severe forms of hearing loss, hearing aids are often the best and most cost-effective option. A hearing aid is defined by the U.S. Food and Drug Administration (FDA) as "any wearable instrument or device designed for, offered for the purpose of, or represented as aiding persons with or compensating for, impaired hearing."[11,14] Essentially, hearing aids consist of a directional microphone, amplifier, microprocessor, and speaker. Over the last approximately four decades, the efficacy of hearing aids has increased, while their size has decreased. Starting with the digitization of signal in the 1980s and 1990s, hearing aid technology has advanced greatly with recent advances in battery capability, noise reduction, signal compression, and device compatibility via Bluetooth.[12,15] The FDA has established requirements regulating hearing aid including technical standards, device capability, as well as the requirement of preintervention medical clearance in certain circumstances.

Unfortunately, hearing aid use in the United States can be expensive, with estimates of average cost for a pair of hearing aids in 2013 being approximately $4,700 (range: $3,300–6,000).[3,16] This estimate includes a package of professional consultation with a licensed audiologist, device selection, fitting, and ongoing adjustments. Approximately 3 million hearing aids are dispensed every year in the United States with the largest single provider being the Department of Veteran's Affairs (VA) Medical System, responsible for about 20% of the total volume of hearing aids dispensed.[3,16] The VA's bulk purchasing power allows it to negotiate much lower prices for each aid compared to what is sold privately. In 2014, for example, the VA reported it paid an average of $369 per device, up to $1,900 cheaper than comparable pricing for aids sold in the surrounding area.[4,17] This pricing is separate from the services bundle provided by VA audiologist and otolaryngologists, however, and

thus gives the best "real-world" example of at-cost device pricing. Indeed, much of the criticism leveled at the cost of hearing aids involves the lack of clarity in pricing structure. An inability to separate the actual technology from the service bundle, vertical integration of hearing aid companies with vendors, and changing insurance coverage structures with insurance plans all contribute.

Hearing aids are specifically not covered by Medicare Part A or B in the original language of the statute: "Notwithstanding any other provision of this title, no payment may be made under Part A or B for any expenses incurred for items or services ... where such expenses are for ... hearing aids or examinations therefore."[13,18] Starting at age 65, U.S. citizens covered by Medicare are eligible for an Annual Wellness Check performed by a qualified medical provider which can include screening for hearing or vestibular disorders and testing thereof.[14,19] Audiologists can be reimbursed for performance of testing (audiogram) as directed by a physician or other medical provider. Hearing aids must then be paid for out-of-pocket or with private insurance. An increasingly popular option is Medicare Part C (Medicare Advantage) programs, which allow for recipients to opt out of traditional Medicare coverage and instead have those funds directed toward a private insurer.

Private insurances, however, have only marginally better rates of coverage for hearing health and vary widely in total dollar amount covered often with omission of key services for fitting, support, and continued service. Employer-sponsored health plans, covered by the Employee Retirement Income Security Act of 1974, are similarly variable in their coverage of hearing services and often vary widely between states. Currently, only three states, Arkansas, New Hampshire, and Rhode Island, mandate coverage of hearing aids and hearing services for adults.[4,17] Some federal employees, such as members of Congress, covered by Federal Employee Health Benefits Program have coverage for hearing aids. Members of the military and their families who are covered by TRICARE have access to hearing aid coverage for qualifying hearing loss. These benefits are often accessed through the VA system.

The VA continues to be one of the largest and most important disbursers of hearing aids in the United States, and audiological services are one of the highest-demand services within the VA itself.[15,20] The VA covers audiological services and hearing aids if hearing loss is determined to be related to military service and is the single largest reason for service-connected coverage within the VA system.[4,17]

A cost-effective alternative for those with mild, minimally bothersome hearing loss are personal sound amplification products (PSAPs). The FDA differentiates a PSAP from a hearing aid as a "wearable electronic product that is not intended to compensate for impaired hearing, but rather is intended for non-hearing impaired consumers to amplify sounds in certain environments."[16] Classically, these have included devices used for bird-watching, hunting, sports watching, and others. They often consist of a simple directional microphone and an amplifier. PSAPs are not subject to FDA regulation as medical devices and thus are available essentially as over-the-counter (OTC) options for amplification. Costs of these devices generally range from approximately $25 to $300. For those with minimally bothersome hearing loss, mild hearing loss, or inability to afford more expensive options for treatment of SNHL, PSAPs

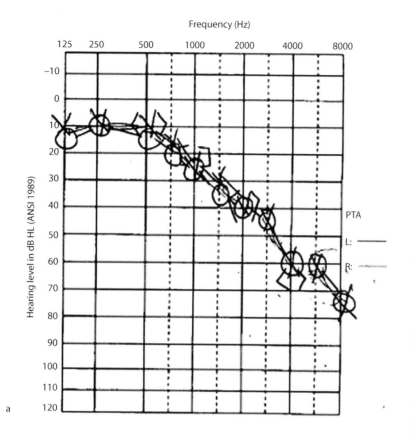

**Fig. 7.2** (a, b) Audiometric results for presbycusis.

|  | SRT | | Word recognition | | |
|---|---|---|---|---|---|
|  | dB | Mask | % | Mask | SL |
| Right | 25 |  | 96 |  | +35 |
| Left | 30 |  | 100 |  | +35 |

may represent a viable alternative for therapy in certain situations. In 2017, the Over the Counter Hearing Aid Act was signed into law, designed to provide greater public accessibility and affordability with OTC hearing aids. The impact of this on access to amplification will surely be substantial, but difficult to quantify this early on.

Despite their high initial cost and continuing cost of maintenance, hearing aids have been shown to mitigate the economic effects of hearing loss, when controlled for demographic data. A 2010 study of the income from 48,000 households showed clear gap in income between normal hearing individuals and those with hearing loss. This gap widened with increasing severity of hearing loss. The authors also questioned whether using hearing aids would help to close the income gap. While the income differential for hearing loss households starts at $2,000 for individuals with mild loss, it increases to $31,000 for profound loss.

When treated with a hearing aid, there is no income differential for people with mild to moderate hearing loss, meaning complete salary equity. After that, it increases to a loss of $1,000 a year to only $11,000 for those with profound loss, a $20,000 salary gain per year from use of hearing aids.[10] This indicates that, while hearing aids may be expensive, they may be cost-effective on both microeconomic and macroeconomic levels compared to the cost of nonintervention.

## 7.3.2 Asymmetric Sensorineural Hearing Loss

Individuals complaining of long-standing or gradually occurring unilateral hearing loss should undergo audiological evaluation. Asymmetrical sensorineural hearing loss (ASNHL) is often defined as (1) a 10-dB difference at three continuous

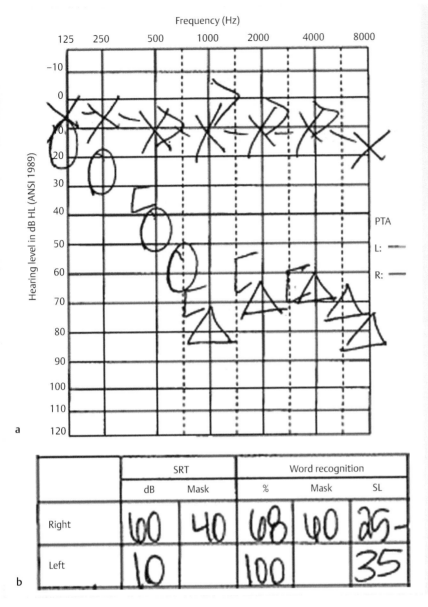

a

| | SRT | | Word recognition | | |
|---|---|---|---|---|---|
| | dB | Mask | % | Mask | SL |
| Right | 60 | 40 | 68 | 40 | 25- |
| Left | 10 | | 100 | | 35 |

b

frequencies, (2) 15-dB difference at two continuous frequencies, (3) 15-dB difference a 3,000 Hz, (4) 15% difference between ears in WRSs, or (5) greater than 10-dB difference between ears across the average of multiple frequencies.[21] Patients found to have ASNHL should be referred to an otolaryngologist for further evaluation (▶ Fig. 7.3).

While in most cases of ASNHL an underlying etiology is never found, about 2% of patients will have an IAC and/or cerebellopontine angle (CPA) tumor and thus require thorough evaluation. The most common IAC/CPA tumor (92%) is VS (see the following text), which is benign but could cause tinnitus, imbalance, or even facial nerve weakness, hydrocephalus, or even life-threatening brainstem compression.

MRI imaging is considered standard of care to evaluate for IAC/CPA pathology in patients with ASNHL and has been shown to be cost-effective in some studies (▶ Fig. 7.4).[21,22] The standard protocol for MRI includes pre- and postcontrast T1-weighted images with submillimeter slices through the IAC and CPA.

However, although most patients with VS will have asymmetric hearing, most patients who present with asymmetric hearing will not have VS. According to estimates, from less than 0.1 to 3% of patients with asymmetric hearing loss will have evidence of VS by MRI.[23,24,25] Therefore, the clinician must have a reasonable index of suspicion to warrant further workup of potential retrocochlear pathology.

Throughout the 1980s and 1990s, the ABR was the standard screening modality for detecting retrocochlear pathology. However, the sensitivity was relatively poor for tumors less than 1 cm. With the growing use of gadolinium-enhanced MRI in the 1990s, detection of even small tumors improved to nearly

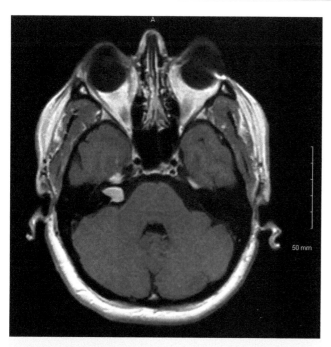

**Fig. 7.4** MRI T1 gadolinium enhanced axial image of an internal auditory canal and cerebellopontine angle vestibular schwannoma.

100% and remains the gold standard method for the diagnosis of VS. Given improvements in resolution and decreased cost of MR, most neurotologists do not consider ABR a cost-effective screening tool for CPA pathology.[26]

Because of the relative frequency of ASNHL, the potential morbidity of VS tumors, and relatively low yield of costly MRI, investigators have sought a most cost-effective way to radiographically evaluate these patients.

Gadolinium-enhanced MRI has been shown to be cost-effective, though high-resolution T2-weighted imaging may also be a reasonable and cost-effective alternative.[21,26] While many otolaryngologists order gadolinium-enhanced MRI scans for initial testing, there is evidence to support T2-weighted MR as a more cost-effective initial screen for CPA pathology. Not only does this decrease cost, but also associated risks of gadolinium (including allergy, nephrogenic systemic fibrosis, and central nervous system deposition) can be avoided.

Many authors have also suggested strategies to more effectively screen patients.[27,28] Over 20 years ago, Fisher and colleagues, citing cost concerns of increasing usage of MRI screening for asymmetric hearing loss, suggested stratifying patients into categories based on risk, particularly in those with unexplained ASNHL.[29] A similar study was published only a few years later by Astor et al adding unilateral low-frequency tinnitus and imbalance as potential risk factors for the presence of a tumor.[27,30] For the general population, Saliba et al described the "Rule of 3,000" where interaural threshold asymmetries on audiogram were found to be most sensitive at 3,000 Hz.[28,31]

These findings were corroborated by Ahsan and colleagues.[29,32] In an effort to cut costs, or in situations where wait time for MRI is unacceptably high, ABR has re-emerged as a reasonable and cost-effective modality for patients with low to moderate suspicion of VS.[30,33]

In our practice (DHC and ENA), we stratify patients into "lower risk" and "higher risk" patients. This is largely based on history, age, and audiogram results. Patients with lower clinical suspicion of retrocochlear pathology are offered a follow-up audiogram in 1 year to rule out atypical progression or an ABR. MRI is discussed, but with proper education most patients understand the likely low yield of imaging. Patients at higher risk are sent for MRI.

Ultimately, the burden of proof lies on the physician, and in a litigious society such as that found in United States, gadolinium-enhanced T1-weighted MRI remains the standard of care. However, with proper counseling as to the reasoning behind a rationale diagnostic algorithm, personal and anecdotal experience shows that the vast majority of patients will agree to alternative methods of investigation, including observation. This is especially true as patient out-of-pocket costs rise.

## Treatment

Depending on the hearing status of both ears, treatment for ASNHL can include traditional hearing aid amplification, contralateral routing of signal (CROS) hearing aids, bone-anchored hearing device (BAHD), or, in some rare cases, a cochlear implant.

In situations of unilateral hearing loss, CROS aids are a popular option for treatment. CROS aids route signal from the hearing-impaired side to the hearing side to rehabilitate the users' sound field. These systems are similar to slightly more expensive in price compared to regular hearing aids. Most CROS aids that previously relied on a hardware connection to route signal to the hearing side now use Bluetooth connection.

BAHD rehabilitation relies on bone conduction and direct stimulation of the cochlea fluid. When compared to CROS users, BAHD users showed increased ease of conversation, listening in reverberant conditions and background noise, and less aversion to noise.[20,34] While there are no studies directly comparing the cost efficacy of CROS devices to BAHD, their profile should be similar to that of conventional hearing aids as they are similar in price and are governed by the same regulations and patterns of disbursement.

## 7.3.3 Sudden Sensorineural Hearing Loss

SSNHL affects 5 to 20 adults per 100,000 population per year. SSNHL is defined as rapid-onset subjective hearing loss over 3 days in one or both ears. The patient may experience associated tinnitus in the affected ear(s). Patients with suspected SSNHL should be evaluated in a timely fashion by a physician. A history and physical examination, including tuning fork tests, should be performed. CHL (such as cerumen impaction) should be ruled out by inspection of the ear canals and with tuning fork testing. An audiological evaluation and urgent referral to an otolaryngologist is warranted in SSNHL for further evaluation and treatment. Although there is some controversy about the cost-effectiveness of MRI in SSNHL, MRI should be performed to evaluate for retrocochlear pathology. The incidence of VS detected by MRI in patients with SSNHL is approximately 4%.[35] CT imaging of the temporal bone and laboratory testing are not recommended routinely.[36] Patients with rapidly progressive or fluctuating unilateral or bilateral SSNHL may have autoimmune hearing loss. The same general diagnostic algorithm can be followed initially for these patients. Routine laboratory testing is not recommended in cases of SSNHL, though directed testing for Lyme disease titers and syphilis (rapid plasma regain [RPR]) may be cost-efffective.[37] Laboratory testing for autoimmune hearing loss should be reserved for cases with high suspicion for AIED (autoimmune inner ear disease) such as younger patients with bilateral or recurrent disease or a known history of systemic autoimmune disease.[38] In cases of suspected autoimmune SSNHL, serologic tests such as antinuclear antibody (ANA), erythrocyte sedimentation rate (ESR), Lyme titers, and RPR have low diagnostic yield, though, and are not currently recommended.

## Treatment

Treatment of SSNHL includes oral or transtympanic steroids in the acute phase to potentially rescue or preserve inner ear function.

## 7.3.4 Conductive Hearing Loss

CHL can be caused by any condition that blocks sound from the ear canal to the inner ear. History, physical examination including tuning fork testing, and audiological evaluation are necessary. Patients with CHL from all causes except manageable cerumen impaction should be referred to an otolaryngologist. Several important causes of CHL such as middle ear effusion, cholesteatoma, and otosclerosis can usually be diagnosed by history, physical examination, and audiological evaluation alone (both diseases are further described later). In the cases where a diagnosis is not apparent at this point, imaging can be considered. Noncontrast CT of the temporal bone is generally the imaging modality of choice in the cases where imaging is warranted.[39]

## 7.3.5 Otitis Media with Effusion

Otitis media with effusion (OME) is an infectious or inflammatory condition of the middle ear with fluid behind an intact TM. Most patients with OME are young children, though OME can happen at any age. There is usually a proceeding upper respiratory infection, adenoid hypertrophy, or allergy flare-up causing mucosal inflammation that results in eustachian tube dysfunction. Acute OME is usually associated with signs of an acute ear infection. OME may also be chronic with the effusion lasting several months or longer. Patients may complain of hearing loss in the affected ear. The diagnosis is made on physical examination and should include evaluation with pneumatic otoscopy. A persistent unilateral middle ear effusion warrants referral to an otolaryngologist for evaluation for a nasopharyngeal or skull base mass obstructing ventilation of the middle ear via the eustachian tube. Evaluation should begin with directed history and physical examination including nasal endoscopy to evaluate the nasopharynx. In the case of negative findings with persistent effusion, CT or MRI may be considered.[40]

In children where the presence of middle ear effusion is uncertain, tympanometry should be performed. Age-appropriate audiogram should be performed if OME lasts for greater than 3 months. A referral to an otolaryngologist is appropriate for OME that lasts greater than 3 months for evaluation for surgical intervention.[41]

## 7.3.6 Chronic Otitis Media

Chronic otitis media encompasses several conditions including a dry, long-standing TM perforation, a chronically draining ear, and cholesteatoma. History should include detailed questions of prior ear trauma (which can cause a TM rupture), any ear surgery including pressure equalization tubes, recurrent childhood infections, foul smelling and/or bloody ear drainage, barotrauma, and hearing loss.

During the physical examination, particular attention should focus on the state of the TM, the presence of areas of retraction with or without keratin debris, and the health of the middle ear mucosa. A tuning fork examination should be done to evaluate for CHL, and if detected, an audiogram should be obtained.

Referral to an otolaryngologist is warranted in all cases of chronic otitis media. The decision to obtain a CT of the temporal bones to further evaluate the chronic otitis media should be left to the discretion of the otolaryngologist.[42] In cases of TM perforation following barotrauma or acute otitis media (where the patient is not suffering from chronic drainage and otomicroscopic evaluation reveals a dry healthy middle ear), no imaging is required. No further testing is generally warranted for chronic otitis media. ▶ Fig. 7.5 demonstrates the audiogram of a patient with left-sided cholesteatoma and ▶ Fig. 7.6 demonstrates an axial non-contrast-enhanced CT scan demonstrating soft-tissue density material in the middle ear and mastoid with ossicular erosion.

Treatment for chronic otitis media includes observation, medical management with aural toilet and ototopical medications, and surgical removal of disease from middle ear and mastoid and usually reconstruction of the TM (tympanoplasty with mastoidectomy).

## Bone-Anchored Hearing Devices

BAHDs were first introduced by Tjellstrom in 1977 and have gained popularity since then.[16,43] The device consists of a percutaneous osseointegrated screw and abutment as well as an

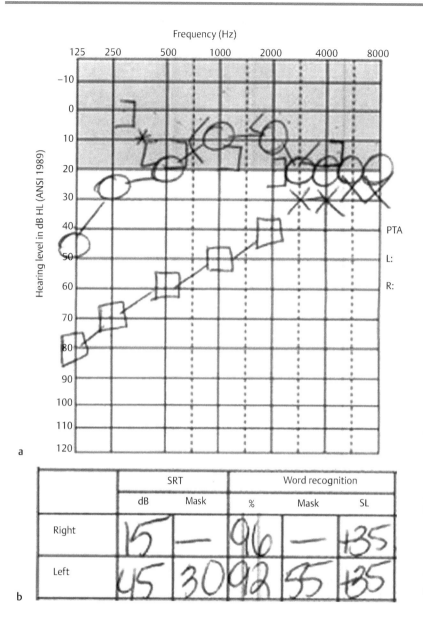

**Fig. 7.5** (a, b) Audiometric results for left-sided cholesteatoma.

|  | SRT | | Word recognition | | |
|---|---|---|---|---|---|
|  | dB | Mask | % | Mask | SL |
| Right | 15 | — | 96 | — | +35 |
| Left | 45 | 30 | 92 | 55 | +35 |

external sound processor that sits just posterosuperior to the auricle, camouflaged within the hairline. By vibrating the skull through the implanted screw, the sound signal is able to bypass the malfunctioning or absent external or middle ear (in the case of CHL), and even traverse the skull to stimulate the contralateral cochlear (in the case of unilateral sensorineural deafness). Utility has been demonstrated in cases of unilateral deafness and an inability to tolerate conventional hearing aids due to recurrent otitis externa, cerumen impaction, or recurrent otitis media. Thus, the hearing rehabilitation provider must often decide whether to treat with conventional hearing aids or progress to using a BAHD. Whereas newer modifications of BAHDs have allowed for transcutaneous passive and active devices (ones that do not require an abutment that comes through the skin), economic efficacy data for those devices are sparse.

Monksfield et al performed a cost-effectiveness study comparing a BAHD with use of a digital hearing aid in the United Kingdom.[17,44] Each subject served as his or her own control and were given a preoperative and postoperative questionnaire to establish an HUI. Seventy patients underwent placement of a BAHD. Total cost per patient for BAHD placement was $8,534 with a recurring annual maintenance fee of $1,506. The total average cost to provide a BAHD with inclusion of maintenance fees over the average projected lifetime of the cohort was $32,145 (95% confidence interval [CI]: $30,395–33,803). In the control group, 39 of 70 patients (56%) were using hearing aids. Total cost of hearing aid placement with replacement every 5 years was $1,241 (95% CI: $966–1,533). Mean incremental cost for obtaining a BAHD (the cost of a BAHD minus the cost of hearing aids) was $30,906 (95% CI: $29,193–32,654). The mean

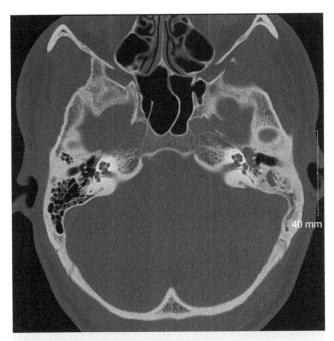

**Fig. 7.6** Axial non-contrast-enhanced CT of left-sided cholesteatoma corresponding to the audiometric results in ▶ Fig. 7.5.

quality-adjusted life years (QALY) gain with BAHD was 1.89. A total accounting of costs and applying in incremental cost-effectiveness ratio (ICER) equation showed a cost of $26,415 per QALY. This indicates that BAHD placement is cost-effective according to the standards put forth by the National Institute for Health and Care Excellence (NICE). Additionally, a number of different factors may increase the calculated cost-effectiveness when translated to the U.S. market. The study taking place though United Kingdom's single-payer market shows a lower cost for hearing aids compared to the United States where the average cost for one hearing aid is $2,400 and up to 84% of individuals obtain two aids.[18,45] The authors admit that a private provider may be able to drive down maintenance costs for BAHD over the life of the device as well. Colquitt et al performed a systematic review comparing the cost-effectiveness of BAHD versus hearing aids including 12 different studies.[19,46] This review was complicated by poor constitutive study quality and heterogeneity. The authors performed a cost-effectiveness analysis with cost of intervention and HUI. This showed an overall ICER of $75,491 to $161,949 and was deemed to not be cost-effective, in contrast to the Monksfield et al study. This may be due to a smaller computed QALY benefits and the assumption of more adverse outcomes requiring treatment in their calculation.

Recently, minimally invasive ponto surgery (MIPS) has become much more popular for BAHD placement. This technique requires a skin punch with placement of the device abutment without incision, skin graft, or any other invasive technique. It can be done under local anesthetic only and has been described as being completed in a clinical setting without need for general anesthesia in the operating room. Sardiwalla et al compared cost in a Canadian setting among 18 patients undergoing MIPS or open approaches.[17,47] MIPS was on average $456.83 cheaper than an open BAHD placement. This also did not capture indirect costs saved by a less invasive approach, with less morbidity, requiring less expensive operating room (OR) time, equipment, and personnel. Such factors would undoubtedly improve costs compared to traditional techniques.

## 7.3.7 Otosclerosis

Otosclerosis is caused by abnormal bone remodeling most commonly centered on the fissula ante fenestram leading to stapes footplate fixation. This stapes fixation causes a predominantly low-frequency CHL. Otosclerosis is a hereditary disease with incomplete penetrance affecting mostly Caucasians. Estimates in a northern European population show prevalence to be about 1.41/1,000 individuals with a strong female predilection.[17,48] About 60% of affected individuals have a relative also affected by the disease.[49]

Patients usually present with a progressive CHL or mixed hearing loss beginning between the second and fourth decade. The hearing loss is usually unilateral, although it can be bilateral (as noted histologically or on radiologic imaging). Often, the patient will have family members who also developed hearing loss at a young age or have a diagnosis of otosclerosis. Pertinent physical examination findings include a normal TM with no middle ear effusion. Rarely, the promontory will appear reddish (known as Schwartz's sign) indicating active otosclerosis, which is called otospongiosis. Tuning fork examination, in particular Rinne's test at multiple frequencies (256, 512, 1,024 Hz), should be performed and will classically reveal a negative Rinne (bone conduction stronger than air conduction), which suggests about a 25-dB ABG (air–bone gap) with 512-Hz tuning fork. An audiogram should be performed to look for CHL, SSHL, or mixed hearing loss. Tympanometry will often reveal a type A tympanogram.

Of note, acoustic reflexes are usually absent (▶ Fig. 7.7). CT of the temporal bone can support a diagnosis of otosclerosis by demonstrating otosclerotic foci and by ruling out other causes of CHL, such as superior semicircular canal dehiscence, ossicular discontinuity, or tympanosclerosis. However, the diagnosis of otosclerosis can still be made clinically and does not require imaging. A referral should be placed to an otolaryngologist for further management.[50,51,52]

### Surgical Intervention: Stapedotomy/Stapedectomy

Treatment options include observation, hearing aid amplification, and surgery. Surgery for otosclerosis involving a fixed stapes footplate includes removing the fixed portion and replacing it with a prosthesis. John Shea popularized an inner ear fenestration technique with removal of the stapes suprastructure and placement of a prosthesis, first performed in 1956.[16,53] Results are usually excellent, with the ability in experienced hands to

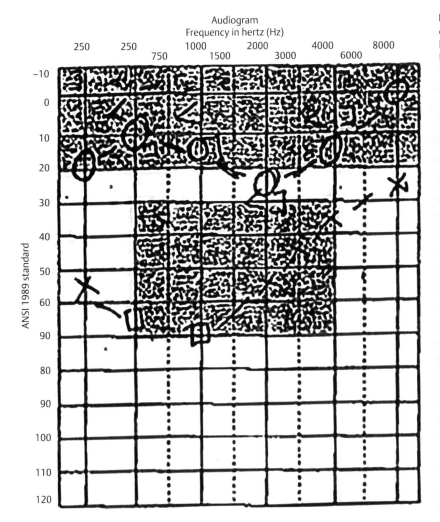

Audiogram
Frequency in hertz (Hz)

**Fig. 7.7** Audiometric results for left-sided otosclerosis. Pure-tone thresholds reveal a left-sided conductive hearing loss with absent left-sided acoustic reflexes.

completely resolve the conductive component of the hearing loss. This procedure is not without risks, however, and can result in a total hearing loss from trauma to the very sensitive inner ear environment. Because otosclerosis poses no health risk aside from hearing loss, surgical intervention is considered to be elective. This raises a dilemma concerning treatment strategies: to treat their hearing loss noninvasively with lifetime use of hearing aids or intervene surgically and risk complications.

Savvas and Maurer examined the cost-effectiveness of stapedotomy to treat CHL from otosclerosis, comparing this to lifelong use of hearing aids.[10,54] They performed a retrospective analysis of 164 cases of primary stapedectomy in a German population. In Germany, a lump sum is disbursed for patients undergoing stapedotomy, totaling €2128. This includes costs for surgery, anesthesia (local or general), a 3- to 5-day inpatient hospital cost (typical in Germany), postoperative care, and audiological evaluation. The total cost of all 164 patients was €348,992. Need for revision surgery occurred in 10% of patients totaling €34,048, which was added to the total cost, resulting in a total surgical cost of €383,040. Using an average cost of a hearing aid of €696 (average cost of most basic

model), factoring need for replacement every 5 years as well as an average age of 50 years at the time of intervention and an estimated lifespan of 80 to 85 years, the authors calculated the total cost of hearing aids to be €3,480 over the course of the patients lifetime. If the 164 patients who had surgery had chosen a hearing aid instead, the total cost would have been €570,720, almost €200,000 more expensive. When calculated with average price of the more popular, more advanced hearing aids (€6,800 lifetime cost), this difference climbs to €732,160.

In some cases of otosclerosis (~10% of cases), the focus of disease can extend into the cochlea, termed retrofenestral otosclerosis, which then causes SNHL. This results in a mixed hearing loss that is termed advanced otosclerosis. In the cases in which the hearing loss is bilateral and severe with poor word discrimination, consideration should be given to placement of a cochlear implant. Merkus et al suggested an algorithm based on high-resolution CT scan findings, pure-tone average, and speech discrimination to decide whether cochlear implantation, stapedotomy, or hearing aids use would be the more efficacious first-line approach.[21,55] While they did not perform a direct cost analysis of this decision algorithm, choosing an appropriate initial intervention is more likely to prevent waste, revision approaches, and economic inefficiency. The differences in cost for stapedotomy versus cochlear implantation are significant. The economic considerations of cochlear implantation for SNHL are discussed separately at the end of this chapter.

# 7.4 Acoustic Neuroma/Vestibular Schwannoma

Vestibular Schwannomas (VS, also known as acoustic neuromas) are benign, generally slow-growing tumors along the cochleovestibular nerve within the IAC and/or CPA. They typically arise from the Schwann cells of the vestibular nerves, and account for roughly 10% of all brain neoplasms and approximately 80% of all CPA tumors. Patients with VS classically present with unilateral otologic symptoms such as asymmetric hearing loss or unilateral tinnitus. Imbalance, and occasionally vertigo, frequently accompanies presentation and, in rare cases, patients may present with facial nerve weakness. In roughly 10% of patients, the hearing loss can be sudden. The vast majority of tumors are unilateral and sporadic.

Patients with bilateral VS have, by definition, neurofibromatosis type 2 (NF2). (Patients with NF2 present a unique and challenging management dilemma, which is beyond the scope of this chapter. Interested readers are referred to an excellent manuscript by Slattery.[56])

## 7.4.1 Diagnosis

Patients are often diagnosed after presenting with unilateral hearing loss, tinnitus, or dizziness and being evaluated with MRI of the IACs. See the section 7.3.2 (Asymmetric Sensorineural Hearing Loss) for discussion of evaluation.

## 7.4.2 Treatment

Once diagnosed, many management options exist for patients, including observation (or "wait-and-scan"), stereotactic radiotherapy, and microsurgical excision. The "best" modality is a source of great controversy, and must be tailored to the individual while allowing for patient input in the decision-making process.

As we have learned more about the natural history of VS, observation has become an increasingly more popular preference for patients with small and medium-sized tumors. In 2009, Verma and colleagues published their evaluation of cost-effectiveness comparison between observation and active management in Toronto, Canada.[31,57] Assuming no increase in active treatment complications arose from continued tumor growth during the period of observation (such as brainstem compression, hydrocephalus, facial nerve weakness), they found an economic advantage to observed tumors. In their model-based approach to cost-effectiveness, Gait and colleagues concluded that observation should be considered the optimal treatment for small and medium-sized tumors.[32,58] Overall, observation is generally considered to be the most cost-effective management of VS, though this may not be optimal medically for more than half of the patients. Moreover, younger patients diagnosed with VS may have decades of MRI ahead of them, the economic cost of which (assuming no side effects from gadolinium) can be substantial.[33,59]

Traditionally, microsurgery has been the mainstay and most common treatment modality for patients with VS. Although the number of patients undergoing surgery for VS has been decreasing in recent years, it remains an excellent option for the right patient. This is particularly true for patients with tumor extension into the CPA, younger patients, patients with brainstem compression, patients with intractable dizziness, or with patients with the potential to preserve hearing. With respect to surgical approach, Semaan et al found that patients undergoing the translabyrinthine approach had significantly shorter hospital length of stay and total adjusted costs than patients undergoing the retrosigmoid approach (though patients with retrosigmoid approaches had larger tumors).[60]

Stereotactic radiotherapy (i.e., Gamma Knife) is a relatively noninvasive, often single treatment modality that has shown great success (as defined by control of tumor growth) in the short- and long-term management of VS. In their 2014 study, Zygourakis et al found that observation was the most cost-effective treatment, though for patients undergoing active treatment, radiotherapy was more cost-effective in patients older than 45 years and less cost-effective in patients younger than 45 years.[61]

Many authors have found the cost of stereotactic radiotherapy to be less than the total cost of open surgery for VS, though most did not account for long-term follow-up.[62,63] In one of the few studies that did look at long-term follow-up, Banerjee and colleagues found the cost of follow-up after radiosurgery to be greater than that of microsurgery, due to the cost of serial imaging and clinical follow-up.[38,64]

In one of the few studies to examine long-term socioeconomic impact of VS, Tos and colleagues investigated a consecutive cohort of 748 patients who underwent all three management modalities.[65] Deterioration of vocational status, ability to handle daily chores, and several aspects of psychosocial well-being were reported both by patients operated on and by patients observed for VS, with deterioration being only slightly worse in the operated patients, especially when comparing observed patients with patients operated on for a small tumor.

Ultimately, the "best" management option for patients with VS relies on numerous factors including patient age, symptoms, general health, tumor size, personality, and experience of the providers. Whereas all clinicians should keep cost efficacy in mind when deciding the optimal treatment, it should not be at the expense of individual outcomes. This is clearly an area ripe for additional research.

## 7.5 Newborn Hearing Evaluation

Congenital bilateral hearing loss occurs in 1 to 5 per 1,000 live births. Universal newborn hearing screening significantly lowers the age of diagnosis of congenital hearing loss and improves auditory outcomes for children. Hearing screening in newborns has been shown to be cost-effective and is considered standard of care. All newborns should be screened by either OAE or ABR in the first few days of life prior to being discharged from the hospital after birth.[66,67] Patients with abnormal results on initial screening should be referred to audiological evaluation for repeat testing at 2 to 8 weeks of life. Patients with abnormal repeat testing results should be referred for prompt evaluation by an otolaryngologist. Early diagnosis and treatment of congenital hearing loss is crucial for hearing and speech development.[68] Despite implementation of universal newborn hearing screening programs, unfortunately, many children are lost to follow-up with subsequent delay in hearing loss diagnosis. History of children with concern for hearing loss should focus on prenatal, perinatal, and postnatal risk factors, including for risk factors for intrauterine cytomegalovirus (CMV), rubella, toxoplasma or syphilis infection, prematurity, need for neonatal intensive care admission, need for extracorporeal membrane oxygenation (ECMO) treatment, and administration of ototoxic medications (such as aminoglycoside antibiotics) and family history. Physical examination should seek to identify physical characteristics associated with syndromic causes of hearing loss. While newborn hearing screening has been shown to be cost-effective, further testing to determine the cause of hearing loss has not been evaluated for cost-effectiveness. A proposed sequence of testing for newborn hearing loss is outlined below. Children found to have bilateral SNHL should undergo testing for CMV, if possible. If CMV is not considered a cause of SNHL, they should then be referred for genetic counseling. Genetic screening may identify the cause of syndromic and nonsyndromic SNHL. In patients with negative genetic testing, imaging with MRI or CT should be obtained. MRI is more costly and requires sedation in children, while CT may be associated with minimal increase in risk of brain and blood cancer. A proposed algorithm for imaging in children with bilateral moderate to profound SNHL is to obtain a noncontrast fast spin-echo T2-weighted MRI. Directed laboratory testing is controversial as the yield of each test is below 1%. Laboratory testing, such as complete blood count, platelet count, ANA, ESR, rheumatoid factor, thyroid-stimulating hormone, blood urea nitrogen, creatinine, urinalysis, blood glucose, fluorescent treponemal antibody, rapid plasma reagent, and lipid panel, should be reserved when clinical suspicion of an associated cause of hearing loss is raised by medical or family history. Patients with SNHL should also be referred for ophthalmologic evaluation to correct any causes of decreased visual acuity and to search for findings associated with syndromic SNHL.[69] Electrocardiogram should be performed in cases of bilateral severe to profound SNHL without identified genetic cause to rule out prolonged QT syndrome as seen in Jervell Lange–Nielsen syndrome.[39]

## 7.6 Cochlear Implants for Profound Sensorineural Hearing Loss

*David Young, Matthew M. Dedmon, Nicolas-George Katsantonis, and Marc L. Bennett*

Cochlear implantation has become the standard of care for hearing restoration in children and adults for whom traditional amplification has proven inadequate in restoring function. Despite this being the standard in developed countries, the literature suggests that market penetrance of eligible patients hovers at 3 to 4% of the nearly 12 million people worldwide who would meet criteria for implantation.[70] Compared with traditional methods of amplification, cochlear implants have much higher material costs, as well as other direct costs associated with the surgical placement of the implant and pre- and postoperative care.

Given both the higher relative costs and the substantial unmet need worldwide, the costs associated with cochlear implantation in both children and adults have been the subject of much scrutiny from government and private payers, as well as from patients and physicians.

## 7.7 Cost–Utility Analysis

While value in health care has traditionally been defined as outcome achieved per dollar spent, there is much nuance in how these factors are defined and measured.[71] There have been numerous papers over the last 20 years examining cost–utility factors as they relate to cochlear implantation, and cost–utility analysis (CUA) in this area remains a subject of active investigation.[72] The concept of measuring cost is initially intuitive but can become increasingly convoluted as one tries to accurately describe the potential direct and indirect expenses related to an intervention. For cochlear implantation, direct costs include things such as the cost of the implant itself, the cost of the implantation surgery, as well as pre- and postoperative visits with audiologists and physicians. Most cost analyses also factor in additional direct costs such as surgical complications, device failures, need for upgrades, cost of reimplantation, and warranty costs. Many of these factors have a strong correlation to the duration of cochlear implantation, and they may therefore be substantially higher in studies looking at children who may have a cochlear implant for 70+ years compared to older adults who would have a shorter duration of implantation. Figures also vary considerably by country where the study was performed given the inherent variability in costs of devices and health care around the world. This leads to a wide variation in total direct costs with reported literature values ranging from $63,622 to $126,523 depending on the exact methods used.[9,73]

While direct costs are more easily measured and typically included in CUA, indirect costs are more nebulous, but no less important when considering costs on a public health scale. One important point is that indirect costs also consider the costs to the patient and to society if they do not receive an implant. Indirect costs include things such as personal productivity, income levels, and educational costs (especially in children). While most cochlear implant studies do not include a robust analysis of the indirect costs and savings resulting from implantation, some have attempted to do this, especially with evaluating pediatric implants. When considering a pediatric cochlear implant recipient, estimates of lost wages and follow-up care alone totaled nearly $50,000, but when adding in things like educational savings resulting from regular school placement versus a school for the deaf, a 2000 study by Cheng et al noted a lifetime net cost savings of over $175,000.[74] When considered along with all the other direct and indirect costs associated with a lifetime of implantation, studies concluded that unilateral cochlear implantation in children actually provided a net savings of anywhere from $2,000 to greater than $50,000.[73,74]

## 7.8 Outcome Measurements

Just as cost measures can vary widely between studies, the methods used for calculating patient outcomes are similarly variable. Generally speaking, studies use either a form of direct elicitation by surveying patients and families directly about their current health and how they value it, or a general preference-based method that calculates utility indirectly. Directly eliciting responses from patients regarding their QOL is straightforward and ubiquitous in the medical literature.

Whether direct or indirect methods are used, they ultimately attempt to arrive at a measure of utility for the intervention in question on a scale from 0 to 1. This measure of utility is further translated into a measure known as QALY, derived simply by multiplying the measured utility by the remaining life expectancy. While other interventions may impact both the quality and duration of life, cochlear implantation only impacts the QOL domain. Consider a 70-year-old patient with profound SNHL; if one estimates a remaining life expectancy of 20 years and current utility measures of 0.5, then the patient has 10 QALYs remaining. If a cochlear implant is found to increase that utility factor from 0.5 to 0.75, then that would yield 15 QALYs remaining, or an overall gain of 5 QALYs.[75,76]

From all of this—the direct and indirect costs, the utility, and the ultimate QALYs of an intervention—one can calculate the cost per QALY. This begets the question: what is a given society willing to pay per QALY? In cost analysis literature, this concept is known as the willingness-to-pay (WTP) threshold and is contingent upon the values and available resources in any given society. Within the United States and much of the western world, the generally accepted value has been suggested to be at or near $50,000 per QALY gained. This cost per QALY is one of the key values that large payers look at when determining whether a given intervention will be covered. While this number has been the paradigm for many years, some authors are advocating to change this threshold or establish a range of acceptable levels.[77,78,79]

The cost–utility literature surrounding cochlear implantation not only must contain the inherent variability of measuring costs and outcomes but also must further take into account a wide variety of implantation candidates. Eligible patients range from prelingually deaf children to profoundly deaf older adults. In addition, patients can be candidates for cochlear implantation in both unilateral and bilateral situations. Given the significant variation in outcome and cost measures between these groups, they will be considered separately.

## 7.9 Unilateral Pediatric Implantation

The literature surrounding unilateral pediatric implantation is robust and includes a number of well-designed trials from multiple countries. All the pediatric QOL measures are modified to allow parents to respond by proxy for their children, but the measures employed are similar to their adult counterparts. A key cost–utility study was performed in 2000 by Cheng et al in which they evaluated utility by using pre- and postimplantation questionnaires for parents of 160 children undergoing unilateral implantation. Average age at implantation was just under 6 years and the postoperative surveys were done 2 years after implantation using three different measures: a visual analog scale, time trade-off, and the HUI3. The life expectancy for these pediatric patients was high (78 years), and the costs are therefore buffered by a high lifetime savings primarily attributed to educational savings and increased earning potential. Depending on the utility calculation from the three instruments, the overall cost per QALY ranged from $5,197 to $9,029 per QALY, a number well below the WTP threshold.[74]

A 2006 paper by Barton et al from the United Kingdom used larger sample sizes to compare 406 implanted children with 1,823 nonimplanted children.[80] The study was powered not only to look at cochlear implant versus traditional amplification, but also to compare utility for different levels of hearing loss. Baseline utility values decreased with worsening levels of hearing loss, and between-group comparisons showed overall utility values for implanted children fell in the range of nonimplanted children with severe to profound hearing loss. When analyzing cost, the authors considered some various scenarios: 15 years versus lifetime of cochlear implant use, implantation at age 3 versus age 6, and hearing loss levels of 105, 115, and 125 dB. In all possible arrangements, these variables showed a cost-effectiveness value less than the $50,000 per QALY WTP threshold, ranging from $15,000 (125-dB hearing loss, lifetime use, implanted at age 3) to $48,000 (105-dB hearing loss, implanted at age 6 with 15 years of use). Compared to the Cheng et al study, these numbers are higher across the board, likely relating to different underlying measures of direct and indirect costs and educational savings.[80]

Another important study is the 2013 paper by Semenov et al. This was a prospective study following 175 patients using the HUI questionnaire at various time points. This trial was further stratified by age at implantation and found significantly increased gains in utility with earlier implantation. Their results showed cochlear implant cost-effectiveness values ranging from $14,000 to $19,000 per QALY.[73] This demonstrated a net cost savings for pediatric cochlear implantation, with costs well below the established WTP threshold of $50,000, even when indirect cost savings were eliminated.

## 7.10 Bilateral Pediatric Implantation

Bilateral implantation has been more controversial in terms of its cost-effectiveness. The gain in utility going from nonhearing to unilateral implantation is impressive, but measuring the improvement after the addition of a second implant is more challenging. The costs involved can also vary depending on whether measurements are derived from sequential implantation situations (two different operations) or simultaneous, bilateral implantation situations. A 2011 systematic review found a range of values for bilateral pediatric implantation, ranging from $31,000 to $94,000 per QALY, although this review was limited by the overall quality of the evidence available. The largest of the included studies used nonimplanted volunteers made up of clinicians and students and other volunteers who were asked a number of questions regarding perceived QOL in various scenarios. They found a CUA value of approximately $35,000 per QALY, but also performed a probability analysis and found low probability that this number was true.[81]

More recent population-based studies, one from 2016 in Australia by Foteff et al and another from Spain by Pérez-Martín et al in 2017, compared cost–utility differences between groups of nonimplanted patients, unilateral cochlear implant patients, and bilateral implant patients. The Australian group found values for unilateral pediatric cochlear implantation of $16,341 per QALY compared with hearing aids alone, consistent with other studies mentioned earlier. For bilateral pediatric implantation, they found a level of $27,000 per QALY compared to hearing aids. They did not report numbers comparing unilateral with bilateral cochlear implantation.[82,83]

## 7.11 Unilateral Adult Implantation

The literature has consistently found unilateral implantation in adults to be a cost-effective intervention.[84,85,86] Almost universally, these studies compare unilateral implantation to traditional bilateral hearing aids. Much of this work has been done in European nations. Studies from the United Kingdom from the 1990s until the present have found a range of values, with the earliest papers showing a lower cost at $15,000 per QALY. More recent data from the United Kingdom was more than twice that amount at $36,000, but still well below accepted WTP thresholds.[72,85,87] The most recent data come from Australia in a 2016 study by Foteff et al where they showed a much lower cost–utility at just under $9,000 per QALY when considering their entire cochlear implant cohort that included unilateral implantation as well as simultaneous bilateral implantation. The values ranged from $7,000 per QALY among unilateral implants to just under $20,000 per QALY for the bilateral implant group. All of these numbers represent the relative cost-effectiveness compared with traditional hearing aids.[82]

As noted earlier, all these papers suffer from a heterogeneity not only of population but also of measures of both costs and outcomes. An element that becomes increasingly important in the adult literature is the question of remaining life expectancy. A paper from the Netherlands by Smulders et al looked at incremental costs depending on life remaining and found an exponential drop from more than $300,000 per QALY assuming 2 years of life remaining to levels below WTP thresholds at just 5 years of life remaining (~$20,000–50,000 per QALY)\, with gradually decreasing incremental costs as life expectancy increases.[88]

Another issue that is particularly pertinent to adult cochlear implantation is the duration of deafness. The U.K. Cochlear Implant Study Group in 2004 looked at cost-effectiveness and what criteria would predict better outcomes in terms of speech perception and overall QOL. They found that postlingually deafened adults who had been profoundly deaf for less than 30 years showed improvements in speech perception and QOL (measured by the HUI3) that would meet standard WTP thresholds with costs just under $30,000 per QALY. This changed substantially when looking at adults who had been profoundly deaf for more than 40 years as their net benefit greatly exceeded the WTP levels with total costs approaching $70,000 per QALY.[89]

Overall, the current data presented in the literature strongly suggest that unilateral implantation in adults is cost-effective. Notable exceptions include older adults with very limited life expectancy as well as those who have had profound deafness for greater than 40 years.

## 7.12 Bilateral Adult Implantation

The cost-effectiveness of bilateral adult implantation remains a hotly debated topic. Broadly speaking, the literature has often studied unilateral or bilateral implantation compared to no intervention, or alternatively compared to traditional amplification. These studies almost universally find the interventions to be cost-effective, but few studies have examined the incremental cost-effectiveness for bilateral cochlear implantation compared with unilateral cochlear implantation. Studies that directly compare bilateral versus unilateral cochlear implantation typically find that the bulk of the benefit comes from placing of the first implant.

Again, the data primarily come from the United Kingdom in a 2002 study by Quentin et al[90] and a 2006 study by Summerfield et al.[91] Cost-effectiveness of bilateral cochlear implantation compared to no intervention was measured at approximately $24,000 per QALY assuming a life expectancy of 22 years. When compared to unilateral implantation, the cost-effectiveness of the second implant was measured at $57,000 per QALY in 2002. In the 2006 study, the same Summerfield et al looked at cost-effectiveness of bilateral versus unilateral cochlear implantation by placing a second device in adult patients who had previously undergone implantation and comparing their utility measures. In this study, the cost-to-utility ratio exceeded $100,000 per QALY with the addition of the second implant. The authors noted some issues with their chosen survey instruments, namely, increased tinnitus in two subjects significantly altered the result given that hearing is only one part of the instruments used.[90]

The heterogeneity in outcomes is a lingering problem and many may not be adequately designed to detect the benefits derived from a second implant. A 2016 study from the Netherlands used five different survey instruments and found a range of values. For three instruments, they found the second implant became cost-effective after 5 years. The remaining two instruments suggested that cost-effectiveness was not achieved within the patients' lifetime. This further underscores the difficulty in evaluating more nuanced outcomes such as sound localization and improved hearing in noise using the currently validated survey instruments.

Based on results from the most recent literature, and accounting for the heterogeneity of results, it is difficult at this time to draw reliable conclusions on the incremental value of adding a second cochlear implant. The potential cost–utility benefits of bilateral cochlear implantation remain an ongoing area of research.

## 7.13 Conclusion

In an era where health care expenditures are coming under increasing levels of scrutiny, clinicians must become more aware of which interventions will truly provide value to patients and are also sustainable from a cost perspective. The literature overwhelmingly supports unilateral cochlear implantation in both children and adults as a highly cost-effective intervention. In children, the personal and societal savings may even provide a net gain over the child's lifetime. The value of bilateral implantation when compared to unilateral implantation remains controversial. While the literature strongly suggests this is a cost-effective intervention in children, it remains an open question in the adult population.

## References

[1] Lin FR, Niparko JK, Ferrucci L. Hearing loss prevalence in the United States. Arch Intern Med 2011;171(20):1851–1852

[2] Chien W, Lin FR. Prevalence of hearing aid use among older adults in the United States. Arch Intern Med 2012;172(3):292–293

[3] Gopinath B, Rochtchina E, Wang JJ, Schneider J, Leeder SR, Mitchell P. Prevalence of age-related hearing loss in older adults: Blue Mountains Study. Arch Intern Med 2009;169(4):415–416

[4] Bagai A, Thavendiranathan P, Detsky AS. Does this patient have hearing impairment? JAMA 2006;295(4):416–428

[5] Lin FR, Ferrucci L. Hearing loss and falls among older adults in the United States. Arch Intern Med 2012;172(4):369–371

[6] Genther DJ, Frick KD, Chen D, Betz J, Lin FR. Association of hearing loss with hospitalization and burden of disease in older adults. JAMA 2013;309(22): 2322–2324

[7] Lin FR, Yaffe K, Xia J, et al; Health ABC Study Group. Hearing loss and cognitive decline in older adults. JAMA Intern Med 2013;173(4):293–299

[8] Brewster KK, Ciarleglio A, Brown PJ, et al. Age-related hearing loss and its association with depression in later life. Am J Geriatr Psychiatry 2018;26(7): 788–796

[9] Chen JM, Amoodi H, Mittmann N. Cost-utility analysis of bilateral cochlear implantation in adults: a health economic assessment from the perspective of a publicly funded program. Laryngoscope 2014;124(6):1452–1458

[10] Kochkin S. MarkeTrak VIII: The efficacy of hearing aids in achieving compensation equity in the workplace. Hear J 2010;63(10):19–24

[11] Hauk L. Cerumen impaction: an updated guideline from the AAO-HNSF. Am Fam Physician 2017;96(4):263–264

[12] Agrawal Y, Platz EA, Niparko JK. Prevalence of hearing loss and differences by demographic characteristics among US adults: data from the National Health and Nutrition Examination Survey, 1999–2004. Arch Intern Med 2008;168(14):1522–1530

[13] Chou R, Dana T, Bougatsos C, Fleming C, Beil T. Screening for hearing loss in adults ages 50 years and older: a review of the evidence for the U.S. Preventive Services Task Force Ann Intern Med 2011;1;54(5):347–3–55

[14] FDA. CFR - Code of Federal Regulations Title 21. Available at: https://www.accessdata.fda.gov/scripts/cdrh/cfdocs/cfCFR/CFRSearch.cfm?fr=801.420. Accessed June 15, 2018

[15] Blazer DG, Domnitz S, Liverman CT, et al. Hearing technologies: expanding options. National Academies Press; 2016. Available at: https://www.ncbi.nlm.nih.gov/books/NBK385313/. Accessed June 15, 2018

[16] Strom KHR. 2013 hearing aid dispenser survey: dispensing in the age of Internet and Big Box Retailers—Hearing Review. 2014. Available at: http://www.hearingreview.com/2014/04/hr-2013-hearing-aid-dispenser-survey-dispensing-age-internet-big-box-retailers-comparison-present-past-key-business-indicators-dispensing-offices/. Accessed June 15, 2018

[17] Blazer DG, Domnitz S, Liverman CT, et al. Improving affordability of services and technologies. Washington, DC: National Academies Press; 2016. Available at: https://www.ncbi.nlm.nih.gov/books/NBK385307/. Accessed June 15, 2018

[18] Legal Information Institute. 42 CFR 411.15—Particular services excluded from coverage. Ithaca, NY: Legal Information Institute. Available at: https://www.law.cornell.edu/cfr/text/42/411.15. Accessed June 15, 2018

[19] Koh HK, Sebelius KG. Promoting prevention through the Affordable Care Act. N Engl J Med 2010;363(14):1296–1299

[20] Office of the Inspector General. Audit of VA's Hearing Aid Services. Available at: https://www.va.gov/oig/pubs/VAOIG-12-02910-80.pdf. Accessed June 15, 2018

[21] Hojjat H, Svider PF, Davoodian P, et al. To image or not to image? A cost-effectiveness analysis of MRI for patients with asymmetric sensorineural hearing loss. Laryngoscope 2017;127(4):939–944

[22] Jiang ZY, Mhoon E, Saadia-Redleaf M. Medicolegal concerns among neurotologists in ordering MRIs for idiopathic sensorineural hearing loss and asymmetric sensorineural hearing loss. Otol Neurotol 2011;32(3):403–405

[23] Dawes PJ, Mehta D, Arullendran P. Screening for vestibular schwannoma: magnetic resonance imaging findings and management. J Laryngol Otol 2000;114(8):584–588

[24] Wong BYW, Capper R. Incidence of vestibular schwannoma and incidental findings on the magnetic resonance imaging and computed tomography scans of patients from a direct referral audiology clinic. J Laryngol Otol 2012;126(7):658–662

[25] Pena I, Chew EY, Landau BP, Breen JT, Zevallos JP, Vrabec JT. Diagnostic criteria for detection of vestibular schwannomas in the VA population. Otol Neurotol 2016;37(10):1510–1515

[26] Fortnum H, O'Neill C, Taylor R, et al. The role of magnetic resonance imaging in the identification of suspected acoustic neuroma: a systematic review of clinical and cost effectiveness and natural history. Health Technol Assess 2009;13(18):iii–iv, ix–xi, 1–154

[27] Crowson MG, Rocke DJ, Hoang JK, Weissman JL, Kaylie DM. Cost-effectiveness analysis of a non-contrast screening MRI protocol for vestibular schwannoma in patients with asymmetric sensorineural hearing loss. Neuroradiology 2017;59(8):727–736

[28] Pan P, Huang J, Morioka C, Hathout G, El-Saden SM. Cost analysis of vestibular schwannoma screening with contrast-enhanced magnetic resonance imaging in patients with asymmetrical hearing loss. J Laryngol Otol 2016; 130(1):21–24

[29] Fisher EW, Parikh AA, Harcourt JP, Wright A. The burden of screening for acoustic neuroma: asymmetric otological symptoms in the ENT clinic. Clin Otolaryngol Allied Sci 1994;19(1):19–21

[30] Astor FC, Lechtenberg CL, Banks RD, et al. Proposed algorithm to aid the diagnosis of cerebellopontine angle tumors. South Med J 1997;90(5):514–517

[31] Saliba I, Bergeron M, Martineau G, Chagnon M. Rule 3,000: a more reliable precursor to perceive vestibular schwannoma on MRI in screened asymmetric sensorineural hearing loss. Eur Arch Otorhinolaryngol 2011;268(2):207–212

[32] Ahsan SF, Standring R, Osborn DA, Peterson E, Seidman M, Jain R. Clinical predictors of abnormal magnetic resonance imaging findings in patients with asymmetric sensorineural hearing loss. JAMA Otolaryngol Head Neck Surg 2015;141(5):451–456

[33] Koors PD, Thacker LR, Coelho DH. ABR in the diagnosis of vestibular schwannomas: a meta-analysis. Am J Otolaryngol 2013;34(3):195–204

[34] Niparko JK, Cox KM, Lustig LR. Comparison of the bone anchored hearing aid implantable hearing device with contralateral routing of offside sig-

nal amplification in the rehabilitation of unilateral deafness. Otol Neurotol 2003;24(1):73–78

[35] Plontke SK. Diagnostics and therapy of sudden hearing loss. GMS Curr Top Otorhinolaryngol Head Neck Surg 2018;16:Doc05

[36] Stachler RJ, Chandrasekhar SS, Archer SM, et al; American Academy of Otolaryngology–Head and Neck Surgery. Clinical practice guideline: sudden hearing loss. Otolaryngol Head Neck Surg 2012;146(3, Suppl):S1–S35

[37] Wilson YL, Gandolfi MM, Ahn IE, Yu G, Huang TC, Kim AH. Cost analysis of asymmetric sensorineural hearing loss investigations. Laryngoscope 2010;120(9):1832–1836

[38] Suzuki Y, Tokunaga S, Ikeguchi S, et al. Induction of coronary artery spasm by intracoronary acetylcholine: comparison with intracoronary ergonovine. Am Heart J 1992;124(1):39–47

[39] DeMarcantonio M, Choo DI. Radiographic evaluation of children with hearing loss. Otolaryngol Clin North Am 2015;48(6):913–932

[40] Leonetti JP. A study of persistent unilateral middle ear effusion caused by occult skull base lesions. Ear Nose Throat J 2013;92(4–5):195–200

[41] Rosenfeld RM, Shin JJ, Schwartz SR, et al. Clinical Practice Guideline: otitis media with effusion (update). Otolaryngol Head Neck Surg 2016;154(1, Suppl):S1–S41

[42] Tatlipinar A, Tuncel A, Öğredik EA, Gökçeer T, Uslu C. The role of computed tomography scanning in chronic otitis media. Eur Arch Otorhinolaryngol 2012;269(1):33–38

[43] Lustig LR, Arts HA, Brackmann DE, et al. Hearing rehabilitation using the BAHA bone-anchored hearing aid: results in 40 patients. Otol Neurotol 2001;22(3):328–334

[44] Monksfield P, Jowett S, Reid A, Proops D. Cost-effectiveness analysis of the bone-anchored hearing device. Otol Neurotol 2011;32(8):1192–1197

[45] Cassel C, Penhoet E, Saunders R. Policy solutions for better hearing. JAMA 2016;315(6):553–554

[46] Colquitt JL, Jones J, Harris P, et al. Bone-anchored hearing aids (BAHAs) for people who are bilaterally deaf: a systematic review and economic evaluation Health Technol Assess 2011;15(26):1–200

[47] Sardiwalla Y, Jufas N, Morris DP. Direct cost comparison of minimally invasive punch technique versus traditional approaches for percutaneous bone anchored hearing devices. J Otolaryngol Head Neck Surg 2017;46(1):46

[48] Sakihara Y, Parving A. Clinical otosclerosis, prevalence estimates and spontaneous progress. Acta Otolaryngol 1999;119(4):468–472

[49] Rudic M, Keogh I, Wagner R, et al. The pathophysiology of otosclerosis: review of current research. Hear Res 2015;330(Pt A):51–56

[50] Révész P, Liktor B, Liktor B, Sziklai I, Gerlinger I, Karosi T. Comparative analysis of preoperative diagnostic values of HRCT and CBCT in patients with histologically diagnosed otosclerotic stapes footplates. Eur Arch Otorhinolaryngol 2016;273(1):63–72

[51] Karosi T, Csomor P, Sziklai I. The value of HRCT in stapes fixations corresponding to hearing thresholds and histologic findings. Otol Neurotol 2012;33(8):1300–1307

[52] Lagleyre S, Sorrentino T, Calmels MN, et al. Reliability of high-resolution CT scan in diagnosis of otosclerosis. Otol Neurotol 2009;30(8):1152–1159

[53] Häusler R. General history of stapedectomy. Adv Otorhinolaryngol 2007;65:1–5

[54] Savvas E, Maurer J. Economic viability of stapes surgery in Germany. J Laryngol Otol 2009;123(4):403–406

[55] Merkus P, van Loon MC, Smit CF, Smits C, de Cock AFC, Hensen EF. Decision making in advanced otosclerosis: an evidence-based strategy. Laryngoscope 2011;121(9):1935–1941

[56] Slattery WH. Neurofibromatosis type 2. Otolaryngol Clin North Am 2015;48(3):443–460

[57] Verma S, Anthony R, Tsai V, Taplin M, Rutka J. Evaluation of cost effectiveness for conservative and active management strategies for acoustic neuroma. Clin Otolaryngol 2009;34(5):438–446

[58] Gait C, Frew EJ, Martin TPC, Jowett S, Irving R. Conservative management, surgery and radiosurgery for treatment of vestibular schwannomas: a model-based approach to cost-effectiveness. Clin Otolaryngol 2014;39(1):22–31

[59] Coelho DH, Tang Y, Suddarth B, Mamdani M. MRI surveillance of vestibular schwannomas without contrast enhancement: clinical and economic evaluation. Laryngoscope 2018;128(1):202–209

[60] Semaan MT, Wick CC, Kinder KJ, Stuyt JG, Chota RL, Megerian CA. Retrosigmoid versus translabyrinthine approach to acoustic neuroma resection: A comparative cost-effectiveness analysis. Laryngoscope 2016;126(Suppl 3):S5–S12

[61] Zygourakis CC, Oh T, Sun MZ, Barani I, Kahn JG, Parsa AT. Surgery is cost-effective treatment for young patients with vestibular schwannomas: decision tree modeling of surgery, radiation, and observation. Neurosurg Focus 2014;37(5):E8

[62] Caruso JP, Moosa S, Fezeu F, Ramesh A, Sheehan JP. A cost comparative study of Gamma Knife radiosurgery versus open surgery for intracranial pathology. J Clin Neurosci 2015;22(1):184–188

[63] Wellis G, Nagel R, Vollmar C, Steiger H-J. Direct costs of microsurgical management of radiosurgically amenable intracranial pathology in Germany: an analysis of meningiomas, acoustic neuromas, metastases and arteriovenous malformations of less than 3 cm in diameter. Acta Neurochir (Wien) 2003;145(4):249–255

[64] Banerjee R, Moriarty JP, Foote RL, Pollock BE. Comparison of the surgical and follow-up costs associated with microsurgical resection and stereotactic radiosurgery for vestibular schwannoma. J Neurosurg 2008;108(6):1220–1224

[65] Tos T, Caye-Thomasen P, Stangerup S-E, Tos M, Thomsen J. Long-term socio-economic impact of vestibular schwannoma for patients under observation and after surgery. J Laryngol Otol 2003;117(12):955–964

[66] Nikolopoulos TP. Neonatal hearing screening: what we have achieved and what needs to be improved. Int J Pediatr Otorhinolaryngol 2015;79(5):635–637

[67] Keren R, Helfand M, Homer C, McPhillips H, Lieu TA. Projected cost-effectiveness of statewide universal newborn hearing screening. Pediatrics 2002;110(5):855–864

[68] Fulcher A, Purcell AA, Baker E, Munro N. Listen up: children with early identified hearing loss achieve age-appropriate speech/language outcomes by 3 years-of-age. Int J Pediatr Otorhinolaryngol 2012;76(12):1785–1794

[69] Prosser JD, Cohen AP, Greinwald JH. Diagnostic evaluation of children with sensorineural hearing loss. Otolaryngol Clin North Am 2015;48(6):975–982

[70] Saunders JE, Francis HW, Skarzynski PH. Measuring success: cost-effectiveness and expanding access to cochlear implantation. Otol Neurotol 2016;37(2):e135–e140

[71] Porter ME. What is value in health care? N Engl J Med 2010;363(26):2477–2481

[72] McKinnon BJ. Cost effectiveness of cochlear implants. Curr Opin Otolaryngol Head Neck Surg 2014;22(5):344–348

[73] Semenov YR, Yeh ST, Seshamani M, et al; CDaCI Investigative Team. Age-dependent cost-utility of pediatric cochlear implantation. Ear Hear 2013;34(4):402–412

[74] Cheng AK, Rubin HR, Powe NR, Mellon NK, Francis HW, Niparko JK. Cost-utility analysis of the cochlear implant in children. JAMA 2000;284(7):850–856

[75] Phillips C, Thompson G. What Is a QALY.pdf. Hayward Medical Communications. 1998. Available at: http://www.vhpharmsci.com/decisionmaking/Therapeutic_Decision_Making/Advanced_files/What%20is%20a%20QALY.pdf. Accessed April 5, 2018

[76] CDC. Concept | HRQOL | CDC. Available at: https://www.cdc.gov/hrqol/concept.htm. Accessed April 5, 2018

[77] Hirth RA, Chernew ME, Miller E, Fendrick AM, Weissert WG. Willingness to pay for a quality-adjusted life year: in search of a standard. Med Decis Making 2000;20(3):332–342

[78] Braithwaite RS, Meltzer DO, King JT Jr, Leslie D, Roberts MS. What does the value of modern medicine say about the $50,000 per quality-adjusted life-year decision rule? Med Care 2008;46(4):349–356

[79] Dakin HA, Devlin NJ, Odeyemi IAO. "Yes", "no" or "yes, but"? Multinomial modelling of NICE decision-making. Health Policy 2006;77(3):352–367

[80] Barton GR, Stacey PC, Fortnum HM, Summerfield AQ. Hearing-impaired children in the United Kingdom, IV: cost-effectiveness of pediatric cochlear implantation. Ear Hear 2006;27(5):575–588

[81] Lammers MJW, Grolman W, Smulders YE, Rovers MM. The cost-utility of bilateral cochlear implantation: a systematic review. Laryngoscope 2011;121(12):2604–2609

[82] Foteff C, Kennedy S, Milton AH, Deger M, Payk F, Sanderson G. Cost-utility analysis of cochlear implantation in Australian adults. Otol Neurotol 2016;37(5):454–461

[83] Pérez-Martín J, Artaso MA, Díez FJ. Cost-effectiveness of pediatric bilateral cochlear implantation in Spain. Laryngoscope 2017;127(12):2866–2872

[84] Berrettini S, Baggiani A, Bruschini L, et al. Systematic review of the literature on the clinical effectiveness of the cochlear implant procedure in adult patients. Acta Otorhinolaryngol Ital 2011;31(5):299–310

[85] Bond M, Elston J, Mealing S, et al. Systematic reviews of the effectiveness and cost-effectiveness of multi-channel unilateral cochlear implants for adults. Clin Otolaryngol 2010;35(2):87–96

[86] Turchetti G, Bellelli S, Palla I, Berrettini S. Systematic review of the scientific literature on the economic evaluation of cochlear implants in adult patients. Acta Otorhinolaryngol Ital 2011;31(5):319–327

[87] Summerfield AQ, Marshall DH. Cochlear Implantation in the UK 1990–1994 Report by the MRC Institute of Hearing Research on the Evaluation of the National Cochlear Implant Programme: Main Report. London: HMSO; 1995

[88] Smulders YE, van Zon A, Stegeman I, et al. Cost-utility of bilateral versus unilateral cochlear implantation in adults: a randomized controlled trial. Otol Neurotol 2016;37(1):38–45

[89] UK Cochlear Implant Study Group. Criteria of candidacy for unilateral cochlear implantation in postlingually deafened adults II: cost-effectiveness analysis. Ear Hear 2004;25(4):336–360

[90] Quentin Summerfield A, Barton GR, Toner J, et al. Self-reported benefits from successive bilateral cochlear implantation in post-lingually deafened adults: randomised controlled trial. Int J Audiol 2006;45(Suppl 1): S99–S107

[91] Summerfield AQ, Marshall DH, Barton GR, Bloor KE. A cost-utility scenario analysis of bilateral cochlear implantation. Arch Otolaryngol Head Neck Surg 2002;128(11):1255–1262

# 8 Cranial Nerve VIII: Vestibular Disorders

*Gavriel D. Kohlberg and Ravi N. Samy*

## Abstract

Dizziness is a common patient complaint and may be challenging to diagnose a definitive cause. Only a fraction of vertigo or imbalance cases are attributable to peripheral (i.e., vestibular nerve and inner ear) pathology. It is critical to consider and evaluate for central, cardiogenic, ophthalmologic, and proprioceptive causes of dizziness. A history focusing on nature of dizziness, its duration, and associated symptoms is essential. Examination includes complete head and neck examination, neurologic examination, and neurotologic maneuvers such as head-impulse test, Dix–Hallpike test, and the head shake test. There are many inner ear function tests available for evaluation of the dizzy patient and can be used to evaluate for specific vestibular disorders. Imaging including CT of the temporal bones and MRI of the internal auditory canals and brain may be useful for ruling out pathology.

*Keywords:* benign paroxysmal positional vertigo, meniere's disease, vestibular neuronitis, superior semicircular canal dehiscence, superior semicircular canal dehiscence, central vertigo

## 8.1 Vestibular Anatomy and Physiology

The vestibular system is comprised of three semicircular canals, the utricle, the saccule, and the superior and inferior vestibular nerves, which join together with the cochlear nerve to form the eighth vestibulocochlear cranial nerve. The superior, posterior, and lateral semicircular canals are three orthogonally positioned canals that sense rotational acceleration. The utricle senses horizontal acceleration, while the saccule senses vertical acceleration. Each of the vestibular organs contains a gelatinous material that deflects hair cells during acceleration or deceleration, resulting in transmission of an electrical signal through the vestibular nerve. Impulses from the superior semicircular canal (SCC), lateral SCC, and utricle travel through the superior vestibular nerve, while impulses from the posterior SCC and saccule travel through the inferior vestibular nerve.

## 8.2 Overview of Dizziness

The body's sense of position and balance relies on the accurate integration of multiple sensory signal inputs within the brain. Information on body position and movement is conveyed through the vestibular system as well as through vision and proprioception. In addition, the sensation of dizziness can be induced as a self-preservation technique—a brain that is not sufficiently perfused will trigger a sense of faintness in order to induce sitting down or lying down in order to increase brain perfusion.

Dizziness is a common patient complaint without a specific definition. As common as dizziness is, it is a fairly imprecise symptom. The differential diagnosis is broad with even the most common etiologies accounting for less than 10% of cases.[1] Dizziness can encapsulate vertigo, disequilibrium, vision changes (e.g., nystagmus), and lightheadedness. Vertigo refers to a sensation of rotational motion. Disequilibrium is a feeling of instability or imbalance. Lightheadedness is the sense of impending faintness.

There are many etiologies for dizziness, and dizziness can be multifactorial as well. Therefore, it is crucial to consider causes of dizziness beyond the vestibular system including neurologic, ophthalmologic, cardiogenic, psychogenic, and proprioceptive (such as peripheral neuropathy from diabetes mellitus).

Vestibular causes of dizziness are usually the result of dysfunction of the semicircular canals or the vestibular nerve.

## 8.3 Epidemiology and Economic Impact of Dizziness

Dizziness and balance disorders are common conditions that result in a substantial number of visits to health care providers. Dizziness accounts for an estimated 5% of all primary care clinic visits and 3% of all emergency room visits.[2,3] This is particularly true in older adults, where up 30% of patients age 60 years and up to 50% of community-dwelling adults older than 80 years have some degree of dizziness.[4] The total cost of evaluation and management of these patients is enormous. In 2008, Saber Terhani and colleagues reported the estimated national cost of patients presenting with dizziness to the emergency department alone exceeded $4 billion.[5] These costs have almost certainly increased since that publication. Individuals with symptomatic balance dysfunction have a 12-fold increase in the odds of falling, with one in three community-dwelling adults older than 65 years falling each year. Ten years of falls result in major injuries with a cost of over $20 billion annually.[6] In general, dizziness and vertigo have a huge negative impact not only on health care resource use but also on work productivity.[7]

## 8.4 History

A general approach should focus on obtaining a thorough history. Timing (onset, duration, evolution, etc.), severity, frequency, triggers, and associated symptoms are likely to clue the clinician as to whether the problem area is central (brain, vestibular nuclei in brainstem, cerebellum, etc.), peripheral (inner ear, cochleovestibular nerve), or nonvestibular (cardiovascular insufficiency, peripheral neuropathy, etc.).

Patients with peripheral inner ear sources of their dizziness tend to have vertigo, or a subjective illusion of movement. Lightheadedness, imbalance and unsteadiness, nausea, and blackouts are generally not seen with peripheral vestibulopathies. Vertigo may be accompanied by hearing loss and is more commonly episodic (rather than constant) when compared to central nervous system causes. For an excellent review of how

**Table 8.1** Timing of common peripheral vestibular disorders

| Duration | Disorder |
| --- | --- |
| s–min | Benign paroxysmal positional vertigo |
| min–h | Meniere's disease<br>Vestibular migraine |
| d–mo | Vestibular neuronitis<br>Labyrinthitis<br>Perilymph fistula |
| mo–y | Superior semicircular canal dehiscence<br>Vestibular schwannoma |

to differentiate the source (central, peripheral, or nonvestibular), the reader is encouraged to see Muncie et al.[8] (For the purpose of this discussion, disorders of the vestibular branch of vestibulocochlear nerve [CN VIII] are considered peripheral [or inner ear] causes of dizziness.)

A complete history of a patient presenting with dizziness must focus on the duration of the dizziness as well as a detailed description of the dizziness. Does the dizziness last for seconds, minutes, hours, or days? Is it intermittent or constant? What is the frequency of each dizziness episode and when did they first begin? Is the dizziness vertigolike or is it a sense of imbalance or of feeling faint? Is the dizziness associated with headaches (e.g., vestibular migraine), hearing loss, aural fullness, or tinnitus? Is the dizziness associated with changes in vision? Is the dizziness positional? Has there been recent barotrauma? A detailed past medical history, medication history, and family and social history should be obtained.

For the smaller percentage of patients with suspected inner ear disorders, their workup and management can be both incredibly challenging and rewarding. Fortunately, duration of symptoms can point toward the likely diagnosis (▶Table 8.1). In addition to history, some simple, targeted "bedside" testing such as the Dix–Hallpike maneuver and head shake test can aid in establishing the correct diagnosis. When available, pure-tone audiometry with speech comprehension testing can be helpful, and may even identify the suspected affected side as the inner ear functions of hearing and balance can be affected in disorders such as Meniere's disease and labyrinthitis. Taken in aggregate, history, limited physical examination, and audiometry can frequently result in the correct diagnosis or at least suggest if the dizziness is central, peripheral, or nonvestibular.

## 8.5 Physical Examination

In addition to the physical examination described earlier for the patient with hearing loss, specific tests help elucidate the diagnosis in dizzy patients.

Testing can be performed in the office for orthostatic hypotension using commonly available sphygmomanometers. During examination of the tympanic membranes (TMs), a fistula test should be performed to examine for pressure-induced vertigo or nystagmus.

Nystagmus should be evaluated with a neutral gaze with and without fixation. Evaluation for gaze-evoked nystagmus to

the right, left, up, and down should also be performed. Ocular alignment, saccades, and smooth pursuit should be tested.

The vestibulo-ocular reflex (VOR) moves the eyes contrary to the head in order to maintain steady vision during head motion. Bilateral vestibular weakness or poorly compensated unilateral vestibular weakness can result in loss of the VOR and lead to symptoms of oscillopsia. Several physical examination maneuvers can test the integrity of the VOR. In the head impulse test (HIT), the examiner rapidly turns the patient's head 30 degrees while the patient attempts to maintain their gaze on a target. In a patient with bilateral vestibular weakness, the patient's eyes do not remain on the target with the test done in either direction. In a patient with a unilateral vestibular weakness, the eyes will lag in returning to the target when head motion is rotated toward the side with vestibular weakness. The post-head-shake nystagmus test can be used to assess for unilateral vestibular weakness. The patient's head is shaken from side to side for 20 seconds at 2 Hz. The head shake is then stopped. In a patient with symmetric vestibular function, there should be no nystagmus. If there is unilateral weakness, there will be fast-phase beating nystagmus away from the weaker side.

The Dix–Hallpike maneuver test is used for posterior canal benign paroxysmal positional vertigo (BPPV). Starting in a sitting position, the patient's head is rotated 45 degrees to one side. The patient is then laid supine with the neck slightly extended. The Dix–Hallpike test is considered positive when it elicits up-beating and torsional nystagmus when the head is tilted toward the affected ear. Nystagmus typically starts at least 1 second after positioning and reaches a maximum at about 10 seconds before fatiguing in less than 60 seconds.

The Romberg test assesses proprioception. The patient first stands in a neutral position with feet slightly apart and arms at the side or folded across the chest. The patient starts with eyes open for 30 seconds and then with eyes closed for 30 seconds. The Romberg test is considered positive if the patient is stable with eyes open and then loses balance with eyes closed. A positive Romberg test occurs in patients with proprioceptive deficits.

The Fukuda stepping test assesses for unilateral peripheral vestibular hypofunction. The patient marches in place with their eyes closed. A rotation to one side may signify an ipsilateral vestibular weakness.

When available, pure-tone audiometry with speech comprehension testing can be helpful, and may even identify the suspected affected side as the inner ear functions of hearing and balance can be affected in disorders such as Meniere's disease and labyrinthitis. Taken in aggregate, history, limited physical examination, and audiometry can frequently result in the correct diagnosis or at least suggest if the dizziness is central, peripheral, or nonvestibular.

If doubt as to the correct diagnosis persists, a variety of tests (behavioral, electrophysiologic, and radiographic) are available to the clinician. Yet judicious use of these tests should be employed. The "shotgun" approach of ordering every test for every patient may only prove to obfuscate the actual diagnosis while only increasing cost.

# 8.6 Laboratory Testing

## 8.6.1 Cost-Effectiveness of Laboratory Testing for Peripheral Vestibular Disorders

There is no clear evidence in the literature pertaining to the cost-effectiveness of the laboratory tests for vestibular disorders described below. The below tests rely on expensive specialized equipment and highly trained operators. Many diagnoses can be made without laboratory testing. Clinicians typically do obtain laboratory testing such as videonystagmography (VNG) prior to performing an ablative procedure on the inner ear (e.g., labyrinthectomy or transtympanic gentamycin injection) in order to confirm the side of vestibulopathy.

## 8.6.2 Videonystagmography/Electronystagmography

VNG and electronystagmography (ENG) are techniques of tracking eye movement in order to assess for nystagmus. VNG and ENG can be used interchangeably. VNG relies on video to capture eye movement, whereas ENG assesses changes in the corneoretinal potentials, which can be translated into eye movements.

VNG generally refers to a series of vestibular tests that rely on quantified measurement of nystagmus: caloric testing, gaze test, Dix–Hallpike maneuver, saccades, positional testing, and smooth pursuit.

## 8.6.3 Caloric Testing

Caloric testing, first described by Barany in 1906, has long been considered the standard method of evaluating the function of an individual's inner ear. The caloric test allows for the assessment of a unilateral vestibulopathy as peripheral or central and for identification of the side of the vestibulopathy. In the caloric test, heated or cooled air or water into the external auditory canal is used to generate endolymphatic flow in the lateral semicircular canal. Each ear is irrigated while the patient lies supine with the head tilted up 30 degrees, placing the lateral SCC in the vertical plane. Cold irrigation causes slow-phase nystagmus toward the irrigated ear, while warm irrigation causes nystagmus away from the irrigated ear. The velocities of irrigation-induced nystagmus with hot and cold stimulus are compared between ears in order to assess for asymmetry between sides. The canal paresis (CP) index is used to quantify asymmetry and is calculated according to the following formula:

$$CP\,(right) = \frac{(RW + RC) - (LW + LC)}{(RW + RC) + (LW + LC)} \times 100$$

where slow-phase velocities are measured for RW = right warm, RC = right cool, LW = left warm, and LC = left cool. Unilateral weakness is considered significant when CP is greater than 20%.

Caloric testing is advantageous as it can localize a lesion to the right or left side. However, as it relies on stimulating the lateral SCC, it is a test of the superior vestibular nerve (innervates the lateral SCC) and not the inferior vestibular nerve. As it relies on comparing the right to the left side, it is not a good test for symmetric bilateral vestibular weakness.

VNG/ENG testing only assesses the lateral semicircular canal and only at low-frequency stimulation. Some have even asserted that caloric testing and ENG/VNG add little value to diagnosis other than to identify central versus peripheral etiology, and laterality when peripheral.[9,10] Such testing can be useful prior to ablative therapy in which the entire malfunctioning vestibular labyrinth is deafferented (chemically or surgically). In their study of cost-effectiveness of workup of unilateral vestibular weakness found on ENG, Gandolfi and colleagues concluded that further workup (MRI) is high cost and low yielding in patients with one isolated abnormality and no other risk factors.[11]

## 8.6.4 Gaze Test

The eyes are assessed for nystagmus as the patient gazes 30 degrees to the right, to the left, up, and down with and without fixation suppression. Nystagmus on gaze test is an abnormal finding that may be of vestibular or central origin. Generally, in an acute unilateral vestibular weakness, there will be nystagmus with the fast phase directed toward the unaffected ear, which will be accentuated with gaze toward the healthy ear and suppressed with gaze toward the affected ear. With any other type of nystagmus on gaze test, a central cause must be considered.[12]

## 8.6.5 Dix–Hallpike Maneuver

The Dix–Hallpike maneuver (described earlier in the Physical Examination section) can be performed with VNG in order to quantify any associated nystagmus.

## 8.6.6 Saccades

A saccade is a rapid movement of the eye between fixation points. Saccades allow for the rapid capture of an image in the peripheral vision onto the fovea of the retina. Saccades are tested in the horizontal and vertical planes by presenting a series of targets that the patient must fixate on. Each saccade is analyzed for eye movement latency, amplitude, velocity, and accuracy. Abnormalities in saccades are generally attributed to a central cause.

## 8.6.7 Positional Test

The patient is monitored for nystagmus with gaze suppression in the sitting, supine, and right and left ear down positions. Nystagmus is an abnormal finding that may be central or peripheral.

## 8.6.8 Smooth Pursuit

With the patient's head fixed, the patient follows a target moving at about 0.5 Hz and amplitude of 15 degrees from side to side. The patient should be able to smoothly track the target.

Patients with deficiency in smooth pursuit will exhibit corrective saccades in order to recapture the image on the fovea. Impairment of smooth pursuit is generally the result of central causes.

## 8.6.9 Rotary Chair Testing

In rotary chair testing, the patient sits with head tilted 30 degrees forward to place the lateral SCC in the horizontal plane. Chair rotation causes head acceleration, which activates the VOR, inducing nystagmus. The test is performed in the dark to suppress gaze fixation. The rotary chair can rotate at a fluctuating velocity or step from one constant velocity to another. VOR gain is measured as eye velocity/chair velocity. The VOR phase is the difference between time of peak eye velocity and peak chair velocity. Rotational chair testing is advantageous in patients with otologic pathology (such as TM perforation), which can limit caloric testing. It is also superior to caloric testing for assessing for bilateral vestibular weakness as it does not rely on comparison between sides to quantify vestibular function. Like caloric testing, rotational chair testing tests the lateral SCC and, therefore, the superior vestibular nerve. Because both right and left vestibular functions are tested simultaneously, rotational chair testing is not as accurate in diagnosing small unilateral weakness compared to caloric testing. However, the rotational chair test is more physiological and can test response at higher frequency stimulation compared to caloric testing. A study comparing VNG to rotary chair testing found them to have very similar sensitivity and specificity for identifying individuals with peripheral vestibular disorder.[13] Of note, rotary chair equipment is currently expensive ($70,000) compared to VNG equipment ($32,000).[14]

## 8.6.10 Video Head Impulse Test

In the video head impulse test (vHIT), the patient wears a head-mounted device that tracks eye movement as well as head velocity. The clinician then performs the HIT. The output of the device allows for assessment of the VOR through the comparison of head velocity stimulus and eye velocity response. Further study is needed of this relatively new technology to assess for clinical utility and cost-effectiveness compared to VNG and rotary chair. Of note, vHIT is a shorter examination compared to VNG and rotary chair and that does not typically induce nausea, so it may be a more comfortable evaluation compared to VNG and rotary chair testing.[13,15]

## 8.6.11 Electrocochleography

Electrocochleography (ECoG) gained popularity through the later decades of the 20th century as a more reliable method of diagnosing Meniere's disease. However, the clinical utility is limited as potentially more than 50% of patients with Meniere's disease will have normal ECoG.[16] As such, the American Academy of Otolaryngology–Head and Neck Surgery does not even consider ECoG as necessary for the diagnosis.[17]

## 8.6.12 Vestibular Evoked Myogenic Potential Testing

Vestibular evoked myogenic potential (VEMP) testing has recently been a useful addition to the vestibular diagnostic battery. VEMP testing relies on sound-induced activation of saccular and utricular afferents. By measuring the vestibulospinal reflex, a VEMP can be useful in evaluating the integrity of the otolithic and utricular systems. For diagnostic purposes in the evaluation of SCC dehiscence syndrome (SSCDS), thresholds are decreased and amplitudes increased when compared to the normative values. Beyond diagnosis, VEMP can be helpful in monitoring efficacy of intratympanic gentamicin when ablating the vestibular sensors in a faulty inner ear or detecting subclinical contralateral disease in patients with Meniere's disease.

## 8.6.13 Cervical Vestibular Evoked Myogenic Potential

Sound-induced activation of the saccule leads to a reflexive activation of the sternocleidomastoid (SCM) muscles. This reflex turns one's head toward a loud sound presented to a particular ear and is mediated by the inferior vestibular nerve. The reflex is measured by surface electrodes placed onto the SCM. Cervical vestibular evoked myogenic potential (cVEMP) is a test of the inferior vestibular nerve.

## 8.6.14 Ocular Vestibular Evoked Myogenic Potential

Sound-induced activation of the utricle leads to a reflexive activation of the ocular muscles to turn the eyes in the direction of a sound stimulus. This reflex is mediated by the superior vestibular nerve and therefore is a test of superior nerve function.

## 8.6.15 Computerized Dynamic Posturography

Computerized dynamic posturography (CDP) can provide a quantitative assessment of the sensory and motor components of postural control, though its use as a first-line diagnostic tool may be limited. It may be helpful in atypical patients with potentially many causes of their dizziness, or in ruling out malingering or exaggeration in medicolegal cases. Likewise, rotary chairs are similarly expensive and of limited widespread diagnostic use other than determining degree of bilateral vestibulopathy.

## 8.6.16 Radiology

Though frequently employed, imaging such as CT and MRI of the head and temporal bones plays a very limited role in the diagnosis of peripheral vestibular disease. As the vast majority of vestibular dysfunctions are limited to the membranous labyrinth, current technologies are limited in their resolution and ability to detect disease. Ahsan and colleagues found the diagnostic yield of brain CT for dizziness in the emergency room to be 0.74% for clinically significant pathology requiring intervention.[18] The same study found a 12.2% yield for MRI. There is a role for imaging for patients with acute dizziness, but imaging should be limited to patients with acute dizziness and other neurological signs or symptoms of stroke. Moreover, imaging is not 100% sensitive and some serious or life-threatening pathology can be missed. A high index of suspicion by history must guide the decision to obtain imaging emergently. Until then, unnecessary imaging will continue to account for a substantial portion of emergency room budgets.

In the setting of chronic dizziness, imaging may be even less useful than in acute setting. Nonetheless, imaging can be useful and even necessary to rule in or rule out important conditions. As mentioned earlier, T1 gadolinium-enhanced MRI remains the gold standard for identifying vestibular schwannoma or other retrocochlear pathology. It can also help identify any mass lesions involving the labyrinth roughly 1 mm or bigger. In addition, recent studies have shown MRI-detectable endolymphatic hydrops in patients with suspected Meniere's disease.[19] Nonetheless, the decision to image should be based on focused clinical suspicion.

# 8.7 Treatment

In the acute phase, supportive care and vestibular-suppressant medication can be helpful. However, no medication has been found to be effective for long-term management of vestibular dysfunction.[20] Ultimately, maximizing both outcome and cost-effectiveness is completely dependent on identifying the correct diagnosis. Once an individual diagnosis is established, or at least highly suspected, proper therapeutic interventions can be initiated.

## 8.7.1 Benign Paroxysmal Positional Vertigo

Benign paroxysmal positional vertigo (BPPV) is characterized by several seconds of spinning dizziness brought on by specific head movements such as rolling over in bed. BPPV can occur at any age, though most commonly it presents in the fourth decade of life. BPPV is more common in women than in men. The sensation of vertigo should not last more than 1 minute. Episodes may occur frequently, followed by a quiescent period.[21] This condition may represent 8% of all patients with dizziness, and likely represents the most common form of peripheral vestibulopathy.

BPPV is believed to be due to free-floating otoconia within the labyrinth, most commonly within the posterior semicircular canal. It is easily diagnosed through a Dix–Hallpike maneuver (posterior canal BPPV) or supine roll test (lateral canal BPPV) in which the clinician observes the patients' eyes and the patient is asked to endorse or deny vertigo. If present, the nystagmus associated with BPPV is latent (occurring after a few seconds) and fatigable (in <60 seconds and with repeated maneuvers). Patients with symptoms concerning for BPPV should undergo a Dix–Hallpike maneuver to confirm the diagnosis. No further testing or referrals are needed for the evaluation of BPPV. BPPV can be treated by the Epley maneuver, which can be performed in the clinic, by the patient themselves, and during vestibular rehabilitation.[22] Recurrent BPPV or BPPV unresponsive to standard therapy should be referred to an otolaryngologist for further evaluation.

In very rare cases of refractory BPPV, surgical options have been described (e.g., singular neurectomy, posterior semicircular canal occlusion) with varying degrees of success and hearing preservation.

## 8.7.2 Meniere's Disease

Meniere's disease is characterized by episodes or "attacks" of vertigo, hearing loss, and tinnitus. Vertigo generally lasts for about 20 minutes to several hours followed by a longer period of malaise. Patients are largely asymptomatic between episodes. Otologic symptoms are generally unilateral fluctuating low-frequency hearing loss, nonpulsatile tinnitus, and aural fullness. Patients may also complain of gait and postural instability, sudden drop attacks (crisis of Tumarkin), and nausea.[19] The exact incidence is not known, though it is estimated to be approximately 15.3 per 100,000 population.[23] Little data exist regarding the cost of treating Meniere's disease, though one recent study estimated the cost at roughly $900 million per year, with substantial indirect costs.[24] While some patients present with classic symptoms of Meniere's disease with no other complaints, often symptoms are not classic. In all cases, especially those with atypical complaints, other vestibular and neurologic diagnoses must be considered. A detailed history concerning dizziness, hearing loss, and otologic symptoms should be ascertained. In addition, history related to vestibular migraine, transient ischemic attack or stroke, retrocochlear lesions (e.g., vestibular schwannoma), and autoimmune inner ear disease should be obtained. Physical examination may reveal a unilateral vestibular weakness with HIT. Neurologic examination is mandatory to look for signs of central pathology.

An audiological evaluation should be performed. While a gadolinium-enhanced MRI of the brain is not always considered mandatory, there should be a low threshold to obtain an MRI to rule out central pathology including vestibular schwannoma or other retrocochlear pathology (e.g., endolymphatic sac tumor) and stroke. Though advances in 3-T MRI with gadolinium have allowed for visualization of endolymphatic hydrops, at this time this is not part of the routine diagnostic evaluation.

Likewise, ENG or VNG to demonstrate unilateral vestibular weakness is not necessary for diagnosis, though procurement of such testing is imperative prior to surgical intervention.[25]

ECoG may demonstrate elevated summating potential (SP)/ action potential (AP) ratios in patients with Meniere's disease, though this is not a necessary test and has been shown to have low accuracy.[16,26] Patients with suspected Meniere's disease should be referred to an otolaryngologist for further management.

Because there is no definitive test for Meniere's disease, the diagnosis may not always be certain prior to treatment. If clinical suspicion is high based on history of fluctuating unilateral hearing loss, tinnitus, aural fullness, and vertigo episodes along with ipsilateral low-frequency sensorineural hearing loss, some clinicians may proceed with first-line treatments (e.g., low-sodium diet, use of diuretic, and possibly steroids) and reevaluate the patient in 6 to 8 weeks for improvement. If the diagnosis is not certain, further testing such as VNG, ECOG, and MRI may be helpful to confirm laterality, to rule in Meniere's disease, and to rule out retrocochlear masses.

The treatment of Meniere's disease is controversial, though the vast majority of patients can be successfully managed medically with a sodium-restricted diet with or without a diuretic.[27] In refractory cases, intratympanic or open surgical procedures can provide relief of vestibular symptoms, though no intervention as of yet has shown to successfully prevent the hearing loss associated with Meniere's disease.

### 8.7.3 Vestibular Neuronitis

Vestibular neuritis stems from an imbalance in tonic vestibular activity thought to be caused by a viral inflammation of the vestibular nerve. Patients presenting with acute-onset vertigo lasting hours to days should be evaluated for vestibular neuritis, labyrinthitis, as well as life-threatening causes of acute vestibular syndrome such as posterior circulation stroke. History, physical examination, and additional testing are aimed at confirming the diagnosis of vestibular neuritis while ruling out central causes of dizziness, such as cerebellar hemorrhage and infarction. Patients with vestibular neuritis often will have associated nausea, vomiting, sweating, and malaise. Symptoms usually develop over hours, last for several days, and then subside over weeks.[28]

Physical examination during the acute event should demonstrate spontaneous nystagmus that is horizontal and torsional. The direction of the nystagmus should not change with gaze direction. In nystagmus that changes direction with change in gaze direction, or in vertical nystagmus, a central cause should be considered. Inability to stand, dysarthria, incoordination, numbness, and weakness are all suggestive of a central cause rather than vestibular neuritis. The HIT should be performed to demonstrate a unilateral vestibular weakness. The diagnosis of vestibular neuritis can be made on the basis of history and physical examination alone. Viral studies are not indicated. While caloric testing will demonstrate a unilateral vestibular weakness, ENG or VNG is not required. MRI of the brain should be performed in the cases where there are associated neurological signs or symptoms suggestive of a possible central cause, or in patients with risk factors for stroke.[29] Clinicians should exclude brainstem and cerebellar strokes as they may present similarly initially, but with dire consequences. Patients with symptoms or signs of hearing loss should undergo audiological evaluation. Patients with associated hearing loss are considered to have labyrinthitis rather than vestibular neuritis. These patients should undergo MRI of the brain in order to rule out vestibular schwannoma or other retrocochlear pathology.[30]

Patients with vestibular neuronitis (vestibular neuritis) experience a single severe attack of vertigo without hearing loss that lasts days with slow, nonlinear improvement over the course of weeks to months. These patients should be administered steroids, vestibular suppressants, and/or antiemetics in the acute phase, but should discontinue their vestibular suppressants as soon as possible to allow for central compensation.[31] Beside a limited course of vestibular physical therapy to expedite central compensation, no other intervention is indicated.

### 8.7.4 Labyrinthitis

Labyrinthitis is similar to vestibular neuronitis, except patients will also have hearing loss. It is usually thought to be serous or aseptic, though suppurative labyrinthitis can be seen as a rare sequela of acute otitis media. For nonbacterial labyrinthitis, the workup and treatment are similar to vestibular neuronitis (steroids, supportive care), with the exception of possibly more aggressive treatment of the hearing loss. When hearing loss occurs without vestibular symptoms, it is referred to as idiopathic sudden sensorineural hearing loss.

### 8.7.5 Vestibular Schwannoma

See section 7.4 (Acoustic Neuroma/Vestibular Schwannoma).

### 8.7.6 Perilymph Fistula

Perilymph fistula is a very rare condition that occurs when perilymph of the inner ear escapes into the middle ear. Almost exclusively a sequelae of head trauma or barotrauma (including valsalva induced), the unusual constellation of symptoms can make diagnosis difficult as it may mimic other peripheral or central pathologies including traumatic brain injury. It may present with fluctuating imbalance, fluctuating hearing loss, and even memory issues with word recall difficulties. Conservative management includes bed rest and steroids, though in rare cases operative exploration and repair of the round and oval windows may be necessary.

### 8.7.7 Superior Semicircular Canal Dehiscence

Patients with a dehiscence in the bone overlying the SCC may experience a constellation of symptoms termed superior semicircular canal dehiscence syndrome (SSCDS), or Minor's syndrome. The most common cochlear symptoms experienced by patients are hyperacusis, autophony, pulsatile tinnitus, and aural fullness. Patients may also experience disequilibrium or sound-/pressure-induced vertigo. Symptoms are caused by the ability of bone-conducted sound to access the inner ear via the dehiscent area of the SCC (considered a mobile third window). History should focus on hearing and dizziness symptoms. Patients should have at least one of the following symptoms to be considered for SSCDS: bone conduction hyperacusis in the form of autophony (audible eye movements, footsteps, etc.), sound-induced vertigo, pressure-induced vertigo (while coughing, sneezing, bearing down during a bowel movement), or pulsatile tinnitus. During the physical examination, eye movements can be elicited by loud noise or pneumatic otoscopy. Patients with suspicion for SSCD should undergo audiological evaluation. Audiogram will often demonstrate a large air–bone gap in the low frequencies with bone conduction normal or better than normal (negative). Unlike otosclerosis, however, acoustic reflexes will be present. Patients with suspected SSCDS based on history should be referred to an otolaryngologist for further evaluation. VEMP testing should be performed. Patients with SSCDS have lower-than-normal thresholds for cVEMP thresholds and higher-than-normal oVEMP response amplitudes.

Patients with suspicion for SSCD should undergo high-resolution CT that is reformatted in the plane of the superior SCC in order to evaluate for radiographic dehiscence of the superior SCC (►Fig. 8.1). ECoG may also be performed and should demonstrate elevated SP/AP ratio in SSCDS. A proposed diagnostic criteria for SSCDS requires (1) high-resolution CT demonstrating SCC dehiscence; (2) at least one of the following symptoms: bone conduction hyperacusis, sound-induced

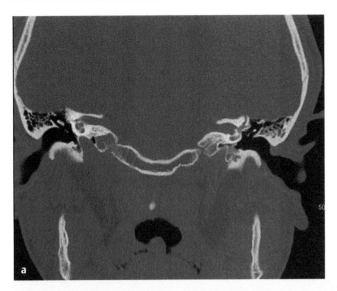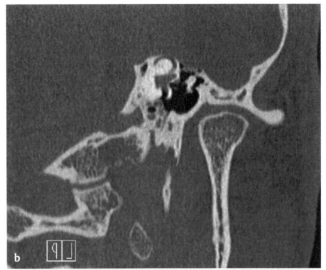

**Fig. 8.1** (a) Coronal non-contrast enhanced CT of left sided superior semicircular canal dehiscence. (b) Poschl view of same dehiscence.

vertigo, pressure-induced vertigo, and pulsatile tinnitus; (3) at least one of the following demonstrations of a mobile third window: negative bone conduction thresholds on audiogram, low cVEMP thresholds or high ocular vestibular evoked myogenic potential (oVEMP) amplitudes, or elevated SP/AP ratio in the absence of sensorineural hearing loss.[32]

Of note, the rate of radiographic SCCD is 9%.[33] However, the rate of histological SCCD is 0.5%.[34] The rate of SSCDS is therefore no higher than 0.5% and vastly lower than the radiographic rate. Therefore, incidental finding of superior SCCD on CT with no clinical symptoms does not warrant further evaluation, but patients should be educated on the potential for cochlear or vestibular symptoms to develop over time.

SCCD results from fistulous connection formed between the dura of the temporal lobe and the membranous SCC. Once diagnosed, the current standard treatment involves surgical repair of the dehiscence with marked improvement or resolution of their symptoms and improvement in health-related quality of life compared with nonoperated patients with SCCD.[35] Recent evidence has suggested that transmastoid repair may offer significant advantages (decreased pain, lower complication rate, shorter hospital stay, lower revision rate) over the traditional subtemporal craniotomy approach.[36]

## 8.8 Vestibular Physical Therapy

For many dizzy patients, irrespective of the specific cause of peripheral disease, physical therapy can be both extremely helpful and cost-effective. This specialized treatment, known as vestibular physical therapy, is a broad concept that incorporates both postural training and central compensation and can be effective for many causes of vertigo, generalized dizziness, or even unsteadiness. Vestibular therapy is able to be effective by using central nervous system adaptation to sensory loss or mismatch. Also known as "balance retraining," vestibular therapy is a program of guided exercises consisting of head, body, and eye movement designed to stimulate the vestibular system in different ways. It can be useful as either a primary or an adjunct

treatment not only for all of the above-listed conditions, but also for multifactorial dizziness, presbystasis (age-related global balance impairment), and post-head injury. However, few patients with these treatable conditions are actually referred for therapy.[37,38] Vestibular rehabilitation is simple, relatively inexpensive, and simple for all patients to perform, including elderly patients. Following initial assessment and plan creation by a physical therapist, most therapy is done by the patient themselves at their own home with periodic interval reassessment. In some cases, locating a suitably trained and available therapist may prove difficult, in which case home exercises (by booklet) or even web-based home instruction is beginning to show promise.[39,40,41,42]

## 8.9 Central Vertigo

The sensation of vertigo can be caused by central pathology as well as peripheral pathology. Therefore, consideration of central causes of vertigo is essential. Causes of central vertigo include vestibular migraine, vascular disorders, stroke, neoplasms, disorders of the craniovertebral junction, multiple sclerosis, seizure, cerebellar ataxia, and normal-pressure hydrocephalus. It is paramount that history and physical examination evaluate for central causes of vertigo. Referral to neurologist or other specialist should be performed if the above symptoms are identified.

## 8.10 Conclusion

Disorders of the peripheral vestibular system can be challenging to diagnose and to manage. However, there certainly remains a close association between how well a condition is defined and understood and the therapeutic options for that condition. Poorly understood vestibular disorders lack effective and cost-effective models, and therefore research should focus on better elucidating the underlying mechanisms of a disease. Much has changed over the past decades in the understanding of vestibular disorders, but what has not changed, as

Fife explains, "is the necessity of obtaining a basic history."[43] In the end, the most cost-effective mechanism is education.[44] As we increase efforts to inform and educate physicians on the intricacies that differentiate causes of dizziness, we may see an improvement in the timeliness, quality, and cost of care for these patients.

# References

[1] Newman-Toker DE, Edlow JA. TiTrATE: a novel, evidence-based approach to diagnosing acute dizziness and vertigo. Neurol Clin 2015;33(3):577–599, viii

[2] Sloane PD. Dizziness in primary care. Results from the National Ambulatory Medical Care Survey. J Fam Pract 1989;29(1):33–38

[3] Kerber KA. Vertigo and dizziness in the emergency department. Emerg Med Clin North Am 2009;27(1):39–50, viii

[4] Fernández L, Breinbauer HA, Delano PH. Vertigo and dizziness in the elderly. Front Neurol 2015;6:144

[5] Saber Tehrani AS, Coughlan D, Hsieh YH, et al. Rising annual costs of dizziness presentations to U.S. emergency departments. Acad Emerg Med 2013;20(7):689–696

[6] Agrawal Y, Ward BK, Minor LB. Vestibular dysfunction: prevalence, impact and need for targeted treatment. J Vestib Res 2013;23(3):113–117

[7] Benecke H, Agus S, Kuessner D, Goodall G, Strupp M. The burden and impact of vertigo: findings from the REVERT patient registry. Front Neurol 2013;4:136

[8] Muncie HL, Sirmans SM, James E. Dizziness: approach to evaluation and management. Am Fam Physician 2017;95(3):154–162

[9] Salman SD. The evaluation of vertigo and the electronystagmogram. J Laryngol Otol 1981;95(5):465–469

[10] Bakr MS, Saleh EM. Electronystagmography: how helpful is it? J Laryngol Otol 2000;114(3):178–183

[11] Gandolfi MM, Reilly EK, Galatioto J, Judson RB, Kim AH. Cost-effective analysis of unilateral vestibular weakness investigation. Otol Neurotol 2015;36(2):277–281

[12] Hullar TE, Zee D, Minor L. Evaluation of the patient with dizziness. In: Niparko JK, ed. Cummings Otolaryngology: head and Neck Surgery. 5th ed. Philadelphia, PA: Mosby Elsevier; 2010:2305–2327

[13] Eza-Nuñez P, Fariñas-Alvarez C, Fernandez NP. Comparison of three diagnostic tests in detecting vestibular deficit in patients with peripheral vestibulopathy. J Laryngol Otol 2016;130(2):145–150

[14] Phillips JS, Mallinson AI, Hamid MA. Cost-effective evaluation of the vestibular patient. Curr Opin Otolaryngol Head Neck Surg 2011;19(5):403–409

[15] Alhabib SF, Saliba I. Video head impulse test: a review of the literature. Eur Arch Otorhinolaryngol 2017;274(3):1215–1222

[16] Kim HH, Kumar A, Battista RA, Wiet RJ. Electrocochleography in patients with Meniere's disease. Am J Otolaryngol 2005;26(2):128–131

[17] Committee on Hearing and Equilibrium guidelines for the diagnosis and evaluation of therapy in Ménière's disease. American Academy of Otolaryngology–Head and Neck Foundation, Inc. Otolaryngol Head Neck Surg 1995;113(3):181–185

[18] Ahsan SF, Standring R, Osborn DA, Peterson E, Seidman M, Jain R. Clinical predictors of abnormal magnetic resonance imaging findings in patients with asymmetric sensorineural hearing loss. JAMA Otolaryngol Head Neck Surg 2015;141(5):451–456

[19] Gürkov R. Ménière and friends: imaging and classification of hydropic ear disease. Otol Neurotol 2017;38(10):e539–e544

[20] Rascol O, Hain TC, Brefel C, Benazet M, Clanet M, Montastruc JL. Antivertigo medications and drug-induced vertigo. A pharmacological review. Drugs 1995;50(5):777–791

[21] Baloh RW, Honrubia V, Jacobson K. Benign positional vertigo: clinical and oculographic features in 240 cases. Neurology 1987;37(3):371–378

[22] Hilton M, Pinder D. The Epley (canalith repositioning) manoeuvre for benign paroxysmal positional vertigo. Cochrane Database Syst Rev 2004(2):CD003162

[23] Wladislavosky-Waserman P, Facer GW, Mokri B, Kurland LT. Meniere's disease: a 30-year epidemiologic and clinical study in Rochester, Mn, 1951–1980. Laryngoscope 1984;94(8):1098–1102

[24] Tyrrell J, Whinney DJ, Taylor T. The cost of Ménière's disease: a novel multi-source approach. Ear Hear 2016;37(3):e202–e209

[25] Lopez-Escamez JA, Carey J, Chung WH, et al; Classification Committee of the Barany Society. Japan Society for Equilibrium Research. European Academy of Otology and Neurotology (EAONO). Equilibrium Committee of the American Academy of Otolaryngology–Head and Neck Surgery (AAO–HNS). Korean Balance Society. Diagnostic criteria for Ménière's disease. J Vestib Res 2015;25(1):1–7

[26] Syed I, Aldren C. Meniere's disease: an evidence based approach to assessment and management. Int J Clin Pract 2012;66(2):166–170

[27] Coelho DH, Lalwani AK. Medical management of Ménière's disease. Laryngoscope 2008;118(6):1099–1108

[28] Goudakos JK, Markou KD, Franco-Vidal V, Vital V, Tsaligopoulos M, Darrouzet V. Corticosteroids in the treatment of vestibular neuritis: a systematic review and meta-analysis. Otol Neurotol 2010;31(2):183–189

[29] Jeong SH, Kim HJ, Kim JS. Vestibular neuritis. Semin Neurol 2013;33(3):185–194

[30] Baloh RW. Clinical practice. Vestibular neuritis. N Engl J Med 2003;348(11):1027–1032

[31] Hamid M. Medical management of common peripheral vestibular diseases. Curr Opin Otolaryngol Head Neck Surg 2010;18(5):407–412

[32] Ward BK, Carey JP, Minor LB. Superior canal dehiscence syndrome: lessons from the first 20 years. Front Neurol 2017;8:177

[33] Williamson RA, Vrabec JT, Coker NJ, Sandlin M. Coronal computed tomography prevalence of superior semicircular canal dehiscence. Otolaryngol Head Neck Surg 2003;129(5):481–489

[34] Carey JP, Minor LB, Nager GT. Dehiscence or thinning of bone overlying the superior semicircular canal in a temporal bone survey. Arch Otolaryngol Head Neck Surg 2000;126(2):137–147

[35] Remenschneider AK, Owoc M, Kozin ED, McKenna MJ, Lee DJ, Jung DH. Health utility improves after surgery for superior canal dehiscence syndrome. Otol Neurotol 2015;36(10):1695–1701

[36] Ziylan F, Kinaci A, Beynon AJ, Kunst HPM. A comparison of surgical treatments for superior semicircular canal dehiscence: a systematic review. Otol Neurotol 2017;38(1):1–10

[37] Jayarajan V, Rajenderkumar D. A survey of dizziness management in General Practice. J Laryngol Otol 2003;117(8):599–604

[38] Yardley L, Donovan-Hall M, Smith HE, Walsh BM, Mullee M, Bronstein AM. Effectiveness of primary care-based vestibular rehabilitation for chronic dizziness. Ann Intern Med 2004;141(8):598–605

[39] Yardley L, Barker F, Muller I, et al. Clinical and cost effectiveness of booklet based vestibular rehabilitation for chronic dizziness in primary care: single blind, parallel group, pragmatic, randomised controlled trial. BMJ 2012;344:e2237

[40] Essery R, Kirby S, Geraghty AWA, Yardley L. Older adults' experiences of internet-based vestibular rehabilitation for dizziness: a longitudinal study. Psychol Health 2017;32(11):1327–1347

[41] Geraghty AWA, Essery R, Kirby S, et al. Internet-based vestibular rehabilitation for older adults with chronic dizziness: a randomized controlled trial in primary care. Ann Fam Med 2017;15(3):209–216

[42] van Vugt VA, van der Wouden JC, Bosmans JE, et al. Guided and unguided internet-based vestibular rehabilitation versus usual care for dizzy adults of 50 years and older: a protocol for a three-armed randomised trial. BMJ Open 2017;7(1):e015479

[43] Fife TD. Dizziness in the outpatient care setting. Continuum (Minneap Minn) 2017;23(2, Selected Topics in Outpatient Neurology):359–395

[44] Edlow JA, Newman-Toker D. Using the physical examination to diagnose patients with acute dizziness and vertigo. J Emerg Med 2016;50(4):617–628

# 9 Cranial Nerves IX, X, XII: Dysphagia

*Erica E. Jackson and Anna M. Pou*

**Abstract**

Intact motor and sensory function of cranial nerves IX (glosso-pharyngeal), X (vagus), and XII (hypoglossal) are paramount to a normal voice and swallow. Paralysis of one or all of these cranial nerves can lead to hoarseness, taste and sensory disturbances, and dysphagia/aspiration, affecting all phases of swallowing to varying degrees. Pain in the head, neck, face, and oral cavity can be another symptom. Multiple cranial neuropathies such as these can be life-threatening and difficult to treat. History and physical examination typically confirm the diagnosis of paraly-sis of these nerves with the etiology typically due to pathology in the lower brainstem, skull base, or extracranial course of the nerves. Workup includes imaging of the brain, brainstem, skull base, and neck in addition to swallowing studies. Treatment is based on etiology and severity of symptoms. Regardless of treatment, all of these patients will require speech and swal-lowing therapy and some will possibly require a percutaneous gastrostomy and/or tracheostomy.

*Keywords:* dysphagia, aspiration, high vagal lesion, vocal cord medialization, cricopharyngeal dysfunction, laryngeal closure

## 9.1 Normal Swallowing Mechanism

The act of swallowing is a complex coordination of events that relies on intact sensory and motor input and intact structures. Cranial nerves V, VII, IX, X, and XII are involved in a normal swallow. There are four phases of swallowing: oral preparatory, oral, pharyngeal, and esophageal. The oral preparatory and oral phases are voluntary and the pharyngeal and esophageal phases are involuntary. In the oral preparatory phase of swallowing, the food is mixed with saliva and chewed, using the lips, cheeks, muscles of mastication, and tongue. The bolus is prepared and voluntarily moved by the tongue posteriorly to the pharynx. The pharyngeal phase is initiated when the bolus reaches the faucial arches and is triggered by the superior laryngeal nerve. The following occurs during the pharyngeal phase: respiration stops, the soft palate elevates to contact the posterior pha-ryngeal wall preventing material from entering the nasal cav-ity, the larynx elevates and glottic closure occurs at all three sphincters (epiglottis/aryepiglottic folds, false vocal cords, and true vocal cords), contraction of the constrictor muscles occur moving the bolus forward, and relaxation of the cricopharyn-geus muscle allowing the bolus to enter into the esophagus and finally the stomach.

## 9.2 Initial Workup

Most patients with swallowing disorders typically pres-ent to their primary care physician complaining of choking with foods. The first test for suspected dysphagia should be a modified barium swallow ($220). If aspiration is suspected with signs of fever and cough, a posteroanterior (PA) and lateral chest X-ray may also be obtained ($30) prior to the swallow study to evaluate for aspiration pneumonia or pneumonitis. Following the initial evaluation, the patient should be referred to an oto-laryngologist. If a devastating neurologic disorder or neoplasm is suspected, referral should be made immediately.

### 9.2.1 Symptoms

Patients presenting with paralysis of cranial nerves IX, X, and XII typically report change in taste, severe dysphagia to both solids and liquids including difficulty forming and moving the food bolus toward the pharynx, aspiration with liquids with possible history of pneumonia, and nasal regurgitation. Changes in ver-bal speech include breathy dysphonia (change in voice quality) and dysarthria (speech not well articulated). These symptoms are due to lack of both motor and sensory inputs with decrease sensation palate, pharynx, larynx, and esophagus. Dyspnea on exertion and weakened cough due to loss of positive end expi-ratory pressure (CN X palsy) can contribute to the poor overall status of these patients, including weight loss.[1]

### 9.2.2 History

Evaluation of every patient should begin with a thorough his-tory. The physician needs to ascertain the following: the dura-tion and progression of symptoms; any precipitating event; recent history of head and neck trauma or surgery; personal or family history of genetic, neuromuscular, or connective tissue disorders; history of muscle weakness; history of head and neck cancer, and history of tobacco and alcohol use. The most com-mon causes of multiple lower cranial nerve palsies are trauma to the skull base, tumors of the skull base, and neuromuscular disorders.[1] While interviewing the patient, attention is paid to the quality of his or her voice and speech. The voice may be breathy, particularly with a high vagal lesion, and difficult to project. It may sound "wet" due to pooling of secretions in the larynx and hypopharynx (▶ Fig. 9.1). Dysarthria, including slurred speech, may also be present due to hypoglossal nerve palsy unless the patient has compensated for it already.

### 9.2.3 Examination

A complete head and neck examination is performed on every patient. Special attention should be given to any mass or lesion found that is suspicious for a neoplasm.

A complete cranial nerve examination is to be done with special attention paid to cranial nerves IX, X, and XII. The glossopharyngeal nerve plays an important role in the phar-yngeal phase of swallowing. Glossopharyngeal nerve palsy is best demonstrated with asking the patient to say "ahh" and observing for palate rise. Also, the gag reflex can be tested by

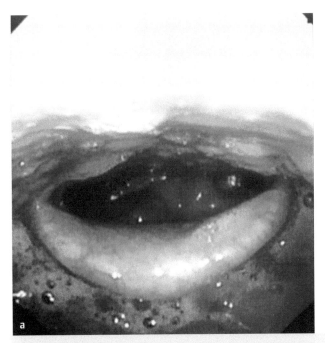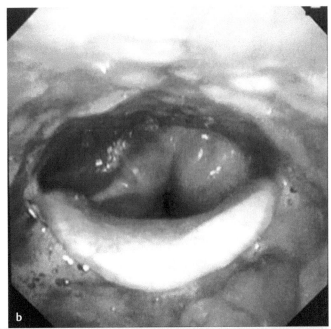

**Fig. 9.1** Bilateral vocal cord paralysis. **(a)** Pooling of secretions in the vallecula. **(b)** Fixed cords in the paramedian position.

touching the palate with a tongue blade. The patient with CN IX palsy will display a decrease gag reflex due to decreased palatal sensation and decreased palatal elevation. Decreased contact of the palate to posterior pharyngeal wall can lead to an incomplete velopharyngeal seal, which leads to nasal regurgitation of foods. The patient can also present with poor pharyngeal constrictor muscle contraction. This can be assessed on flexible fiberoptic laryngoscopy (FFL) in which a small flexible endoscope is passed through the nose and used to view the throat from above. The patient is instructed to carry out a forceful "eee" while watching the pharyngeal walls for contraction (pharyngeal squeeze). This can be graded as normal or abnormal, and when poorly functioning, it can indicate an aspiration risk.

The hypoglossal nerve innervates the tongue muscles and therefore plays a vital role in the oral preparatory and oral phases of swallowing where it facilitates formation of and movement of the bolus. The hypoglossal nerve is examined by asking the patient to protrude his or her tongue and move it side to side. Patients with CN XII palsy will have deviation of the tongue to the weak side as well as muscle wasting and fasciculations. One can also ask the patient to push their tongue against their cheek to check strength.

The vagus nerve plays an important role in the pharyngeal phase of swallowing, of which glottic closure is the hallmark. Vagal lesions above the nodose ganglion result in deficits of both the recurrent and superior laryngeal nerves, which leads to unilateral vocal fold paralysis and decreased sensation to the supraglottic larynx, respectively. This may lead to "silent" aspiration in which aspiration occurs asymptomatically due to loss of cough reflex. Loss of the vagal contribution to the pharyngeal plexus may also cause incoordination of the pharyngeal constrictors and incomplete relaxation of the cricopharyngeus

muscle during swallowing. Similar to CN IX injury with subsequent pharyngeal plexus injury, patients with CN X injury will show decreased gag reflex and the uvula may be deviated to the side of the lesion. The voice is assessed for breathiness, pitch, and projection.

The larynx is best evaluated using FFL ($115), which can be performed in the office or at the bedside. It should be part of every dysphagia and dysphonia workup done by an otolaryngologist. When testing laryngeal movement and sensation, an anesthetizing agent should not be sprayed through the nostril as this could show a false-positive loss of sensation; the agent should be placed on a pledget and placed in the nasal cavity only in order to prevent anesthetizing the pharynx and larynx.

Injury to the recurrent laryngeal nerve typically presents with voice complaints and a paralyzed vocal cord being visualized in the paramedian position leading to an incomplete glottic closure. Over time, this can lead to atrophy, which will cause bowing and flaccidity of the vocal fold. The fold will typically be shortened with anterior displacement of the arytenoid. Many can accommodate to this deficit, but when there is also a loss of sensation as in a high vagal injury mentioned earlier, this often leads to significant aspiration.

The tip of the scope should be used to test laryngeal sensation. If the patient is insensate when touching the pharyngeal wall and supraglottis, it suggests superior laryngeal nerve involvement. Pooling of secretions in the ipsilateral pyriform sinus and post cricoid areas can be seen, indicating pharyngeal weakness. If severe, this can result in a suboptimal laryngeal examination. Frank "silent" aspiration of saliva can also be detected when it is freely aspirated into the tracheobronchial tree. Again, pharyngeal squeeze is useful in assessing pharyngeal muscular contraction and when absent signifies a higher risk of aspiration.

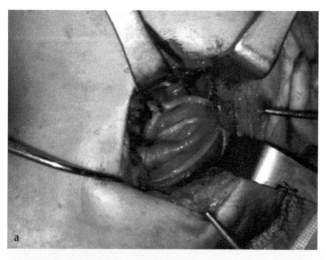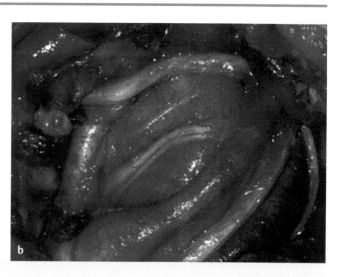

**Fig. 9.2** (a, b) Neck lipoma stretching cranial nerves X, XI, and XII.

## 9.3 Differential Diagnosis

Lesions/palsies of lower cranial nerves have many causes: genetic, vascular, traumatic, iatrogenic, infectious, immunologic, metabolic, nutritional, degenerative, or neoplastic. Some of the causes include motor neuron disorders, amyotrophic lateral sclerosis (ALS), ischemic stroke, aneurysm, vasculitis, skull base fracture, carotid surgery and neck dissection, varicella zoster, Guillain–Barré syndrome, multiple sclerosis (MS), diabetes, vitamin B deficiency, and skull base neoplasms such as paraganglioma tumors (▶ Fig. 9.2). The work up described in the following section will be helpful in determining the exact cause and subsequent treatment.

## 9.4 Workup

### 9.4.1 Imaging

Imaging is essential in the evaluation of dysphagia. The first test is a modified barium swallow study (MBSS), which is a "live" fluoroscopic view of bolus passing through the throat (see the following text) to determine the degree of dysphagia/aspiration and where the abnormality lies. Both CT and MR imaging of the skull base and neck may be used to assess for intracranial, skull base, or neck pathology.

### 9.4.2 Modified Barium Swallow Study

If an MBSS has not been previously done by the referring physician, one must be ordered as the initial test. MBSS is the gold standard for diagnosing and treating dysphagia (▶ Fig. 9.3). A speech pathologist and a radiologist perform this test jointly in the radiology suite. This is a dynamic study that tests three consistencies of food: thin (liquid), thick (puree), and solid foods. All phases of swallowing are evaluated. Each phase of swallowing is closely analyzed and therapeutic maneuvers are taught to the patient during the test and their effectiveness is

determined. A diet is then recommended to the patient and dysphagia exercises are taught. If the patient aspirates all consistencies, particularly if silent aspiration is present, a percutaneous gastrostomy or jejunostomy tube is recommended for nutrition while the patient is undergoing rehabilitation or surgical treatment for dysphagia. The disadvantages of the MBSS include the need to travel to the radiology suite, the need for specialized personnel, and its inability to always provide information about the subtle abnormalities of the palate, vocal folds, pharyngeal musculature, and sensation.

### 9.4.3 Fiberoptic Endoscopic Evaluation of Swallowing

Fiberoptic endoscopic evaluation of swallowing (FEES) is also used to evaluate dysphagia, but it is limited to the pharyngeal phase of swallowing. It is complimentary to the MBSS. The examination includes a standard FFL examination. The patient ingests dyed foods of varying consistencies. Retention of substances in the valleculae and hypopharynx is noted as well as aspiration of dyed foods. Sensory testing can be added by producing pulsed air stimuli via the fiberoptic scope, referred to as fiberoptic endoscopic evaluation of swallowing and sensory testing (FEESST). This test is sensitive in providing information about structural abnormalities of the palate, pharyngeal wall, and vocal folds. It can also be performed in the office or at the bedside when patients are unable to travel to the radiology suite or when other resources are not available. It is also useful in following effectiveness of treatment.

### 9.4.4 Imaging of Brain

MRI of the brain with and without gadolinium ($235) may be used to evaluate for central nervous system pathology such as demyelinating diseases and tumors.

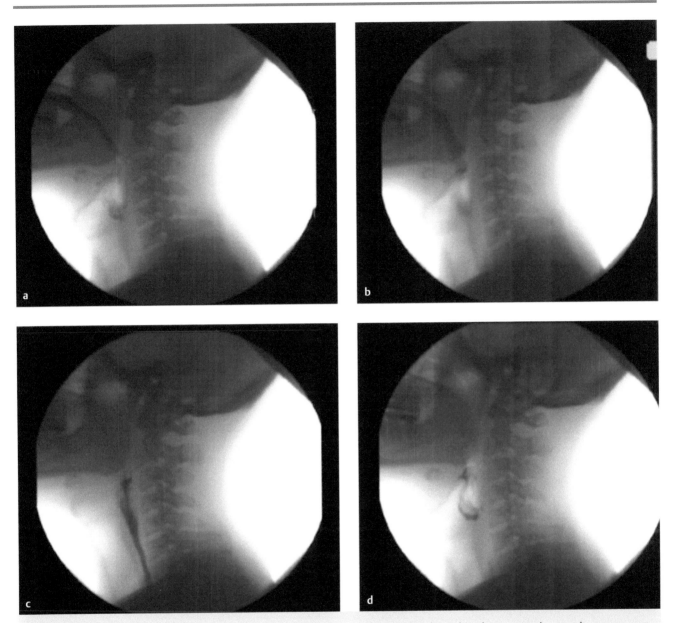

**Fig. 9.3** (a–d) Modified barium swallow study of a 50-year-old patient with cranial nerve X and XII palsies due to a parapharyngeal space sarcoma.

### 9.4.5 Imaging Skull Base

In order to determine the etiology of lower cranial nerve palsies, imaging of the brainstem, skull base, and neck may be necessary. Imaging should be multiplanar, using thin sections (0.5–0.6 mm). If the etiology is suspected to come from a skull base lesion, both CT ($205) and MRI ($325) should be obtained as these images are complimentary.[2] A noncontrast CT of the mastoids, temporal bone, and entire skull base is recommended (▶ Fig. 9.4). MRI with and without gadolinium will provide soft-tissue detail. If there is a contradiction to MRI, then the imaging required is a CT scan with contrast. In this case, a noncontrast CT is not necessary.[2]

High-resolution CT is the modality of choice in defining bony anatomy of the skull base and is the gold standard for evaluation of skull base fractures. MRI should include axial and coronal images using fast-spin echo T1- and T2-weighted images with fat suppression, postcontrast images with a slice thickness of 3 mm or less. In addition, short tau inversion recovery (STIR) images should be obtained as they have better fat suppression. MRI is better for diagnosing inflammatory lesions because they have higher water content and higher T2-weighted intensity signal.[3]

### 9.4.6 Imaging of Neck

CT scan with contrast of the neck ($205) is first done, followed by an MRI with and without gadolinium if needed. Close attention is paid to the oral cavity, pharynx, larynx, and trachea

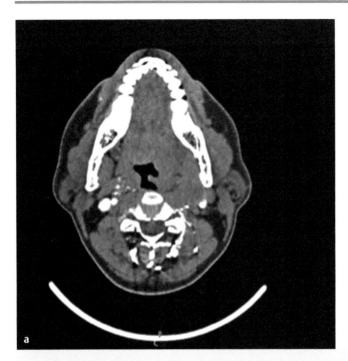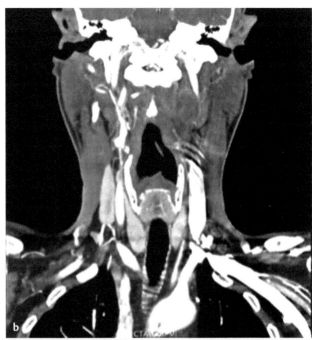

**Fig. 9.4** (a, b) CT scan depicting a 55-year-old patient with parapharyngeal space mass causing cranial nerve X and XII palsies.

passages as well as the cartilaginous framework of the larynx. Any mass lesions that could cause mass effect or dysfunction of any nerves or muscles of swallowing should be excluded.

## 9.5 Nonsurgical Treatment

### 9.5.1 Dysphagia and Voice Therapy

Following assessment by MBSS and speech therapy, a program can be individualized based on each patient's swallowing deficits. The goal of therapy is to prevent aspiration and create a safe and effective mechanism to swallow by overcoming the effects of each cranial neuropathy. Therapists use a variety of techniques including changes in diet consistency, postures when swallowing, and different maneuvers elicited during each swallow.

In patients with hypoglossal nerve paralysis and dysfunction of the oral phase of swallowing, a "head back posture" can be employed. This posture uses gravity to push the bolus into the pharyngeal phase.[4] Others with poor pharyngeal phase can benefit from smaller volume feeds at a slower pace with multiple dry swallows after each bite, thus preventing aspiration.[5] Oftentimes, patients with CN X deficits will lack laryngeal sensation affecting the patient's ability to sense the bolus and activate the swallow. Techniques to enhance sensation have been employed such as the downward pressure on the tongue with a spoon or the use of carbonated boluses.[6] Overall there are numerous techniques utilized by speech therapists to maximize a patient's ability to safely swallow. Success requires patient participation in therapy and dedication to home exercises.

## 9.6 Surgical Management

### 9.6.1 Tracheostomy

The surgical management of aspiration should be as simple as possible because many patients are in poor medical condition. One should also remember that no single procedure is absolutely indicated in all patients. Although tracheostomy does not prevent aspiration (and in some patients may actually produce aspiration), it does facilitate pulmonary toilet for those who are actively aspirating. Initially, the patient may require a cuffed tracheostomy tube for mechanical ventilation and frequent suctioning, but upon recovery, the patient should be decannulated if possible to reduce aspiration risk. In patients who are neurologically devastated, a gastrostomy or jejunostomy tube should be established for feeding.[7]

### 9.6.2 Passy–Muir Valve

In patients who cannot be decannulated, a Passy–Muir valve (PMV) is a speaking valve that can be used to assist with voice and swallowing by increasing subglottic pressure. Studies have shown that aspiration during swallow of liquids was significantly less in adults with the PMV in place than in those without the PMV. The benefit of the PMV should be evaluated in selected patients who aspirate. A modified barium swallow can be done with and without the use of a PMV in order to determine if its use decreases aspiration. If so, it can be placed during meals.[8,9,10]

## 9.6.3 Treatment of the Cricopharyngeus Muscle

Aspiration can be worsened when there is failure of the cricopharyngeus muscle (CPM) to relax during the pharyngeal phase of swallowing as seen in high vagal lesions. A cricopharyngeal myotomy may be performed as a primary procedure or in conjunction with other procedures such as vocal cord medialization. A database search reviewing 567 articles from 1990 to 2013 compared outcomes of cricopharyngeal dilation, botulinum toxin injections (Botox), and myotomy in treating cricopharyngeal dysfunction.[11] Logistic regression analysis of patient outcomes showed that there was a significantly higher success rate with myotomy than Botox injections and that dilatation had an intermediate success rate not statistically different from either myotomy or Botox injections. In addition, endoscopic myotomy had a higher success rate compared to open ($p$ = 0.0025).

The patient's overall condition must be taken into consideration when deciding the method in which the CPM will be addressed as Botox injections can be done in the office by an experienced clinician. A retrospective study of 36 patients was conducted to assess the effectiveness and safety of office-based injections of Botox in the CPM under electromyography guidance in patients with CPM dysfunction despite maximal swallowing therapy.[12] MBSS, FEES, Disability Rating Scale, penetration–aspiration score, and National Institutes of Health Swallowing Safety Scale were used in the evaluation of dysphagia. The total success rate was 63.9%, which was defined as patients no longer requiring gastrostomy tube feeds and those who demonstrated improvement in disability rating. Botox injections were more successful in patients with CN IX and X palsies ($p$ = 0.006). The complication rate was very low, with only one patient showing temporary unilateral vocal fold paralysis.

## 9.6.4 Vocal Cord Medialization and Arytenoid Adduction

See Chapter 10, Cranial Nerve X: Dysphonia.

## 9.7 Treatment of Velopharyngeal Insufficiency

The velopharyngeal sphincter is formed from the muscles of the soft palate and lateral and posterior pharyngeal walls. Its function separates the nasal and oral cavities during speech and swallowing. Incomplete closure can result in hypernasal speech and or nasal regurgitation of foods. Nonsurgical treatment includes speech therapy and a palatal lift obturator, but this more often requires surgical treatment. Procedures such as posterior pharyngeal flap and sphincter pharyngoplasty have been traditionally used successfully, but they carry significant perioperative morbidity. More recently, this has been treated with the injection of fat and biomaterials such as hyaluronic acid (HA) and calcium hydroxyapatite into posterior velopharynx to add bulk and decrease the velopharyngeal gap.[13,14] A study in 2017 evaluated 25 consecutive patients who were injected with HA and dextranomer copolymer from 1 January, 2011 to December, 2014. The amount injected ranged from 2.5 to 4.1 mL for larger gaps. The procedures were performed in clinic using local anesthesia, monitored anesthesia care, and general anesthesia. Overall, 19/25 patients had improvement in their perceptual nasal resonance after their first injection. There was improvement in 6 of 12 patients complaining of nasal regurgitation, 2 did not improve, and there were no data on the remaining 4. Nineteen of 25 needed only one injection to reach the final result. Those with benign causes and good lateral wall motion had better outcomes than those whose velopharyngeal insufficiency was due to malignancy. Complication rate was minimal and consisted of postoperative neck pain, odynophagia, and retropharyngeal fluid collection in two patients requiring drainage. Histologic studies have demonstrated that HA acts as a transport medium and dissipates from the site of injection within several weeks and the tissue bulking effect is primarily driven by an immunologic response to the dextranomer microsphere, which stimulates collagen and synthesis and influx of fibroblasts and myofibroblasts to create a consolidate bulking of tissue.[15]

## 9.8 Definitive Surgical Treatment

The patient who has intractable, life-threatening aspiration that does not respond to conservative treatment may be a candidate for one of several procedures designed to completely prevent soilage of the tracheobronchial tree. This often occurs in neurologically devastated patients resulting from cerebrovascular accidents, brainstem infarction, ALS, and MS or patients following extensive head and neck or skull base surgery.

### 9.8.1 Laryngeal Closure Procedures

Laryngeal closure procedures may be divided into glottic, supraglottic, and subglottic. All require a permanent tracheostomy and have the potential for recurrence of aspiration. In the glottic closure, mucosa of the free edge of the true and false vocal cords is stripped and they are sutured to one another. Normal speech is sacrificed with glottic closure. The closure is potentially reversible. Closure at the glottic level has been unreliable in patients with mobile true vocal cords, likely due to persistent laryngopharyngeal movement placing excessive tension on the closure.

Closure of the supraglottis is performed by stripping the mucosal edges of the epiglottis, arytenoids, and aryepiglottic folds and then suturing them together through an infrahyoid pharyngotomy. It should be noted that glottic and supraglottic closures have a relatively high failure rate and recurrence of aspiration is not uncommon.

### 9.8.2 Partial Resection of the Cricoid Cartilage

Krespi et al described a technique of partial resection of the cricoid to reduce aspiration in patients undergoing extensive resections of the tongue base and pharynx many years ago. A permanent tracheostomy is required for airway. The technique consists of a submucosal dissection of and removal of the posterior lamina of the cricoid cartilage. The cricoarytenoid joints and posterior cricoarytenoid muscle and its innervation are preserved. It is performed with a CPM. The result is a decreased anteroposterior laryngeal dimension and enlarged hypopharyngeal inlet. Phonation is preserved.[16] Over time, additional methods of closing the larynx have been developed but are based on the above principles. In a recent study by Kimura et al, it was found that the quality of life of patients with severe dysphagia and vocal dysfunction was significantly improved following the Kano procedure ($p < 0.05$). The quality of life of family caregivers was also significantly improved ($p < 0.05$). Nine patients who underwent the Konno method were evaluated for oral intake and activities of daily living using the functional oral intake scale and the Barthel Index, respectively, as indices of quality of life. Other factors such as inflammation were also analyzed. Seven family caregivers were also queried regarding frequency of sputum suction, mood of family caregivers, and postoperative satisfaction. Postoperative satisfaction was very high.[17]

### 9.8.3 Laryngotracheal Separation

Laryngotracheal separation involves the division of the trachea just below the larynx with either closure of the proximal stump or diversion to the skin or esophagus. The classic Lindeman procedure, named for the author of its initial description, divides the trachea in its upper rings with the proximal stump diverted to the anterior esophagus.[18]

This procedure has largely been abandoned as the anastomosis to the anterior esophagus is technically challenging, which leads to a high leakage rate. Tucker later described the "double-barrel" tracheostomy technique in which the proximal trachea is sutured to the skin of the neck as a controlled fistula.[19]

A variation of the Lindeman procedure that is widely used today is the laryngotracheal separation (LTS). The proximal tracheal stump is closed on itself and may be reinforced with flaps created from the strap muscles. Secretions pool in the blind pouch and empty when the patient assumes a supine position. The closure prevents a high-tension anastomosis to the esophagus that may result if the patient has had a previous high tracheostomy with a resulting short tracheal stump. The fistula rate for LTS is reported as greater than 33% and is even higher in patients with prior tracheostomy. The prevention of aspiration is near 100% with any of the procedures, and successful reversals have been reported for each of the techniques.[20,21,22]

### 9.8.4 Total Laryngectomy

Total laryngectomy (TL) clearly separates the respiratory and digestive tracts, and has for many years been regarded as the procedure of choice for the definitive treatment of the patient with life-threatening aspiration.[23] Some authors feel that it remains the procedure of choice in patients with extremely poor prognoses, other associated medical conditions, or evidence of poor wound healing, as less radical procedures have more frequent complications. A narrow-field laryngectomy may be performed in which the larynx from the hyoid to the lower border of the cricoid is resected, and this spares the hyoid bone, mucosa of the arytenoids and postcricoid region, and strap muscles. The mucosal closure is reinforced using the strap muscles. While TL remains the most reliable and definitive way to achieve complete

cessation of aspiration, it has no potential for reversal and has significant negative stigmata for the patient and family.

Some patients with severe complications of aspiration and poor neurologic function and prognosis may never regain the ability for oral intake. In such patients, a permanent feeding tube should be established with a gastrostomy or jejunostomy tube. The ligation of the parotid and submandibular ducts can effectively reduce salivary flow and decrease the aspiration of oral secretions in the vegetative patient.[24]

### 9.8.5 Laryngeal Stents

Laryngeal stents are completely reversible and their insertion and removal is relatively simple. Multiple sizes are available. Perhaps the most widely used stent is that designed by Eliachar. It is a silicone tube designed to adhere to the configuration of the larynx and upper trachea. Multiple sizes are available. A domelike projection from the superior portion of the tube can be incised to form a one-way valve, allowing air to escape from the airway while still preventing aspiration. Airflow through the valve allows for some functional phonation in alert patients. Leakage around the stent can occur, but it may be rectified with the placement of a larger size. The stent may remain in place for as long as 9 to 12 months. Stent placement is a reasonable first choice to halt aspiration in a seriously ill patient, especially if their condition is potentially reversible.

## 9.9 Conclusion

Chronic aspiration can occur in patients with a wide variety of pathologic processes. The determination of etiology is paramount, as it will guide treatment and determines overall prognosis. Early diagnostic steps should include an MBSS and in-office fiberoptic laryngology by an otolaryngologist. Imaging is indicated for suspected malignancy or nerve palsy. For patients with confirmed dysphagia, options for intervention range from conservative measurements such as speech and swallowing therapy to increasingly aggressive surgical procedures such as vocal cord injection, tracheostomy with/without the use of a Passy–Muir valve, minimally invasive techniques, and definitive complete separation of the respiratory and digestive tracts (laryngeal closure procedures, laryngectomy). The otolaryngologist is often called upon to evaluate these patients and should be thoroughly aware of methods of evaluation and treatment.

Maintaining an airway is essential for life, and some forms of dysphagia with aspiration can be life-threatening if untreated. While there are many diagnostic and treatment options for which a cost analysis could be performed, the paramount importance of the airway equates to fewer decisions about cost-effectiveness and more decisions about preservation of life.

Early intervention and treatment may prevent life-threatening complications and speed up recovery from the primary disease process. In the senior author's experience, these early interventions should include speech and swallowing therapy, vocal cord medialization by injection of a biomaterial, followed with Botox to the CPM, all of which can be done in the outpatient setting, which is coincidentally cost-effective compared to more aggressive procedures.

# References

[1] Finsterer J, Grisold W. Disorders of the lower cranial nerves. J Neurosci Rural Pract 2015;6(3):377–391

[2] Hudgins PA, Baugnon KL. Head and neck: skull base imaging. Neurosurgery 2018;82(3):255–267

[3] Raut AA, Naphade PS, Chawla A. Imaging of skull base: pictorial essay. Indian J Radiol Imaging 2012;22(4):305–316

[4] Calvo I, Sunday KL, Macrae P, Humbert IA. Effects of chin-up posture on the sequence of swallowing events. Head Neck 2017;39(5):947–959

[5] Nascimento WV, Cassiani RA, Santos CM, Dantas RO. Effect of bolus volume and consistency on swallowing events duration in healthy subjects. J Neurogastroenterol Motil 2015;21(1):78–82

[6] Turkington LG, Ward EC, Farrell AM. Carbonation as a sensory enhancement strategy: a narrative synthesis of existing evidence. Disabil Rehabil 2017;39(19):1958–1967

[7] George BP, Kelly AG, Schneider EB, Holloway RG. Current practices in feeding tube placement for US acute ischemic stroke inpatients. Neurology 2014;83(10):874–882

[8] Dettelbach MA, Gross RD, Mahlmann J, Eibling DE. Effect of the Passy-Muir valve on aspiration in patients with tracheostomy. Head Neck 1995;17(4):297–302

[9] Elpern EH, Borkgren Okonek M, Bacon M, Gerstung C, Skrzynski M. Effect of the Passy-Muir tracheostomy speaking valve on pulmonary aspiration in adults. Heart Lung 2000;29(4):287–293

[10] Stachler RJ, Hamlet SL, Choi J, Fleming S. Scintigraphic quantification of aspiration reduction with the Passy-Muir valve. Laryngoscope 1996;106(2, Pt 1):231–234

[11] Kocdor P, Siegel ER, Tulunay-Ugur OE. Cricopharyngeal dysfunction: a systematic review comparing outcomes of dilatation, botulinum toxin injection, and myotomy. Laryngoscope 2016;126(1):135–141

[12] Kim MS, Kim GW, Rho YS, Kwon KH, Chung EJ. Office-based electromyography-guided botulinum toxin injection to the cricopharyngeus muscle: optimal patient selection and technique. Ann Otol Rhinol Laryngol 2017;126(5):349–356

[13] Brigger MT, Ashland JE, Hartnick CJ. Injection pharyngoplasty with calcium hydroxylapatite for velopharyngeal insufficiency: patient selection and technique. Arch Otolaryngol Head Neck Surg 2010;136(7):666–670

[14] Cantarella G, Mazzola RF, Mantovani M, Baracca G, Pignataro L. Treatment of velopharyngeal insufficiency by pharyngeal and velar fat injections. Otolaryngol Head Neck Surg 2011;145(3):401–403

[15] Peck BW, Baas BS, Cofer SA. Injection pharyngoplasty with a hyaluronic acid and dextranomer copolymer to treat velopharyngeal insufficiency in adults. Mayo Clin Proc Innov Qual Outcomes 2017;1(2):176–184

[16] Krespi YP, Pelzer HJ, Sisson GA. Management of chronic aspiration by subtotal and submucosal cricoid resection. Ann Otol Rhinol Laryngol 1985;94(6, Pt 1):580–583

[17] Kimura Y, Kishimoto S, Sumi T. Improving the quality of life of patients with severe dysphagia by surgically closing the larynx. Ann Otol Rhinol Laryngol 2019; 128(2):96–103

[18] Eisele DW, Yarington CT Jr, Lindeman RC, Eisele DW, Yarington CT. Indications for the tracheoesophageal diversion procedure and the laryngotracheal separation procedure. Ann Otol Rhinol Laryngol 1988;97(5, Pt 1):471–475

[19] Tucker HM. Double-barreled (diversionary) tracheostomy: long-term results and reversibility. Laryngoscope 1993;103(2):212–215

[20] Eibling DE, Snyderman CH, Eibling C. Laryngotracheal separation for intractable aspiration: a retrospective review of 34 patients. Laryngoscope 1995;105(1):83–85

[21] Francis DO, Blumin J, Merati A. Reducing fistula rates following laryngotracheal separation. Ann Otol Rhinol Laryngol 2012;121(3):151–155

[22] Zocratto OB, Savassi-Rocha PR, Paixão RM, Salles JM. Laryngotracheal separation surgery: outcome in 60 patients. Otolaryngol Head Neck Surg 2006;135(4):571–575

[23] Topf MC, Magaña LC, Salmon K, et al. Safety and efficacy of functional laryngectomy for end-stage dysphagia. Laryngoscope 2018;128(3):597–602

[24] Klem C, Mair EA. Four-duct ligation: a simple and effective treatment for chronic aspiration from sialorrhea. Arch Otolaryngol Head Neck Surg 1999;125(7):796–800

# 10 Cranial Nerve X: Dysphonia

*Lacey Adkins, Melda Kunduk, and Andrew J. McWhorter*

**Abstract**

The recurrent laryngeal nerve is a branch of the vagus nerve whose paralysis frequently causes a breathy dysphonia and potentially dysphagia. Flexible laryngoscopy is used to make the initial diagnosis, while stroboscopy can provide better evaluation of mucosal wave and glottic closure. Laryngeal electromyography can be used to help confirm the diagnosis. Workup includes imaging along the course of the recurrent laryngeal nerve with serology reserved for select cases. Treatment options include observation while awaiting reinnervation or voice therapy. Injection augmentation can help medialize the vocal fold to provide better closure. Laryngeal framework surgery may also be used if the paralysis fails to resolve. In addition to medialization thyroplasty, further improvement may be gained with arytenoid adduction, adduction arytenopexy, and/or cricothyroid subluxation. Laryngeal reinnervation is another treatment option, helping the vocal fold to regain bulk and tone.

*Keywords:* vocal fold paralysis, laryngeal electromyography, medialization thyroplasty, laryngeal reinnervation

## 10.1 Initial Presentation

Laryngeal innervation ultimately arises from the vagus nerve. The recurrent laryngeal nerve (RLN) and the superior laryngeal nerve (SLN) are the branches of the vagus nerve that provide the motor and sensory innervation. When the mobility is compromised, this commonly results in dysphonia. A patient presenting with dysphonia needs a thorough evaluation. Usually, the patient will initially present to their primary care physician, where the national Medicare nonfacility price is roughly $75.[1] Current American Academy of Otolaryngology guidelines suggest that if dysphonia exists for greater than 4 weeks, they should be referred to an otolaryngologist ($170) for a laryngeal examination.[1,2] The referral should take place even sooner should suspicion for a serious underlying cause exist, such as recent neck or chest surgery, recent intubation, neck mass, or history of tobacco use.[2]

### 10.1.1 Symptoms

When patients have a paralysis or paresis of the vagus nerve or its branches, the resulting dysphonia typically results in a breathy voice. Patients frequently complain of having difficulty with projection or trouble talking over ambient noise. Phonatory dyspnea, vocal fatigue, and a higher pitched voice or paralytic falsetto are also common. They may note a weakened cough or even dyspnea on exertion due to the loss of autopositive end-expiratory pressure. They frequently will have coinciding dysphagia complaints as well, ranging from aspiration with liquids to dysphagia with all consistencies to nasal regurgitation.[3,4]

### 10.1.2 History

The initial otolaryngology assessment should start with a thorough history. Was the dysphonia sudden or gradual? Did it start after a recent surgery? The most common etiology for vocal fold paralysis is iatrogenic, followed by malignancy and idiopathic.[5,6,7] A history of any other neurologic symptoms should also be elucidated. Any associated symptoms such as those previously discussed should also be reviewed.

### 10.1.3 Examination

Next, examine the voice. The clinician should closely listen to the quality of the patient's voice. It should be assessed for any breathiness or evidence of paralytic falsetto. As the patient slowly ascends in pitch by lengthening the vocal folds and reducing their flaccidity, they will demonstrate less breathiness, which is why some patients adopt the paralytic falsetto. When asked to project, patients with paralysis will frequently demonstrate a diplophonic voice (more than one tone is produced at the same time) that may not be present at quieter conversational volumes. The range is also frequently diminished, most commonly at the upper frequencies. The cough is frequently weak and the maximum phonation time is typically less than 10 seconds.[4] Occasionally, when the SLN is involved, innervation to the cricothyroid muscle is affected and the patient may note a lower pitch or monotone voice.[3]

A complete head and neck examination should also be performed, particularly looking for any neck masses or associated cranial neuropathies. With a high vagal lesion that is more proximal along the course of the vagus before it begins to branch, the palate may be weak with a decreased palatal rise demonstrated on the paralyzed side as the pharyngeal branch of the vagus will be involved. Indirect mirror laryngoscopy can also be used to assess for the general mobility of the vocal folds or evidence of pooling of secretions.

Endoscopy ($115), whether flexible or rigid, can provide further information.[1] In addition to evaluating gross movement, a more thorough evaluation of vertical and horizontal movements as well as evidence of vocal fold bowing or atrophy can be seen. With flexible laryngoscopy, the palatal movement and velopharyngeal seal can also be investigated as well as the lateral pharyngeal wall movement. By having the patient hold a loud and high pitch, normal pharyngeal contracture should be evident along the lateral and posterior wall. However, when one side of the pharynx is paralyzed as you would expect with a higher vagal lesion, the muscular bulging is lacking and the posterior midline raphe will frequently be pulled toward the nonparalyzed side.[4] In addition, secretions pooling within a unilateral pyriform also indicates pharyngeal weakness on that side. ▶ Fig. 10.1 is an example of these findings; in the background, you can see an atrophied right vocal fold with bowing as well as secretions within the pyriform sinus, suggestive

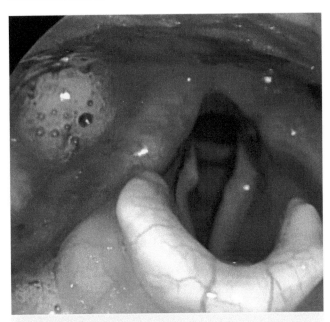

Fig. 10.1 Right unilateral vocal fold paralysis with vocal fold bowing and pooling of secretions within the right pyriform sinus, suggesting a high vagal lesion.

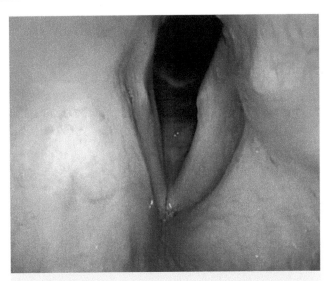

Fig. 10.2 Left vocal fold paralysis with an atrophied vocal fold and ventricle enlargement.

of a high vagal lesion. During the assessment, the tip of the scope can be used to test the laryngeal sensation. If sensation is absent, this points toward SLN involvement, which helps further localize the lesion.

When examining the overall appearance of the vocal folds, note the resting position as well as the contour. Muscle atrophy may cause bowing of the vocal fold, flaccidity, or an enlarged ventricle. ▶ Fig. 10.2 demonstrates this in a patient with a left vocal fold paralysis. The left vocal fold is atrophied and bowed with resulting ventricle enlargement. With the addition of stroboscopy ($180), you can carefully evaluate glottic closure on phonation or mucosal wave asymmetry; however, when the immobile vocal fold is lateralized, it may be difficult to capture a signal.[1] Flaccidity can also be evaluated by having the patient phonate at a low pitch; at a lower pitch, the vocal fold will begin to display lateral buckling and aperiodicity, which will resolve as the patient moves to a higher frequency. It is important to also note any vertical height mismatch that may be present as determined by the paralyzed vocal fold position and arytenoid rotation. While any position is possible, frequently the paralyzed vocal fold is shortened with anterior displacement of the arytenoid.[8]

If a patient has had synkinetic reinnervation or a paresis, the examination findings are more subtle. Symptoms are similar to those found with complete paralysis and rarely associated with swallowing issues. On endoscopy, there typically appears to be hypomobility or bowing of the vocal fold. During the examination, it may be helpful to have the patient perform repeated tasks in hopes of fatiguing the pathologic side and making a vocal fold lag more noticeable.[3] Occasionally, the only examination finding may be asymmetry in vocal fold tension and supraglottic hyperfunction.

The SLN may also be involved, in either its sensory or its motor components. The sensory components are for supraglottic sensation and the motor function provides the innervation for the cricothyroid muscle. When the SLN is involved, the patient will frequently note a lowered pitch and more monotone speech. In addition, it can also cause vocal fatigue and breathiness. Due to the sensory component, patients may also experience choking and throat clearing. On examination, as the patient phonates at higher pitches, the posterior commissure will frequently rotate to the weaker side. With the flaccidity of the paralyzed side, this will cause it to appear shortened with bowing.[3]

## 10.2 Workup

### 10.2.1 Imaging

Once paralysis is identified, an attempt to ascertain the etiology should be made. As malignancy remains one of the most common etiologies, this requires imaging along the course of the paralyzed nerve (from the skull base to the level of the xiphoid process). The etiology will also affect the treatment, as inflammation and compression may cause transient paralysis, while trauma or malignancy may be more permanent. The most commonly used imaging includes chest X-ray (CXR), ultrasound, computed tomography (CT), and magnetic resonance imaging (MRI).

Optimal imaging is debatable and not well supported by evidence. In a survey of members of the American Broncho-Esophagological Association (ABEA), most respondents (70–73%) stated that a CXR or neck/chest CT was always or often needed in paralysis workup. However, the majority also said that MRI was only sometimes required. Ultrasound usage was not surveyed.[9]

One study looked at contrast-enhanced head CT ($165), neck CT ($205), and chest CT ($200), for every patient who had an unknown clinical etiology (or no recent head, neck, or chest surgery that correlated with the onset).[1] They looked at both paralysis and paresis. Routine imaging revealed lesions in 21% of the patients, with thyroid abnormalities being the most common finding. Ultimately, these lesions were thought to have contributed to the immobility in only 6% of the cases.[10] Other studies have shown that CT can identify the cause in 23.5% of patients with an unknown clinical etiology, with lung disease and thyroid disease being the most common causes.[11] Another study showed that a chest CT identified the responsible lesion in 30.9%, the neck CT in 24.5%, and the brain CT in 14.8% of patients.[12] The utility of CT imaging for paresis is much lower, with studies indicating yields ranging from 0 to 2.9%.[13,14]

In comparing CT to CXR ($30), CXR was diagnostic in 59% of the chest lesions and 80% of the cardiovascular lesions. As expected, CXR did not identify mediastinal disease well or lesions involving the skull base or neck. However, all of the chest lesions noted on CXR required contrast-enhanced CT for further evaluation and staging. Since a negative CXR does not exclude a malignancy and positive CXR still requires a CT for workup, it appears to have low utility.[11]

In comparing neck ultrasound ($120) to CT results, ultrasound was able to identify 100% of the cervical lesions and 12% of the chest lesions.[1,11] Another study showed comparable identification rates between a Neck CT and neck ultrasound, 24.5 and 26.2% respectively.[12]

There are few studies regarding MRI. Brain, neck, and chest MRI cost $235, $325, and $465, respectively.[1] In general, they seem to highlight that MRI is best for more "proximal" lesions as they provide better visualization of the skull base.[15] However, they have a high false-positive rate, especially in low-suspicion cases.[16]

## 10.2.2 Serology

Occasionally, serology may be used in the workup. In the survey of ABEA members, most people stated that lab tests could be used; however, 80% stated these should be used occasionally or rarely.[9] The most commonly ordered tests were Lyme titer ($20), rheumatoid factor ($7), erythrocyte sedimentation rate ($5), and antinuclear antibody ($15).[1] Unfortunately, the evidence for these tests is weak, with most of the articles being case reports. The only cross-sectional study that appeared to show any relationship between vocal fold paralysis and a systemic disease found that it was more common in diabetics, 0.44% in nondiabetics and 4 to 5.6% in diabetics.[17] A blood glucose would cost $5 and a hemoglobin A1c costs roughly $10.[1] It is generally felt that given the low likelihood of these serologies being positive and the lack of evidence, they should only be ordered should there be suspicion for a particular disease.

## 10.2.3 Laryngeal Electromyography

Laryngeal electromyography (LEMG) may be performed by the otolaryngologist in conjunction with a neurophysiologist, to confirm vocal fold paralysis, postulate on the site of the lesion, and offer a view on recovery prognosis. According to a recent consensus statement, the optimal time to perform it is between 4 weeks and 6 months after initial insult.[18] Usually, the cricothyroid and thyroarytenoid muscles are tested to help determine SLN and RLN involvement. If both nerves are involved, this suggests a lesion proximal to their branching or a vagal injury.

In LEMG ($150), the change in the negative resting potential of the muscle cells is what produces the electrical activity. The basic component studied is the motor unit action potential (MUAP), which is the electrical summation of all muscle fiber potentials that are innervated by a single motor neuron and initially are bi- or triphasic waves. Immediately after a complete nerve injury, there is electrical silence at rest as well as with attempted movement. However, if the injury is incomplete, some fibers are still intact causing an MUAP with decreased amplitude. As reinnervation occurs, low-amplitude polyphasic MUAPs appear due to disordered reinnervation and muscle fiber atrophy with the amplitude increasing with time.[19] ▶ Fig. 10.3 is an example of LEMG findings for a normally mobile thyroarytenoid (▶ Fig. 10.3a) versus one with paralysis (▶ Fig. 10.3b). Note that normally on contraction, there are multiple motor units firing and that a single MUAP can no longer be distinguished as the baseline is obscured (▶ Fig. 10.3a). This is contrasted to (▶ Fig. 10.3b) where there is a less robust electrical response and a clearly distinguishable baseline.

When the needle is initially inserted, a few fibers will depolarize before quieting down. If this activity is prolonged, this could indicate muscle instability or persistent denervation. At rest, muscle fibers usually have some spontaneous activity and negative deflections that do not propagate but if they are persistently firing and forming spike fibrillations or positive sharp waves, this is suggestive of denervation. Frequently, this can be seen starting 3 weeks after the initial injury, although some studies have indicated that this may happen even sooner.[19]

In LEMG, findings of positive sharp waves, polyphasic MUAPs, or fibrillations are evidence of neurologic impairment. However, when it is paresis as opposed to paralysis, the signal of the remaining muscle activity usually obscures these findings. What may be seen with paresis instead is decreased recruitment, a finding that can also be mimicked by improper needle placement or incomplete muscle contraction.[20] Also, striated muscle will still achieve a maximal interference pattern at only 30% of its maximum contraction because multiple motor units are firing at a high frequency and obscuring the features of a single MUAP, meaning paresis may not be even identified on EMG. With this in mind, LEMG may not be more accurate for diagnosing paresis than physical examination. In fact, a recent survey of laryngologists showed that most of them, 89%, relied on examination alone. The laryngoscopic findings that they thought to have the highest predictive value were motion anomalies such as sluggish motion and decreased tone.[21] However, it has also been shown that there is poor inter-rater agreement when presented with examinations suggestive of paresis, both on the diagnosis itself and on the laterality.[22] When trying to correlate stroboscopy findings with LEMG-confirmed paresis, the examination findings that had the strongest correlation appear to be ipsilateral axis deviation, shorter vocal fold, thinner vocal fold, vocal fold bowing, reduced kinesis, and phase lag.[23]

There are some studies that suggest that LEMG can be used to assess the potential for recovery after paralysis. Criteria that are typically used to define "excellent prognosis" include no fibrillations or positive sharp waves with good motor recruitment. However, even using these criteria there is varied success, with studies indicating recovery in these patients anywhere from 13 to 90%.[24,25,26,27,28,29,30] A recent meta-analysis did reveal that the presence of MUAPs increased the likelihood of recovery by 53% over their absence, while there was insufficient evidence for the

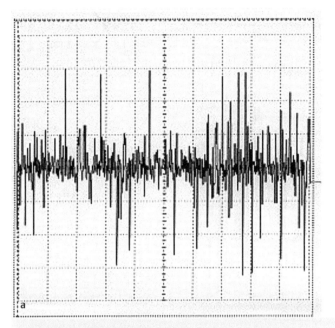
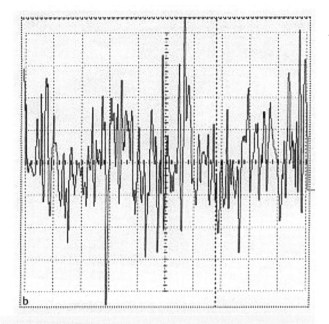

**Fig. 10.3** Laryngeal electromyography thyroarytenoid findings in a normal vocal fold **(a)** and one with paralysis **(b)** during contraction. **(a)** There are multiple motor units firing obscuring the baseline. **(b)** There is a less robust electrical response and a clearly distinguishable baseline.

usefulness of fibrillation potentials and sharp waves. The absence of electrical synkinesis was also found to have a positive predictive value for recovery of 68% and a sensitivity of 93%.[18]

## 10.2.4 Dysphagia Evaluation

When there is vocal fold paralysis, up to half of the patients may have accompanying dysphagia or aspiration.[31,32] This is the result of incomplete glottic closure as well as decreased pharyngeal contracture and sensation. There are multiple ways to evaluate their swallow. Perhaps the most basic in performance and results is a bedside swallow ($85).[1] Theoretically, a wet dysphonic voice on a bedside swallow could indicate penetration or aspiration; however, this test is neither sensitive nor specific.[33] A modified barium swallow (MBS) and flexible fiberoptic endoscopic evaluation of swallowing (FEES) provide more information and are more accurate.

### Modified Barium Swallow

An MBS ($220) allows real-time visualization of bolus transportation by using fluoroscopy.[1] Using this, the effectiveness of any compensatory strategy can also be identified and various consistencies may be trialed as well. In addition to showing aspiration or penetration, it provides further information about pharyngeal movement and contraction, which may help further localize the lesion along the vagus nerve. Specifically, this is measured by the pharyngeal constriction ratio, a measure of the pharyngeal area visible in lateral radiograph when the bolus is held in oral cavity divided by pharyngeal area at the point of maximal contraction.[34] Patients with pharyngeal weakness are at an additional risk for aspiration as this may cause residue in the pharynx, leading to aspiration after swallow. ▶ Fig. 10.4 is an example of an MBS in a patient with vocal fold paralysis. Before the

onset of the swallow (▶ Fig. 10.4a), note that there is no barium within the trachea. As the swallow progresses, one can start to see penetration (▶ Fig. 10.4b) followed by evidence of aspiration (▶ Fig. 10.4c)

### Functional Endoscopic Evaluation of Swallowing

A FEES ($235) allows direct visualization of the pharynx during swallowing.[1] As with flexible laryngoscopy mentioned earlier, any palatal or pharyngeal motor deficits can also be identified. Signs of aspiration or penetration may be seen, but any information about aspiration/penetration during the actual swallow is limited due to the "white out" of the epiglottis tilting. However, FEES is the only way to determine how the patient is handling their secretions and the presence/absence of transient aspiration with secretions. Sensory testing ($180) may be added to the FEES by blowing pulses of air onto the laryngeal mucosa to elicit the laryngeal adductor reflex, with the afferent limb being the internal branch of the SLN and the efferent limb being the RLN.[1] The lowest pulse of air that can elicit the reflex is defined as the threshold, with normal sensation being 4.0 mm Hg and below.[19,20]

## 10.3 Treatment

Once the diagnosis of paralysis is made, there are various treatment options. Depending on the etiology, the nerve has varying potential for reinnervation. Those whose paralysis is due to neoplasm or iatrogenic injury are less likely to recover, while those with idiopathic paralysis are more likely to recover.[35,36] While complete recovery is ideal, voice recovery is not always synonymous with recovery of motion.[35] A recent literature review showed that on average, 39% will have some recovery

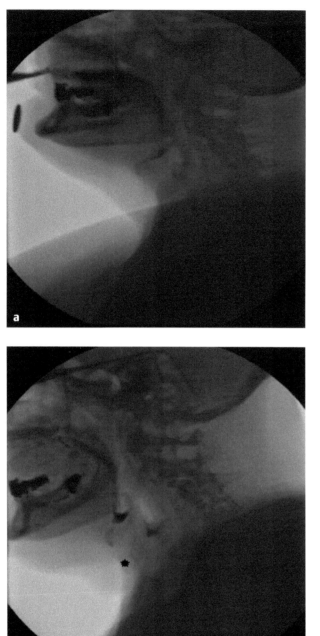
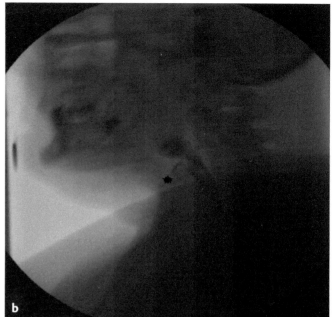

**Fig. 10.4** A modified barium swallow study in a patient with unilateral vocal fold paralysis. Before the swallow onset **(a)**, there is no barium within the laryngeal introitus or trachea. During the swallow **(b)**, you begin to see laryngeal penetration as demonstrated by the *star* and finally aspiration **(c)**, again demonstrated by the *star* highlighting the barium within the trachea.

of motion. In regard to voice recovery, 52% will note a complete voice recovery and 61% will note some degree of recovery.[35] Historically, it had been felt that if there is any recovery, it generally happens within a year after the initial paralysis. In general, about two-thirds of those that recover, recover within the first 6 months. With each additional month, the overall chance of recovery drops.[37] Since the potential for recovery, whether in motion or in sound, is possible with time, some patients may initially choose observation.

### 10.3.1 Voice Therapy

In addition to observation, another noninvasive treatment option is voice therapy ($80 per session).[1] Most commonly, this involves working on abdominal breathing, resonant voice, and hard glottal attacks where the vocal folds are brought together forcibly prior to sound production, all maneuvers that work to try to narrow the glottis while at the same time trying to avoid supraglottic hyperfunction. If there is any dysphagia or

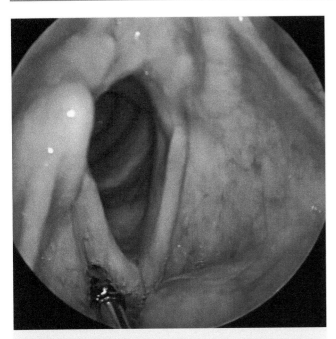

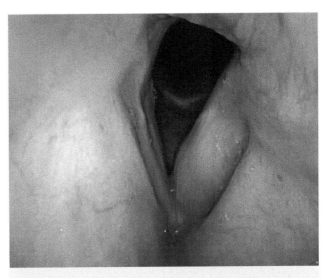

**Fig. 10.6** A patient with left vocal fold immobility undergoing transcutaneous injection medialization with acellular cadaveric dermis that requires over-injection as demonstrated here.

**Fig. 10.5** Peroral injection medialization in a patient with right vocal fold immobility. Note the placement of the needle along the lateral vocal fold, allowing the filler to be injected into the paraglottic space.

aspiration, swallowing therapy techniques such as chin tuck, head turn, and supraglottic swallow can also be used. Patients undergoing voice therapy frequently note a subjective perceptual improvement as well as an improvement in acoustic measurements. However, these results are clouded by coinciding neurological function return with further studies needed.[38,39,40]

## 10.3.2 Injection Medialization

Injection medialization is a more invasive way to provide temporary, and occasionally permanent, improvement by using a paraglottic filler to push the paralyzed vocal fold toward the midline to improve glottal closure. These injections can be performed either under general anesthesia with a direct laryngoscopy ($255 for the physician fee, not including anesthesia or operating room time) or awake in the office ($1035), with both options producing nearly equivalent success (97 vs. 99%) and complications rates (2 vs. 3%).[1,41] There has been a recent growth in the number of injections performed in the office, performed either peroral or percutaneously (transcricothyroid, transthyrohyoid, or transthyroid cartilage).

For peroral injection, visualization can be obtained through flexible fiberoptic laryngoscopy performed by an assistant or through rigid transoral laryngoscopy by the surgeon's non-dominant hand. After appropriate anesthetic, with the tongue held, the peroral needle is inserted through the oropharynx into the lateral aspect of the true vocal fold, as demonstrated in ▶Fig. 10.5, with care being taken to avoid injection into the superficial lamina propria. Depending on the material, it may need to be overinjected so that the vocal fold remains well medialized once the carrier absorbs.

For the percutaneous techniques, flexible laryngoscopy is used simultaneously to allow for visualization. For the transcricothyroid approach, after local anesthetic is applied, the cricothyroid membrane is identified and the needle is inserted inferior to the thyroid ala slightly off of midline toward the side of immobility. Once the needle is seen tenting the infraglottis, it is directed superiorly into the membranous vocal fold. For the transthyroid cartilage approach, the needle is instead inserted through the thyroid cartilage at the level of the true vocal folds. For both techniques, the needle ideally does not enter the airway and instead endoscopic visualization of submucosal movement of the needle back and forth is used to help ascertain proper placement. For the thyrohyoid approach, the needle is inserted at the thyroid notch and directed inferiorly so that it enters the airway at the petiole and is then guided under direct visualization to the correct injection site.[42] The material is then injected under visualization, allowing the vocal fold to swell and push toward the midline. ▶Fig. 10.6 is a patient with left vocal fold immobility, the same patient demonstrated in ▶Fig. 10.2, who is undergoing transcutaneous injection medialization with cadaveric acellular dermis with appropriate over-injection as dictated by the type of filler.

Injection medialization may be either temporary or more permanent depending on the material used. Historically, Teflon was the favored material although this has now largely fallen out of favor due to its long-term complications including foreign body reactions with granuloma formation. Now, there are multiple materials that are regularly used. The most commonly used are carboxymethylcellulose, collagen, and calcium hydroxylapatite in the clinic, and calcium hydroxylapatite and methylcellulose in the operating room.[41] Bovine gelatin is the shortest acting temporary filler, lasting 4 to 8 weeks, and requires a large bore needle with a pressurized injection device. Cadaveric acellular dermis is in a powder form that is then reconstituted for injection and usually lasts for 3 to 6 months; however, some reports indicate an even longer effect. Carboxymethylcellulose is another temporary material that lasts 2 to 3 months and one that is actually Food and Drug Administration (FDA) approved for vocal fold augmentation. Hyaluronic acid gels are a naturally occurring glycosaminoglycan that typically lasts 4 to 6 months. Calcium hydroxylapatite is regarded as a long-term implant that lasts up to 12 months. When injected, fibrosis replaces the gel carrier and microspheres of calcium hydroxylapatite remain. However, due to the loss of the gel carrier, this still needs to be slightly overinjected. Finally, autologous fat, while easily obtained, does have an unpredictable rate and degree of resorption, making it somewhat unpredictable.[42,43]

Temporary vocal fold medialization is done to lessen glottic insufficiency while awaiting return of mobility. Recently, there have been some data to suggest that early injection medialization, defined as anywhere from less than 3 months to less than 6 months from initial paralysis, may reduce the need for future permanent medialization thyroplasty.[44,45,46,47] It is believed that an early injection may influence the final glottal configuration by altering reinnervation (through the vibrotactile feedback caused by resulting glottic contact) or causing fibrosis. It is also thought that synkinetic reinnervation while the vocal fold is already in a favorable position from the injection helps reduce the requirement for further framework surgery.[44] Complications of injection medialization are rare, but include stridor/airway compromise, material migration, abscess formation, and dysphonia. As mentioned earlier, care must be taken to avoid superficial injection as this may cause dysphonia.[8,41]

For permanent medialization, a more permanent injection material may be selected. There are only a few studies comparing the outcomes of "permanent" injection medialization versus the gold standard of medialization thyroplasty and most of them have a relatively short follow-up period. One study compares micronized acellular dermis and calcium hydroxylapatite injection against medialization thyroplasty, with and without arytenoid adduction. At 3 months, the stroboscopy examination, perceptual analysis, and patients' subjective voice assessments were comparable.[48] A follow-up study with a larger cohort then confirmed similar results at 6 months.[49] Autologous fat injection versus medialization thyroplasty at 2 years has comparable acoustic parameters; however, during this follow-up period 20% of the autologous fat cohort required revision with a repeat injection or a medialization thyroplasty.[50]

### 10.3.3 Laryngeal Framework Surgery

#### Medialization Thyroplasty

Medialization thyroplasty ($1,065 for the surgeon's fee), or thyroplasty type I, is the most common laryngeal framework surgery for vocal fold paralysis.[1] It is done under sedation, so the patient can phonate during the procedure, and involves creating a window within the thyroid cartilage, incising the inner perichondrium, undermining the paraglottic space, and placing a permanent implant to medialize the vocal fold. An example is ▶ Fig. 10.7, where you can clearly see the window in the thyroid cartilage with a Silastic implant in place. Popularized

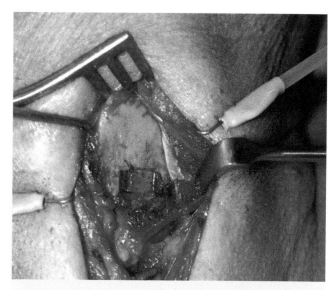

**Fig. 10.7** A patient with a medialization thyroplasty. Notice the window within the anteroinferior aspect of the thyroid cartilage with the implant in place. This allows the implant to enter the paraglottic space to help medialize the vocal fold.

by Isshiki et al in the 1970s, it has undergone modifications since then with multiple implant materials being used.[51] The most frequently reported implants are Silastic, titanium, and Gore-Tex, but there are only a handful of studies directly comparing the outcomes of the materials. One study of 57 patient who either underwent medialization with the Montgomery implant or Gore-Tex showed no difference in patient's self-evaluation; however, there was an improvement in jitter, shimmer, and noise-to-harmonic ratio in those patients with the Montgomery implant.[52] In comparing a hydroxyapatite implant versus titanium, another study of 26 patients showed better glottal closure, maximal phonation time, and voice intensity in those with the titanium implant.[53] A third study compared the titanium implant to silicone, showing an improved Voice Handicap Index in the patients with the titanium implant and a trend toward improvement in their maximum phonation time.[54]

A survey among otolaryngologist showed an average complication rate with medialization thyroplasty of 15%. Among these complications, intubation was required in 0.1% and a tracheostomy in 0.07%. Occasionally, the procedure had to be prematurely terminated (2.2%) or the implant was found to extrude (0.8%). Dysphonia persisted or worsened in 4% and there was a 6% implant revision rate.[55] Other studies have reported overall complication rates varying from 14 to 29%.[56,57]

Usually after this procedure is performed, patients are observed overnight in the hospital. While more research in this area is still required, recent studies have suggested that with appropriate risk stratification, this may be a same-day procedure for some.[58] Patients who may be at a higher risk for complications, and therefore warrant overnight observation, are those on anticoagulation, those undergoing revision surgeries, and those with atrophic or absent laryngeal tissue.[59]

## Arytenoid Adduction

Another laryngeal framework procedure is arytenoid adduction ($1005), where the motion of the action of the lateral cricoarytenoid is mimicked by a suture pulling the muscular process of the arytenoid anteriorly.[1] This helps close the posterior glottic gap. It is frequently performed in conjunction with medialization thyroplasty and indications include a large posterior glottic gap, shortened immobile vocal fold, height mismatch, and a maximum phonation time less than 5 seconds.[42] According to a recent systematic review, the reported outcomes have had mixed results.[60] There appears to be a trend toward better acoustic parameters; however, it was not statistically significant.[61] When comparing laryngoscopy findings, Abraham et al showed that there was improved posterior glottic closure, while Li et al were unable to reproduce these results.[57,62] The addition of arytenoid adduction also has no statistically significant increase in the associated complication rate.[57]

## Adduction Arytenopexy

Adduction arytenopexy ($1005) is another method to close the posterior glottic gap.[1] The cricoarytenoid joint is opened and the arytenoid is affixed in an optimal position along the cricoid facet. Theoretically, this helps avoid the exaggerated medial rotation that may be seen with arytenoid adduction. In a cadaveric study, it was shown to increase the length of the membranous vocal fold in comparison to arytenoid adduction.[63] Patients who have this procedure demonstrate improvement in the mean maximum phonation time and mean intensity with a decrease in glottal airflow. However, this has not been compared to medialization thyroplasty alone or to arytenoid adduction.[64] A cadaveric study did directly compare arytenoid adduction and adduction arytenopexy. While there were only five larynges tested, the adduction arytenopexy resulted in phonation threshold pressures that were 80% of those for arytenoid adduction. The arytenopexy cases also vibrated at a single dominant frequency with its harmonics, while the arytenoid adduction would vibrate at two dominant frequencies.[65]

## Cricothyroid Subluxation

Cricothyroid subluxation is a method to address the shortened immobile vocal fold. The subluxation results in rotation of the anterior commissure away from the midline to the side opposite the paralysis, therefore lengthening the vocal fold. In the original article by Zeitels et al, all nine patients achieved a normal maximum frequency range of more than 2 octaves compared to 22% of patient who underwent medialization thyroplasty alone.[66] However, direct comparison to other medialization techniques is still needed.

## 10.3.4 Laryngeal Reinnervation

More recently, laryngeal reinnervation ($890) has been used to improve tone on the immobile side.[1] It is this resulting increased muscle tone that causes the voice improvement as any functional return of mobility is typically limited by synkinesis. Multiple reinnervation techniques exist, from primary anastomosis, nerve–muscle pedicle transfer to thyroarytenoid, direct nerve transfer to the thyroarytenoid, and anastomosis between the RLN and the donor nerve. Commonly used donor nerves include the ansa cervicalis, phrenic, and hypoglossal. It is believed that reinnervation can help maintain thyroarytenoid muscle tone and bulk, alleviating the long-term vocal fold position changes that may be seen with medialization thyroplasty. Also, as there is no implant, there is less change in vocal fold pliability and mucosal wave.[67] A systematic review comparing the outcomes of the different techniques showed improved perceptual analysis and LEMG improvement for all reinnervation techniques. However, ansa-to-RLN resulted in the greatest improvement in glottal closure and ansa-to-thyroarytenoid neural implantation had the greatest improvement in acoustical analysis for ansa-to-thyroarytenoid neural implantation.[68]

A randomized trial that directly compared laryngeal reinnervation to medialization thyroplasty showed equal perceptual ratings. However, a subgroup analysis showed that patients younger than 52 years who had undergone laryngeal reinnervation had better ratings than the comparable medialization thyroplasty group. In patients older than 52 years, the medialization thyroplasty provided better results. It is speculated that younger patients have better reinnervation results due to their better neuroregenerative potential. However, this was a small study, with 12 people in both arms.[67]

As it takes some time for reinnervation to improve muscle tone, it is occasionally done in conjunction with laryngeal framework surgery. In comparing patients who had undergone nerve–muscle pedicle reinnervation with medialization thyroplasty to those who had a medialization without reinnervation, reinnervation allowed for better long-term voice preservation.[69] Another study compared arytenoid adduction with neuromuscular pedicle to arytenoid adduction, with and without medialization thyroplasty. Both resulted in an improved mean phonation time, jitter, shimmer, harmonics-to-noise ratio, and subjective perception initially. However, over the course of the 2-year follow-up, those who had a neuromuscular pedicle continued to improve, surpassing those values obtained without reinnervation.[70] In fact, the amount of jitter, shimmer, overall grade, and breathiness actually had increased in the second year in those who had not undergone reinnervation. Chhetri et al compared arytenoid adduction alone to those who had also had ansa-to-RLN anastomosis and reported no significant difference in the amount of improvement noted on glottal closure, mucosal wave, airflow, subglottic pressure, and perception.[71]

Few studies specifically mention complications or lack thereof. Both Chhetri et al and Miyauchi et al note no complications in their reinnervation series.[71,72] Blumin and Merati compared complication rates and demonstrated no statistical difference between major (airway compromise, dysphagia, death) and minor complication (wound problems or hematoma) rates between framework surgery and those who underwent reinnervation.[73]

## 10.4 Conclusion

Vagal neuropathy, due to the paralysis of the RLN and/or the SLN, may cause dysphonia and true vocal fold paralysis. Endoscopy and LEMG may be used to confirm the diagnosis, while imaging along the course of the nerve, with selective use of serology, may be used to determine the etiology. There is the potential for spontaneous reinnervation within the first year, but even should mobility not return occasionally synkinetic reinnervation provides enough tone that there is voice recovery. Voice therapy or temporary injection medialization may be used to help improve glottic closure. If the paralysis is deemed permanent, laryngeal framework surgery such as medialization thyroplasty can be performed to help medialize the immobile vocal fold. Laryngeal reinnervation has also been used to provide bulk and tone to the vocal fold with good voice outcomes.

## References

[1] Centers for Medicare & Medicaid Services. Physician Fee Schedule Search. https://www.cms.gov/apps/physician-fee-schedule/search/search-criteria.aspx. Accessed August 1, 2018

[2] Stachler RJ, Francis DO, Schwartz SR, et al. Clinical Practice Guideline: Hoarseness (Dysphonia) (Update). Otolaryngol Head Neck Surg 2018;158(1, Suppl):S1–S42

[3] Rubin AD, Sataloff RT. Vocal fold paresis and paralysis. Otolaryngol Clin North Am 2007;40(5):1109–1131, viii–ix

[4] Richardson BE, Bastian RW. Clinical evaluation of vocal fold paralysis. Otolaryngol Clin North Am 2004;37(1):45–58

[5] Spataro EA, Grindler DJ, Paniello RC. Etiology and time to presentation of unilateral vocal fold paralysis. Otolaryngol Head Neck Surg 2014;151(2):286–293

[6] Rosenthal LH, Benninger MS, Deeb RH. Vocal fold immobility: a longitudinal analysis of etiology over 20 years. Laryngoscope 2007;117(10):1864–1870

[7] Takano S, Nito T, Tamaruya N, Kimura M, Tayama N. Single institutional analysis of trends over 45 years in etiology of vocal fold paralysis. Auris Nasus Larynx 2012;39(6):597–600

[8] Misono S, Merati AL. Evidence-based practice: evaluation and management of unilateral vocal fold paralysis. Otolaryngol Clin North Am 2012;45(5):1083–1108

[9] Merati AL, Halum SL, Smith TL. Diagnostic testing for vocal fold paralysis: survey of practice and evidence-based medicine review. Laryngoscope 2006;116(9):1539–1552

[10] Chen DW, Young A, Donovan DT, Ongkasuwan J. Routine computed tomography in the evaluation of vocal fold movement impairment without an apparent cause. Otolaryngol Head Neck Surg 2015;152(2):308–313

[11] Kang BC, Roh JL, Lee JH, et al. Usefulness of computed tomography in the etiologic evaluation of adult unilateral vocal fold paralysis. World J Surg 2013;37(6):1236–1240

[12] Bilici S, Yildiz M, Yigit O, Misir E. Imaging modalities in the etiologic evaluation of unilateral vocal fold paralysis. J Voice 2018:S0892–1997(18)30089–4

[13] Badia PI, Hillel AT, Shah MD, Johns MM III, Klein AM. Computed tomography has low yield in the evaluation of idiopathic unilateral true vocal fold paresis. Laryngoscope 2013;123(1):204–207

[14] Paddle PM, Mansor MB, Song PC, Franco RA Jr. Diagnostic yield of computed tomography in the evaluation of idiopathic vocal fold paresis. Otolaryngol Head Neck Surg 2015;153(3):414–419

[15] Jacobs CJ, Harnsberger HR, Lufkin RB, Osborn AG, Smoker WR, Parkin JL. Vagal neuropathy: evaluation with CT and MR imaging. Radiology 1987;164(1):97–102

[16] Liu AY, Yousem DM, Chalian AA, Langlotz CP. Economic consequences of diagnostic imaging for vocal cord paralysis. Acad Radiol 2001;8(2):137–148

[17] Schechter GL, Kostianovsky M. Vocal cord paralysis in diabetes mellitus. Trans Am Acad Ophthalmol Otolaryngol 1972;76(3):729–740

[18] Munin MC, Heman-Ackah YD, Rosen CA, et al. Consensus statement: using laryngeal electromyography for the diagnosis and treatment of vocal cord paralysis. Muscle Nerve 2016;53(6):850–855

[19] Sulica L, Blitzer A. Electromyography and the immobile vocal fold. Otolaryngol Clin North Am 2004;37(1):59–74

[20] Sulica L, Blitzer A. Vocal fold paresis: evidence and controversies. Curr Opin Otolaryngol Head Neck Surg 2007;15(3):159–162

[21] Wu AP, Sulica L. Diagnosis of vocal fold paresis: current opinion and practice. Laryngoscope 2015;125(4):904–908

[22] Estes C, Sadoughi B, Mauer E, Christos P, Sulica L. Laryngoscopic and stroboscopic signs in the diagnosis of vocal fold paresis. Laryngoscope 2017;127(9):2100–2105

[23] Woo P, Parasher AK, Isseroff T, Richards A, Sivak M. Analysis of laryngoscopic features in patients with unilateral vocal fold paresis. Laryngoscope 2016;126(8):1831–1836

[24] Sittel C, Stennert E, Thumfart WF, Dapunt U, Eckel HE. Prognostic value of laryngeal electromyography in vocal fold paralysis. Arch Otolaryngol Head Neck Surg 2001;127(2):155–160

[25] Min YB, Finnegan EM, Hoffman HT, Luschei ES, McCulloch TM. A preliminary study of the prognostic role of electromyography in laryngeal paralysis. Otolaryngol Head Neck Surg 1994;111(6):770–775

[26] Wang CC, Chang MH, Wang CP, Liu SA. Prognostic indicators of unilateral vocal fold paralysis. Arch Otolaryngol Head Neck Surg 2008;134(4):380–388

[27] Parnes SM, Satya-Murti S. Predictive value of laryngeal electromyography in patients with vocal cord paralysis of neurogenic origin. Laryngoscope 1985;95(11):1323–1326

[28] Munin MC, Rosen CA, Zullo T. Utility of laryngeal electromyography in predicting recovery after vocal fold paralysis. Arch Phys Med Rehabil 2003;84(8):1150–1153

[29] Wang CC, Chang MH, De Virgilio A, et al. Laryngeal electromyography and prognosis of unilateral vocal fold paralysis: a long-term prospective study. Laryngoscope 2015;125(4):898–903

[30] Smith LJ, Rosen CA, Munin MC. Vocal fold motion outcome based on excellent prognosis with laryngeal electromyography. Laryngoscope 2016;126(10):2310–2314

[31] Bhattacharyya N, Kotz T, Shapiro J. Dysphagia and aspiration with unilateral vocal cord immobility: incidence, characterization, and response to surgical treatment. Ann Otol Rhinol Laryngol 2002;111(8):672–679

[32] Leder SB, Ross DA. Incidence of vocal fold immobility in patients with dysphagia. Dysphagia 2005;20(2):163–167, discussion 168–169

[33] Splaingard ML, Hutchins B, Sulton LD, Chaudhuri G. Aspiration in rehabilitation patients: videofluoroscopy vs bedside clinical assessment. Arch Phys Med Rehabil 1988;69(8):637–640

[34] Leonard R, Rees CJ, Belafsky P, Allen J. Fluoroscopic surrogate for pharyngeal strength: the pharyngeal constriction ratio (PCR). Dysphagia 2011;26(1):13–17

[35] Sulica L. The natural history of idiopathic unilateral vocal fold paralysis: evidence and problems. Laryngoscope 2008;118(7):1303–1307

[36] Mor N, Wu G, Aylward A, Christos PJ, Sulica L. Predictors for permanent medialization laryngoplasty in unilateral vocal fold paralysis. Otolaryngol Head Neck Surg 2016;155(3):443–453

[37] Husain S, Sadoughi B, Mor N, Levin AM, Sulica L. Time course of recovery of idiopathic vocal fold paralysis. Laryngoscope 2018;128(1):148–152

[38] D'Alatri L, Galla S, Rigante M, Antonelli O, Buldrini S, Marchese MR. Role of early voice therapy in patients affected by unilateral vocal fold paralysis. J Laryngol Otol 2008;122(9):936–941

[39] Busto-Crespo O, Uzcanga-Lacabe M, Abad-Marco A, et al. Longitudinal voice outcomes after voice therapy in unilateral vocal fold paralysis. J Voice 2016;30(6):767.e9–767.e15

[40] Mattioli F, Bergamini G, Alicandri-Ciufelli M, et al. The role of early voice therapy in the incidence of motility recovery in unilateral vocal fold paralysis. Logoped Phoniatr Vocol 2011;36(1):40–47

[41] Sulica L, Rosen CA, Postma GN, et al. Current practice in injection augmentation of the vocal folds: indications, treatment principles, techniques, and complications. Laryngoscope 2010;120(2):319–325

[42] Simpson CB, Rosen CA. Operative techniques in laryngology. Berlin: Springer; 2008

[43] Kwon TK, Buckmire R. Injection laryngoplasty for management of unilateral vocal fold paralysis. Curr Opin Otolaryngol Head Neck Surg 2004;12(6):538–542

[44] Friedman AD, Burns JA, Heaton JT, Zeitels SM. Early versus late injection medialization for unilateral vocal cord paralysis. Laryngoscope 2010;120(10):2042–2046

[45] Prendes BL, Yung KC, Likhterov I, Schneider SL, Al-Jurf SA, Courey MS. Long-term effects of injection laryngoplasty with a temporary agent on voice quality and vocal fold position. Laryngoscope 2012;122(10):2227–2233

[46] Yung KC, Likhterov I, Courey MS. Effect of temporary vocal fold injection medialization on the rate of permanent medialization laryngoplasty in unilateral vocal fold paralysis patients. Laryngoscope 2011;121(10):2191–2194

[47] Alghonaim Y, Roskies M, Kost K, Young J. Evaluating the timing of injection laryngoplasty for vocal fold paralysis in an attempt to avoid future type 1 thyroplasty. J Otolaryngol Head Neck Surg 2013;42:24

[48] Morgan JE, Zraick RI, Griffin AW, Bowen TL, Johnson FL. Injection versus medialization laryngoplasty for the treatment of unilateral vocal fold paralysis. Laryngoscope 2007;117(11):2068–2074

[49] Vinson KN, Zraick RI, Ragland FJ. Injection versus medialization laryngoplasty for the treatment of unilateral vocal fold paralysis: follow-up at six months. Laryngoscope 2010;120(9):1802–1807

[50] Hartl DM, Hans S, Crevier-Buchman L, Vaissière J, Brasnu DF. Long-term acoustic comparison of thyroplasty versus autologous fat injection. Ann Otol Rhinol Laryngol 2009;118(12):827–832

[51] Isshiki N, Morita H, Okamura H, Hiramoto M. Thyroplasty as a new phonosurgical technique. Acta Otolaryngol 1974;78(5–6):451–457

[52] Nouwen J, Hans S, De Mones E, Brasnu D, Crevier-Buchman L, Laccourreye O. Thyroplasty type I without arytenoid adduction in patients with unilateral laryngeal nerve paralysis: the montgomery implant versus the Gore-Tex implant. Acta Otolaryngol 2004;124(6):732–738

[53] Storck C, Fischer C, Cecon M, et al. Hydroxyapatite versus titanium implant: comparison of the functional outcome after vocal fold medialization in unilateral recurrent nerve paralysis. Head Neck 2010;32(12):1605–1612

[54] van Ardenne N, Vanderwegen J, Van Nuffelen G, De Bodt M, Van de Heyning P. Medialization thyroplasty: vocal outcome of silicone and titanium implant. Eur Arch Otorhinolaryngol 2011;268(1):101–107

[55] Young VN, Zullo TG, Rosen CA. Analysis of laryngeal framework surgery: 10-year follow-up to a national survey. Laryngoscope 2010;120(8):1602–1608

[56] Cotter CS, Avidano MA, Crary MA, Cassisi NJ, Gorham MM. Laryngeal complications after type 1 thyroplasty. Otolaryngol Head Neck Surg 1995;113(6):671–673

[57] Abraham MT, Gonen M, Kraus DH. Complications of type I thyroplasty and arytenoid adduction. Laryngoscope 2001;111(8):1322–1329

[58] Zhao X, Roth K, Fung K. Type I thyroplasty: risk stratification approach to inpatient versus outpatient postoperative management. J Otolaryngol Head Neck Surg 2010;39(6):757–761

[59] Bray D, Young JP, Harries ML. Complications after type one thyroplasty: is day-case surgery feasible? J Laryngol Otol 2008;122(7):715–718

[60] Siu J, Tam S, Fung K. A comparison of outcomes in interventions for unilateral vocal fold paralysis: a systematic review. Laryngoscope 2016;126(7):1616–1624

[61] Mortensen M, Carroll L, Woo P. Arytenoid adduction with medialization laryngoplasty versus injection or medialization laryngoplasty: the role of the arytenoidopexy. Laryngoscope 2009;119(4):827–831

[62] Li AJ, Johns MM, Jackson-Menaldi C, et al. Glottic closure patterns: type I thyroplasty versus type I thyroplasty with arytenoid adduction. J Voice 2011;25(3):259–264

[63] Zeitels SM, Hochman I, Hillman RE. Adduction arytenopexy: a new procedure for paralytic dysphonia with implications for implant medialization. Ann Otol Rhinol Laryngol Suppl 1998;173:2–24

[64] Franco RA, Andrus JG. Aerodynamic and acoustic characteristics of voice before and after adduction arytenopexy and medialization laryngoplasty with GORE-TEX in patients with unilateral vocal fold immobility. J Voice 2009;23(2):261–267

[65] McNamar J, Montequin DW, Welham NV, Dailey SH. Aerodynamic, acoustic, and vibratory comparison of arytenoid adduction and adduction arytenopexy. Laryngoscope 2008;118(3):552–558

[66] Zeitels SM, Hillman RE, Desloge RB, Bunting GA. Cricothyroid subluxation: a new innovation for enhancing the voice with laryngoplastic phonosurgery. Ann Otol Rhinol Laryngol 1999;108(12):1126–1131

[67] Paniello RC, Edgar JD, Kallogjeri D, Piccirillo JF. Medialization versus reinnervation for unilateral vocal fold paralysis: a multicenter randomized clinical trial. Laryngoscope 2011;121(10):2172–2179

[68] Aynehchi BB, McCoul ED, Sundaram K. Systematic review of laryngeal reinnervation techniques. Otolaryngol Head Neck Surg 2010;143(6):749–759

[69] Tucker HM. Long-term preservation of voice improvement following surgical medialization and reinnervation for unilateral vocal fold paralysis. J Voice 1999;13(2):251–256

[70] Hassan MM, Yumoto E, Sanuki T, et al. Arytenoid adduction with nerve-muscle pedicle transfer vs arytenoid adduction with and without type I thyroplasty in paralytic dysphonia. JAMA Otolaryngol Head Neck Surg 2014;140(9):833–839

[71] Chhetri DK, Gerratt BR, Kreiman J, Berke GS. Combined arytenoid adduction and laryngeal reinnervation in the treatment of vocal fold paralysis. Laryngoscope 1999;109(12):1928–1936

[72] Miyauchi A, Inoue H, Tomoda C, et al. Improvement in phonation after reconstruction of the recurrent laryngeal nerve in patients with thyroid cancer invading the nerve. Surgery 2009;146(6):1056–1062

[73] Blumin JH, Merati AL. Laryngeal reinnervation with nerve-nerve anastomosis versus laryngeal framework surgery alone: a comparison of safety. Otolaryngol Head Neck Surg 2008;138(2):217–220

# 11 Cranial Nerve XI: Spinal Accessory Neuropathy

*Rizwan Aslam*

**Abstract**

Cranial neuropathies can significantly impact a patient's quality of life. Therefore, it is imperative for health care providers to understand the etiology and management of these injuries. In this chapter, we will discuss the clinical presentation and management of neuropathies involving the spinal accessory nerve (SAN), cranial nerve XI. SAN palsy may result in significant pain and deficits in shoulder mobility.

*Keywords:* spinal accessory nerve palsy, spinal accessory nerve neuropathy, spinal accessory nerve paralysis

## 11.1 Introduction

The spinal accessory nerve (SAN) is the main motor innervation of the trapezius and sternocleidomastoid (SCM) muscles. The SAN has a long course through the posterior neck, making it vulnerable to injury. SAN injury has been related to iatrogenic, traumatic, neurologic, and inflammatory injury. Injury may result in shoulder pain (most common) and limited range of motion (ROM). This could result in significant impairment in activities of daily living for patients. Iatrogenic injury during surgery may result in physician stress and management challenges. Early diagnosis and management may decrease these symptoms and reduce further costs. Comprehensive intervention will decrease both physician and patient stress.

## 11.2 Anatomy

The SAN has a long course originating in the upper cervical portions of the spine and terminating in the neck. The SAN pathway begins with two separate parts. The spinal and motor portions include fibers that originate in the ventral horn, typically from the upper four cervical (C1–C4) segments of the spinal cord. These fibers then ascend adjacent to the spinal cord and enter the skull via the foramen magnum. Following passage into the skull, the fibers then join the second or accessory component of the SAN that begins in the nucleus accumbens brain stem nucleus of the medulla in the posterior fossa. The joined components then exit the skull base through the jugular foramen and with a level of variability separate into the two original components. The components are identified as the superior and inferior branches. The superior branch (accessory branch) joins the vagus directly or via the ganglion nodosum and then contributes to the pharyngeal, laryngeal, and cardiac sympathetic fibers. The inferior branch (spinal branch) is a pure motor nerve and innervates the SCM and trapezius muscles.[1] The SAN then travels deep to the posterior belly of the digastric muscle and crosses the internal jugular vein (IJV) near the upper limit of the SCM. This relationship of the SAN and IJV is variable—most commonly the nerve passes over the vein, but it infrequently passes deep and rarely the nerve splits around the vein. The SAN joins the second cervical nerve prior to insertion into the SCM.[2] The nerve then exits from the posterior aspect of the SCM, and takes an oblique path through the posterior triangle of the neck downward and laterally where it inserts into the trapezius muscle.

## 11.3 Pathophysiology

SAN injury may result from multiple causes. Unfortunately, the most common source of neuropathy is tumor invasion or iatrogenic injury related to surgical dissection in the region of the SAN. Because of the SAN's lengthy course around other critical structures from the skull base to the shoulder, it is vulnerable to injury at different locations. If there is malignant invasion anywhere along the nerve, it must be sacrificed for oncologic margins. Additionally, the nerve must be identified, retracted, and sometimes completely skeletonized during a standard surgery to remove cancer from the surrounding neck lymph nodes, referred to as a neck dissection.

Neck dissections can be categorized based on which compartments or "levels" undergo lymph node removal. These levels represent lymph node drainage basins in the submuscular recess along the carotid sheath. Neck levels II to IV are along the IJV from superior near the mastoid tip to inferior at the clavicle. Level V is represented as an area between the posterior border of the SCM, trapezius, and the clavicle.

SAN injury rates following neck dissections vary depending on the extent of disease that requires resection. This decision is frequently made during the surgery based on extent of malignant invasion and the need for oncologic margins.

Traditional radical neck dissection (RND) includes lymphadenectomy of levels II to V plus sacrifice of the SAN, IJV, and SCM in order to obtain oncologic resection of lymph nodes related to malignancies of the head and neck. Unsurprisingly, profound functional deficits have been reported in 60 to 80% of patients undergoing RND.[3]

Modified radical neck dissection (MRND) still involves cervical lymphadenectomy of levels II to V, but aims to preserve at least one of the three critical structures if uninvolved by malignant lymphadenopathy. Reported rates of injury following MRND are about 42.5%.[4]

Furthermore, selective neck dissections of levels II to IV with the aim to preserve all three critical structures without nerve sacrifice still have reported rates of injury as high as 30%. This is likely related to nerve traction or revascularization due to skeletonization.[5]

Level II is an area of contention. This level is at the upper limit of the SCM, the posterior belly of the digastric muscle, and the IJV. The SAN creates a distinction between level IIa and level IIb. Level IIb is posterior to the nerve, and execution of the dissection may require extensive retraction on the nerve. Some experienced surgeons recommend avoiding level IIb unless clinically indicated as it may result in less morbidity. Frequency of postoperative morbidity following neck dissection decreases significantly from RND (46.7%) and MRND (42.5%) to selective neck dissection (25%).[4]

The SAN is also vulnerable at the jugular foramen where it exits the skull base. Tumors such as jugular paraganglioma or meningioma may cause direct damage to the lower cranial nerves, or injury may result from surgical resection or radiation to the area.

SAN injury has many other less common causes. Other surgical procedures can lead to injury including excision of lymph nodes in the posterior triangle, neck mass excision, parotidectomy, carotid surgery, jugular vein manipulation, and facelift.[6]

Traumatic insults can cause SAN. Penetrating and blunt trauma have been associated with SAN injury. Sports injury including hockey stick injury, wrestling, and whiplash can also cause SAN trauma. Neurologic disease processes such as Collet–Sicard syndrome, Vernet's syndrome, poliomyelitis, motor neuron disease, brachial neuritis, and syringomyelia have been associated with SAN injury. Rarely, spontaneous isolated nerve injury has been reported.[7]

During any of the events, the nerve could be transected, devascularized, or stretched. The nerve may become transected when exploring, devascularized when there is extensive skeletonization, or stretched during retraction. Ischemia may lead to segmental demyelinization resulting in loss of nerve function.[8] SAN injury leads to axonal degeneration resulting in muscle atrophy and contractures. This is evidenced by needle electromyography (EMG) and cicatrix formation.[7]

## 11.4 Clinical Presentation

Clinical presentation of patients with SAN injury may range from asymptomatic to significant motor weakness and pain of the shoulder. The type of injury usually defines the sequelae that follow. There is variability of motor contribution from cervical and SAN branches.

Predicting outcomes from the type of nerve injury may be challenging. In 1961, Nahum described the syndrome of pain and shoulder dysfunction as "shoulder syndrome." A majority of the signs and symptoms associated with shoulder syndrome stem from denervation of the trapezius muscle. Shoulder pain is the most common initial symptom. The pain may be radiating to the neck, upper back, and sometimes the ipsilateral arm. Pain can develop secondary to overcompensation of surrounding musculature and brachial plexus traction. Patients may develop weakness with loss of sustained abduction of the shoulder. This limited mobility is the most common initial sign of SAN injury. As a late sequelae, some patients may develop a "frozen shoulder" secondary to adhesive capsulitis with decreased ROM. The classic findings of winged scapula and internal rotation of the humeral head may be seen as well.

## 11.5 Diagnostic Workup

A thorough history and physical examination is compulsory. A detailed history may allow the clinician to establish an early working diagnosis. Sometimes, a careful review of operative reports from neck or skull base surgery is critical to understanding the source of injury related to surgery. Physical examination including ROM and muscle strength is vital in assessing dysfunction. The constant shoulder scale is a validated test that assesses patient symptoms and objective findings on

a scale of 0 to 100. A higher score indicates better function.[9] There are multiple quality of life surveys that can be utilized to assess shoulder function including shoulder disability questionnaire (SDQ), Neck Dissection Impairment Index, and The University of Washington QOL scale.

Objective testing may have a role in evaluation of suspected SAN palsy. While CT and MRI may be helpful for cases of idiopathic SAN weakness to evaluate for skull base or central nervous system pathology, they are typically not useful in postoperative cases of suspected iatrogenic injury.

Alternatively, high-resolution ultrasound (HRUS) and EMG may have a role in evaluating a damaged nerve. HRUS can be utilized to evaluate peripheral nerve complete or partial transection, nerve matter enlargement, laceration, epineural hematoma, and neuroma formation.[10] In a prospective study conducted by Peer et al, HRUS was successful in demonstrating nerve swelling, scar tissue, neuroma, and insufficient surgical repair. These findings were consistent with operative interventions for nerve repair.[11] It can also be utilized to assess for soft-tissue changes involving the muscle, scarring, inflammation, and infection.

Electrophysiological testing such as EMG is the most sensitive test for nerve conduction impairment.[5] It can be used for intraoperative nerve monitoring to minimize chance of injury. It can also be utilized to monitor trapezius recovery as well as for physical therapy (PT) planning.[12]

Following the patient closely with examination and EMG can tell the natural course of what to expect in terms of function.

In a study conducted by Lee et al, the authors examined prospectively the utility of intraoperative nerve monitoring during neck dissections. This study was conducted in order to examine the outcomes following neck dissection in a training environment and correlating those results to postoperative shoulder syndrome. They examined 25 patients undergoing neck dissection with intraoperative nerve monitoring. Testing was performed at the initial identification of the nerve and at the conclusion of the case. Functional shoulder status was also measured postoperatively at 1 month. Similarly, EMG was obtained 1 month postoperatively. EMG studies revealed fibrillation potentials at rest in 40% of patients and positive sharp waves in 64% of patients. They concluded even with nerve monitoring, traction-related denervation still occurs; however, use of nerve monitor may result in less painful forms of shoulder syndrome.[13] In our institution, we do not routinely perform nerve monitoring. Special attention to anatomical detail and meticulous dissection is given in order to preserve and maintain shoulder function.

All of the above diagnostic examinations represent affordable options. Outpatient workup including physical examination will be associated with office fees. Diagnostics HRUS is a simple outpatient procedure, limited mainly by expertise of interpreting physician. EMG testing according to Hospital for Special Surgery takes approximately 30 to 90 minutes. The test includes a nerve conduction study and a needle examination. EMG is typically covered by insurance, and may result in copays of $10 to $50, or coinsurance of 10 to 50% depending on coverage. For those patients without insurance, an EMG may cost anywhere between $150 and $500 depending on the number of sites. There is variability between health care providers, with estimates from Kaiser Permanente and On Site at $247 to $350 per site, respectively.

## 11.6 Treatment

Treatment options range from conservative therapy to surgical interventions. Serial patient clinical and EMG examinations will drive the decision-making toward the appropriate treatment interventions. Conservative therapy can be utilized in the cases where there is minimal discomfort and minimal motor dysfunction. Non-steroidals anti-inflammatory diseases (NSAIDs), transcutaneous nerve stimulation, and regional nerve blocks are short-term solutions that will likely require repeated doses to maintain symptom symptomatic relief.

Patients may also undergo PT. The aim of PT is to improve ROM and achieve a reduction in pain. This is done by maintaining or regaining passive ROM of the shoulder. We recommend early PT consultation on all of our inpatients following neck dissection. A study by Salerno et al emphasized early and prolonged PT, beginning within 1 month of surgery and lasting, on average, 3 months.[14] In this study, all patients had prior neck dissection; those in the PT group were able to obtain zero

position or 165 degrees of flexion, the range necessary for activities of daily living.

Laska and Hannig reported a PT algorithm for a patient with SAN following carotid endarterectomy (▶ Fig. 11.1). They recommended a 30-week protocol, with two sessions per week for 3 weeks, followed by appointments at 16, 18, 22, and 30 weeks postoperatively for a total 10 sessions.[15]

Salerno et al recommended the following exercises[14]:
• Passive forward elevation of the arm in the scapular plane in supine and half sitting positions.
• Passive forward elevation with hands locked in supine and half sitting with subsequent stretching movements.
• External rotation of the elbow at the side and flexed to 90 degrees.
• Internal rotation with the hand behind the back.

Early mobility of the shoulder can help prevent the dreaded frozen shoulder secondary to adhesive capsulitis. Patients can do the following cost-effective maneuvers at home to unload the affected arm: avoid heavy lifting on the affected side, hook the thumb of affected hand or place affected hand in pocket, and utilize an arm sling.[16]

The Akman–Sari orthosis can provide symptomatic relief and is an alternative to surgical intervention. The orthosis provides relief by aligning musculature and subsequently providing pain relief.

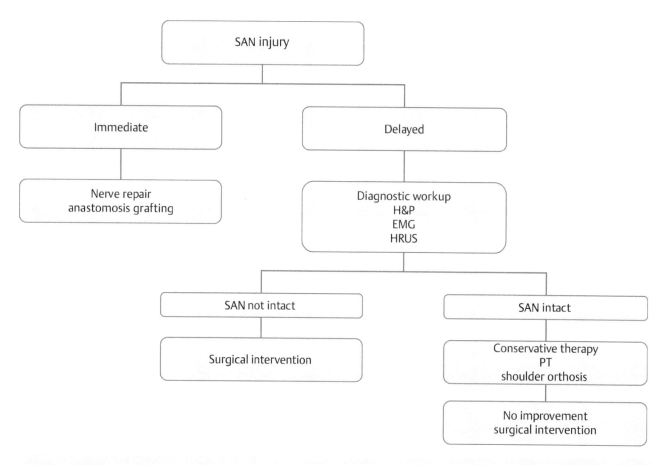

**Fig. 11.1** Physical therapy algorithm for a patient with spinal accessory nerve following carotid endarterectomy.

Indications for nonsurgical management include clinical improvement with serial physical examination, EMG findings indicating electrical regeneration, and mild symptoms of minimal pain and shoulder dysfunction.[17] Some patients may not receive any symptomatic improvement with conservative measures and require surgical intervention.

Indications for surgical management of SAN injury include iatrogenic intraoperative injury, delayed signs of shoulder syndrome, and lack of improvement with conservative therapy and EMG demonstrating degeneration.[10,13] Surgical options include nerve surgery, nerve grafting, and nerve regeneration.

At the initial awareness of injury, one should consider immediate repair if feasible. Primary repair or cable grafting of known injury or planned sacrifice of the nerve may prevent pain and other symptoms in the future. Nerve repair with primary anastomosis can be completed if the approximation is tension free. However, if nerve sacrifice is performed, the distance may not allow for primary repair requiring nerve grafting. Cable grafting utilizing the greater auricular nerve has been described. In a study by Weisberger et al, outcomes of patients with nerve reconstruction were improved compared to those with no reconstruction.[18]

Alternative surgical options include tendon or muscle transfer to stabilize the scapula, and this is employed for patients not responding to nerve repair. One of the widely used surgical techniques is scapulothoracic fusion. The most common technique is the Eden–Lange procedure, which stabilizes the scapula by securing the levator scapulae and rhomboid muscles, which in turn mimic the function of the trapezius. It is indicated in patients with time interval since injury of greater than 20 months, failed surgical reconstruction of the nerve, and delayed diagnosis.

## 11.7 Conclusion

In conclusion, at our institution we feel a thorough understanding of the surgical anatomy, preoperative assessment, and early therapy can help prevent some of the untoward consequences of SAN injury. The management of SAN injury can be achieved in a cost-efficient manner by understanding the pathology and providing early diagnostics and interventions.

# References

[1] Shiozaki K, Abe S, Agematsu H, et al. Anatomical study of accessory nerve innervation relating to functional neck dissection. J Oral Maxillofac Surg 2007;65(1):22–29

[2] Overland J, Hodge JC, Breik O, Krishnan S. Surgical anatomy of the spinal accessory nerve: review of the literature and case report of a rare anatomical variant. J Laryngol Otol 2016;130(10):969–972

[3] Leipzig B, Suen JY, English JL, Barnes J, Hooper M. Functional evaluation of the spinal accessory nerve after neck dissection. Am J Surg 1983;146(4):526–530

[4] Popovski V, Benedetti A, Popovic-Monevska D, Grcev A, Stamatoski A, Zhivadinovik J. Spinal accessory nerve preservation in modified neck dissections: surgical and functional outcomes. Acta Otorhinolaryngol Ital 2017;37(5):368–374

[5] Cappiello J, Piazza C, Giudice M, De Maria G, Nicolai P. Shoulder disability after different selective neck dissections (levels II–IV versus levels II–V): a comparative study. Laryngoscope 2005;115(2):259–263

[6] Millett PJ, Romero A, Braun S. Spinal accessory nerve injury after rhytidectomy (face lift): a case report. J Shoulder Elbow Surg 2009;18(5):e15–e17

[7] Ozdemir O, Kurne A, Temuçin C, Varli K. Spontaneous unilateral accessory nerve palsy: a case report and review of the literature. Clin Rheumatol 2007;26(9):1581–1583

[8] Kierner AC, Burian M, Bentzien S, Gstoettner W. Intraoperative electromyography for identification of the trapezius muscle innervation: clinical proof of a new anatomical concept. Laryngoscope 2002;112(10):1853–1856

[9] Rogers SN, Scott B, Lowe D. An evaluation of the shoulder domain of the University of Washington quality of life scale. Br J Oral Maxillofac Surg 2007;45(1):5–10

[10] Chiou H-J, Chou Y-H, Chiou S-Y, Liu J-B, Chang C-Y. Peripheral nerve lesions: role of high-resolution US. Radiographics 2003;23(6):e15

[11] Peer S, Bodner G, Meirer R, Willeit J, Piza-Katzer H. Examination of postoperative peripheral nerve lesions with high-resolution sonography. AJR Am J Roentgenol 2001;177(2):415–419

[12] Erisen L, Basel B, Irdesel J, et al. Shoulder function after accessory nerve-sparing neck dissections. Head Neck 2004;26(11):967–971

[13] Lee CH, Huang NC, Chen HC, Chen MK. Minimizing shoulder syndrome with intra-operative spinal accessory nerve monitoring for neck dissection. Acta Otorhinolaryngol Ital 2013;33(2):93–96

[14] Salerno G, Cavaliere M, Foglia A, et al. The 11th nerve syndrome in functional neck dissection. Laryngoscope 2002;112(7, Pt 1):1299–1307

[15] Laska T, Hannig K. Physical therapy for spinal accessory nerve injury complicated by adhesive capsulitis Phys Ther 2001;81(3):936–944

[16] Bodack MP, Tunkel RS, Marini SG, Nagler W. Spinal accessory nerve palsy as a cause of pain after whiplash injury: case report. J Pain Symptom Manage 1998;15(5):321–328

[17] Chandawarkar RY, Cervino AL, Pennington GA. Management of iatrogenic injury to the spinal accessory nerve. Plast Reconstr Surg 2003;111(2):611–617, discussion 618–619

[18] Weisberger EC, Kincaid J, Riteris J. Cable grafting of the spinal accessory nerve after radical neck dissection. Arch Otolaryngol Head Neck Surg 1998;124(4):377–380

# 12 Radiology in Cranial Neuropathy

*Richard K. Gurgel, Vanessa Torrecillas, and Richard H. Wiggins, III*

**Abstract**

When patients present with cranial neuropathies, imaging is often a valuable adjunct to the history and clinical examination. Each cranial nerve has a unique relationship to surrounding vascular, bony, and soft-tissue landmarks, and an understanding of the normal anatomy of cranial nerves is essential to interpreting radiographic images. The clinician must choose an appropriate imaging modality for the study of single or multiple cranial neuropathies and possible associated regional anatomy. The cranial nerve in its entirety is often best depicted with magnetic resonance imaging. Computed tomography is frequently a complementary adjunct to depict foramina and surrounding bony structures. This chapter will review common clinical presentations of cranial neuropathies, associated cranial nerve anatomy in brief, relevant radiographic studies, and important imaging findings.

*Keywords:* cranial nerve, cranial neuropathy, magnetic resonance imaging, computed tomography, imaging

## 12.1 Introduction

The skull base is an anatomically complex region encompassing the brain, orbits, cranial nerves (CNs), vessels, soft tissues, and multiple distinct bones. Many parts of this region are not directly accessible for clinical evaluation; thus, imaging plays an critical role in diagnosis and management. While a variety of imaging modalities are available, magnetic resonance (MR) imaging and computed tomography (CT) are the most commonly used studies to evaluate the skull base and CNs. These studies are complementary to each other and often are used in conjunction.[1,2,3,4]

MR imaging with contrast is helpful for the evaluation of the soft tissues surrounding the skull base, central nervous system (CNS), and CNs. MR imaging better characterizes soft tissues and is particularly sensitive in its depiction of intracranial, perineural, and perivascular spread of tumors. In addition, MR images can be acquired in any plane, allowing the examiner to tailor the study to the specific structure in question. For discussion purposes of this chapter, MR is the best modality for evaluation of the CNs themselves. On the other hand, CT is the imaging modality of choice for evaluating bony architecture and CN foramina. It is more sensitive in detecting calcifications within lesions and evaluating bony anatomy and pathology including fractures, erosion/dehiscence, sclerosis, and/or hyperostosis. Because these studies are complementary to each other, both MR and CT are often performed in the evaluation of lesions of the skull base and CNs.[3,4,5,6]

While imaging is often an important and necessary adjunct to the history and physical examination, the physician must be conscious of associated costs to patients. Price varies greatly among different examination types (CT vs. MRI), insurance groups (public vs. private), regional geography, and practice settings (academic vs. private). See ▶Table 12.1 for an example of cost comparison between different imaging modalities adapted from the Healthcare Bluebook website. Cost discrepancies also exist between practice types, as seen in a study comparing upper-tier academic hospitals to private radiology practices where the cost of a noncontrast head CT could range from $211 to $2,015 with the cost at academic centers significantly on the higher end of the spectrum.[7]

In addition, the physician should consider the potential safety issues associated with imaging studies. Measuring radiation exposure is complex, but the most widely accepted mechanism is for measuring effective dose of partial body irradiations.[8] Effective dose is reported in millisieverts (mSv) and is used to compare different types of radiation and imaging studies.[9] For reference, citizens of the United States are exposed to about 3 mSv (range 1–10 mSv) per year from ubiquitous background radiation. In comparison, a noncontrast brain CT may deliver 2 mSv and contrasted brain CT 4 mSv (range 1–10 mSv). This relatively low radiation dose is not thought to dramatically increase cancer risk. However, it should be kept in mind that multiple examinations over short periods of time may cause DNA damage that could lead to increased cancer risk.[10,11]

Similarly, there are concerns currently about the possible effects of gadolinium-based contrast material used in MR imaging studies. Concerns include deposition, impaired clearance from the body, and acute physiologic and hypersensitivity reactions. Deposition has been found to occur in skin, brain, bones, and liver. Elevated gadolinium presence in tissues theoretically can cause toxicity, but gadolinium deposition, even within the perivascular spaces of the brain, has not been associated with any known symptoms, and this is not currently well studied.[12] The only clinical entity that is definitively linked to gadolinium deposition is nephrogenic systemic fibrosis that occurs in some patients with renal dysfunction.[12,13,14] Acute adverse reactions range from mild to severe and include pruritus, edema, nausea/vomiting, chest pain, laryngeal edema, anaphylactic shock, hypotension, and/or seizures. The average acute adverse reaction rate is 0.06 to 0.3% of patients, which is similar or lower than with iodinated contrast agents.[12] Therefore, unintended patient safety outcomes from imaging studies must always be weighed with the clinical usefulness of the examination.

## 12.2 Cranial Nerve I: Olfactory Nerve

The anatomy of the olfactory nerve is unique. It is the shortest CN and does not arise from the brainstem. Instead, the cell bodies of the olfactory neurons are in the olfactory neuroepithelium, which is located in the upper part of the nasal cavity, the nasal septum, and the inner aspect of the superior nasal concha.

**Table 12.1** Cost of imaging techniques

| Study | Fair price ($) | Low end ($) | High end ($) |
|---|---|---|---|
| Noncontrast brain CT | 425 | 203 | 1,856 |
| Contrast brain CT | 503 | 329 | 2,099 |
| Noncontrast brain MRI | 808 | 414 | 3,456 |
| Contrast brain MRI | 921 | 465 | 4,474 |

The cell bodies transmit odor signals to the olfactory nerves, which pass through the cribriform plate of the ethmoid bone to reach the cranial cavity (▶Fig. 12.1). Nerve bundles form the olfactory bulbs and signals are then transmitted through the olfactory tract to the brain.[15,16,17]

MR imaging is the imaging modality best suited for visualizing the olfactory nerve. A standard examination protocol often includes thin-section T2-weighted images in the fast-spin echo mode in the coronal plane. This view allows for assessment of the anatomy of the olfactory apparatus, visualization of parenchymal lesions, and volumetry of the olfactory bulbs. CT is often a helpful clinical tool for evaluating the bony structure of the cribriform plate. It is most useful for the evaluation of craniofacial trauma in the acute setting. It also can be used to characterize bone disruption in chronic settings such as in

cerebral spinal fluid (CSF) leak. Other modalities and imaging techniques, such as X-ray, angiography, and positron emission tomography/CT (PET-CT), are often low yielding in assessing the olfactory nerve and are not often used.[2,4,16,17,18,19]

The clinical importance of the olfactory nerve is exhibited in cases of anosmia. The best first study for the evaluation of isolated anosmia is a sinus CT scan, including coronal plane reconstructions, because it can identify most lesions of the nasal vault and cribriform plate. In more complex cases of anosmia, MR of the brain with close attention to the anterior cranial fossa and sinonasal region can be used. The etiology for anosmia is broad and can include trauma, which transects the cribriform plate (▶Fig. 12.2), congenital disorders like Kallmann's syndrome in which the olfactory bulb is hypoplastic or absent (▶Fig. 12.3 and ▶Fig. 12.4), inflammatory disorders

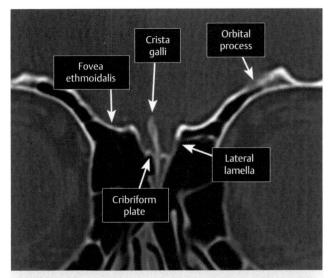

**Fig. 12.1** Coronal thin-section bone algorithm (maximum edge enhancement) CT through the anterior paranasal sinuses demonstrates the complex anatomy surrounding the olfactory bulbs, including the midline crista galli, cribriform plate, lateral lamella, fovea ethmoidalis, and the orbital process (*labeled arrows*).

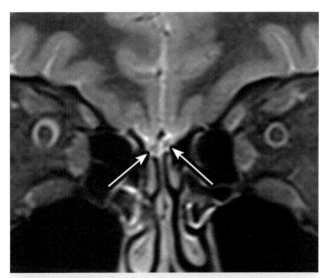

**Fig. 12.3** Coronal thin-section T2-weighted image demonstrates normal bilateral olfactory bulbs (*arrows*).

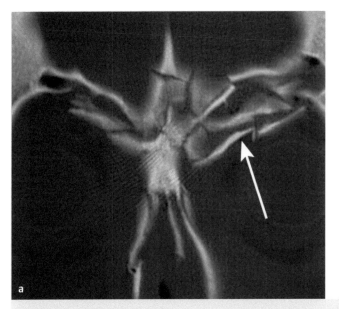

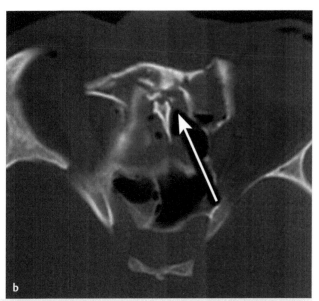

**Fig. 12.2** Axial (**a**) and coronal (**b**) thin-section bone algorithm CT images demonstrate complex orbito-nasal-ethmoid bilateral fractures (*arrows*).

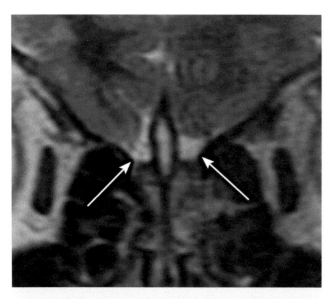

Fig. 12.4 Coronal thin-section T2-weighted image demonstrates absence of the bilateral olfactory bulbs (*arrows*).

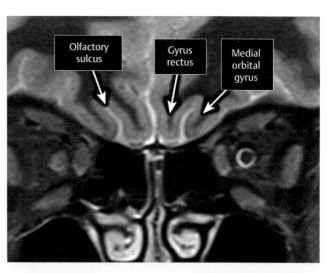

Fig. 12.5 Coronal thin-section T2-weighted image demonstrates the olfactory sulcus, with medial gyrus rectus, and lateral medial orbital gyrus (*labeled arrows*).

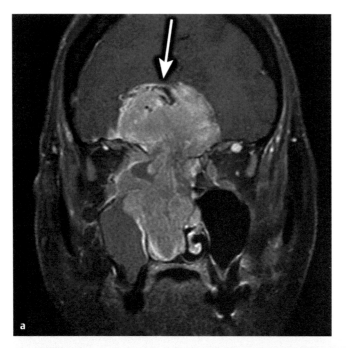
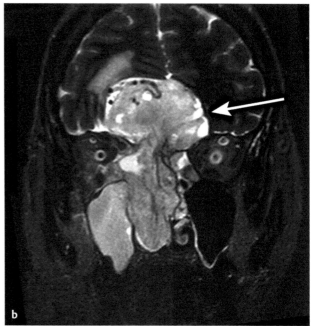

Fig. 12.6 Contrasted MRI coronal images of an esthesioneuroblastoma with T1 postcontrasted (**a**) and coronal T2-weighted (**b**) images demonstrate an enhancing lesions (**a**) with superior vasculature (*arrow*) centered at the cribriform plate, with peripheral cysts (**b**; *arrow*) between the lesion and brain parenchyma.

like sarcoidosis or granulomatosis, and neoplastic disorders, such as meningioma or esthesioneuroblastoma (▶Fig. 12.5 and ▶Fig. 12.6).

## 12.3 Cranial Nerve II: Optic Nerve

The optic nerve is an extension of the CNS and thus is surrounded by CSF and the meninges. Visual information is received by the rod and cone cells, which transmit signals to the retinal ganglion cells in the back of the globe. Retinal ganglion cells coalesce to form the optic nerve, which then passes posteriorly and medially in the orbital cavity to travel through the optic canal. The nerve then assumes a posteromedial direction to reach the optic chiasm where the optic nerves from each eye come together. In the chiasm, the temporal fibers of each optic nerve pass posteriorly and the nasal fibers of each optic nerve cross the midline to join the contralateral optic tract. Nerve fibers in each optic tract then pass visual signals along to the primary visual cortex of the brain through the optic radiations.[15,16,17]

MR is uniquely suited to image the entirety of the visual pathway from the globe to the visual cortex of the brain.

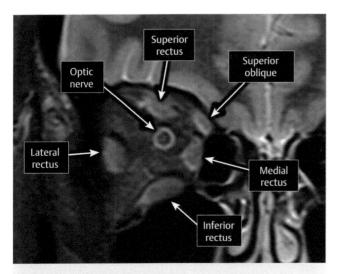

**Fig. 12.7** Coronal thin-section T2-weighted MR image through the orbit, posterior to the globe demonstrating larger anatomic structures (*labeled arrows*).

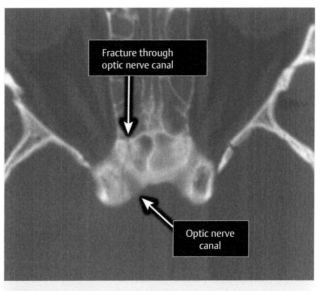

**Fig. 12.8** Axial thin-section bone algorithm CT through the level of the central skull base, demonstrating an acute fracture in the sagittal plane extending through the optic canal (*labeled arrows*).

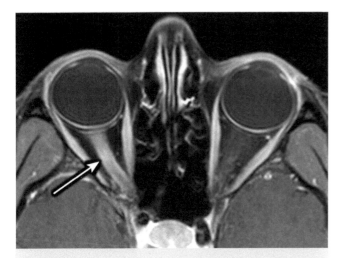

**Fig. 12.9** Axial thin-section T1-weighted postcontrasted image with fat saturation through the orbits demonstrates avid enhancement of the right optic nerve (*arrow*), consistent with optic neuritis.

A standard protocol for imaging the optic nerve, optic chiasm, and surrounding CSF involves T1-weighted axial and coronal images, and heavily T2-weighted images and short-tau inversion recovery (STIR) images. Intracranial portions of the optic nerve can be imaged using standard T1- and T2-weighted images (▶Fig. 12.7).[2,4,16,17,20] Complementary information can be provided by CT, which is a particularly sensitive modality for identifying fractures of the orbit and skull base that may affect the nerve. CT may also be used to evaluate the extraocular muscles, detect conal mass lesions, and characterize edema.[21] Other less common but useful imaging studies include optic coherence tomography (OCT) and orbital B-scan ultrasound. OCT can be used to distinguish retinal pathology versus optic neuropathy. Orbital B-scan ultrasound can be valuable in assessing abnormalities in which the optic nerve is thickened.[21]

In cases of suspected trauma, CT is the most appropriate first choice for imaging. CT allows for assessment of orbital and/or skull base fractures, orbital hematomas, intracranial injuries,

and possible radiopaque foreign bodies (▶Fig. 12.8). If there is no evidence of a metallic foreign body, MR may be useful to assess avulsion of the optic nerve, optic nerve sheath hematoma, axonal injury, or nerve ischemia.[20,21]

Patients with diseases of the visual pathway or surrounding structures will often present clinically with vision loss. The overall differential diagnosis for visual loss is broad, and the type of visual field defect (monocular loss, bitemporal hemianopia, homonymous hemianopia, quadrantanopia, etc.) may help the physician narrow the differential. This section will provide a brief glimpse of optic nerve pathology, specifically demyelinating disorders and neoplasms.

Multiple sclerosis (MS) is a commonly recognized demyelinating disease that is known for lesions that are disseminated in space and time. Many patients with MS suffer visual disabilities at some point in their disease. Specifically, the initial diagnosis of MS may result from the workup for optic neuritis that is seen on MRI as edema and avid optic nerve enhancement (▶Fig. 12.9). Various other autoimmune and infectious processes can also cause an optic neuropathy. Ophthalmic manifestations can be seen in cases of sarcoidosis, and rarely systemic lupus erythematosus. In all the above-listed circumstances, MRI in itself is often not diagnostic of the disease and further serologic studies, neuroimaging, and/or body imaging may need to be performed.[21,22,23]

There are many neoplasms that can involve the visual apparatus either directly or indirectly by compression. For patients with a suspected neoplasm, MR is the imaging modality of choice because it allows for the most complete evaluation of the optic nerve, optic chiasm, and extent of intraorbital and intracranial involvement. However, in many cases, CT is also necessary for differentiating between tumor types as it may reveal findings that are not detected on MR.[20,21,22] For example, MR in conjunction with CT is useful for differentiating between optic nerve gliomas (ONGs) and optic nerve sheath meningiomas (ONSMs). On MRI, ONGs often have a fusiform appearance and the optic nerve may appear kinked at the midorbit. ONGs are typically isointense on T1-weighted images and isointense

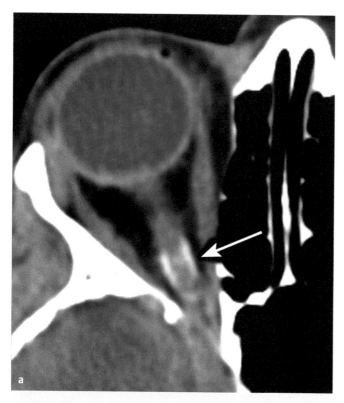
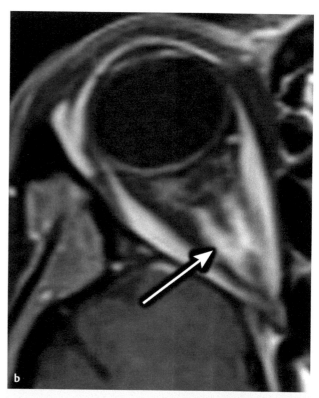

**Fig. 12.10** Axial thin-section standard algorithm CT (**a**) and correlating axial thin-section T1-weighted postcontrasted MR image with fat saturation (**b**) show linear "tram-tracking" calcifications (**a**, *arrow*) along the optic nerve and avid enhancement (**b**; *arrow*) tracking along the optic nerve, consistent with an optic nerve meningioma.

to hyperintense on T2-weighted images (▶Fig. 12.10). In contrast, ONSMs may be tubular, globular, fusiform, or focal on MR. They are hypointense to isointense on T1-weighted images and slightly hyperintense on T2-weighted images. CT is particularly valuable in assessment of ONSMs, as it may show dural tail, CSF cleft, bony erosion, and/or hyperostosis in the region surrounding the lesion. ONSMs also characteristically exhibit tram track or bull's eye signs, which are hyperdense enhancement of meninges surrounding a hypodense nerve, and this can be seen on both MR and CT (▶Fig. 12.11).[20,21,22]

## 12.4 Cranial Nerves III, IV, and VI: Oculomotor, Trochlear, and Abducens Nerves

For the purposes of this chapter, these three ocular nerves will be discussed together. High-yield anatomy of the oculomotor, trochlear, and abducens nerves is reviewed briefly in this section. The oculomotor nerve arises from the anterior surface of the midbrain and extends anteriorly and laterally, passing between the posterior cerebral artery (PCA) and superior cerebral artery (SCA) vessels (▶Fig. 12.12). The nerve then enters the oculomotor cistern within the superior and lateral wall of the cavernous sinus, and then continues superiorly and laterally through the superior orbital fissure. It passes through the annular tendon, and then branches into a superior and inferior division, which then supply a majority of the extraocular muscles including the medial, lateral, dorsal rectus, and

ventral oblique muscles as well as the levator palpebrae superioris muscle.[15,16,17]

The trochlear nerve has the longest intracranial cisternal course and is the only nerve to arise from the dorsal aspect of the midbrain, and it then crosses midline to the contralateral side, traveling lateral to the midbrain (▶Fig. 12.13). The nerve then passes through the lateral wall of the cavernous sinus, exits through the superior orbital fissure, passes superior to the annular tendon, and terminates in the superior oblique muscle.[15,16,17]

The abducens nerve arises from the pontomedullary junction off midline, then extends superiorly to enter the abducens cistern (▶Fig. 12.14). The nerve then passes through the cavernous sinus, then the superior orbital fissure, and ends in the lateral rectus muscle.[15,16,17]

The oculomotor, trochlear, and abducens nerves can be divided into segments. Each nerve has four segments: intra-axial, cisternal, cavernous, and extracranial or intraorbital. The abducens nerve also has a fifth segment, which is intradural. MR is the best imaging modality for visualization of each one of the ocular nerves. Additionally, there are specific MR imaging sequences (thin-section T2-weighted or CSF bright) that can be reconstructed in oblique planes tailored to imaging each nerve segment (▶Fig. 12.2, ▶Fig. 12.3, and ▶Fig. 12.14). Complementary CT can assist to better examine the skull base, osseous borders of the CN foramina, and the orbital walls.[24,25,26,27]

Patients with lesions involving the ocular nerves often will present clinically with diplopia. It is important to note that patients are much less likely to present with an isolated ocular nerve palsy. More often, ocular nerve palsies present in conjunction with multiple other cranial neuropathies, and this

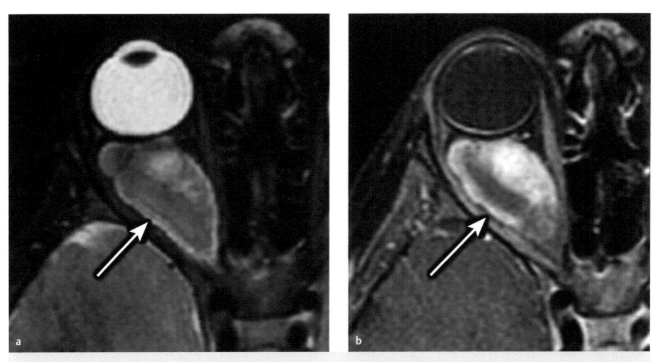

**Fig. 12.11** Axial thin-section T2-weighted (**a**) and correlating axial T1-weighted postcontrasted MR image (**b**), both with fat saturation, demonstrate well-circumscribed enlargement of the optic nerve with enhancement (**b**), without surrounding aggressive changes, consistent with an optic nerve glioma.

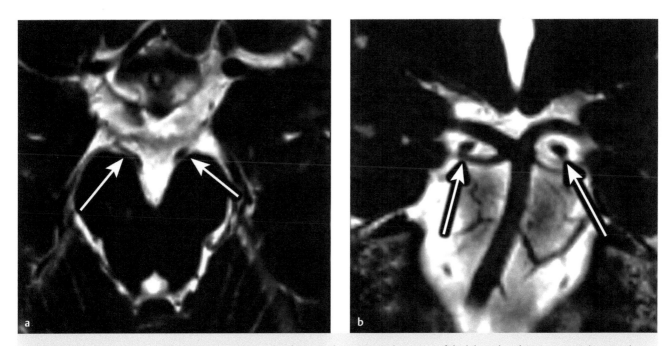

**Fig. 12.12** Axial (**a**) and coronal (**b**) thin-section T2-weighted images demonstrate the origins of the bilateral oculomotor nerves (**a**; *arrows*) arising from the anterior midbrain, and extending between the posterior cerebral artery vessels superiorly and the superior cerebral artery vessels inferiorly in the coronal plane (**b**; *arrows*).

constellation of symptoms may lead the clinician to a more specific diagnosis, and more focused imaging evaluations.

A complete oculomotor nerve palsy causes the eye to stay locked in a "down and out" position. Thirty percent of isolated oculomotor nerve palsies are caused by aneurysms, and these often arise from the origin of the posterior communicating artery (PCOM; ▶Fig. 12.15). Pupillary involvement is classic in these patients. In the cases where an aneurysm is highly suspected, with this clinical presentation, the best first imaging study remains MRI, which can demonstrate a variety of lesions, with an MR angiogram. A CT angiogram and/or a catheter angiogram can also assist with vascular evaluation. Additional causes of an isolated third nerve palsy include lesions near the brainstem. These lesions may include arteriovenous malformations and cavernous hemangiomas, which can bleed and cause palsy, infarctions, brainstem gliomas, schwannomas, demyelinating lesions, or traumatic shearing injuries.[4,24,25,27]

Isolated trochlear nerve palsy is uncommon. However, if it were to occur, the patient would present with an oblique diplopia that worsens when the affected eye looks nasally. Because this nerve has the longest cisternal segment, it is most likely to be affected by shearing or stretching forces as the result of trauma, and head trauma is the commonest cause of injury.[25] Conventional MR imaging may demonstrate atrophy of the superior oblique muscle with prolonged injury, but high-resolution MR imaging is needed to visualize the nerve itself. Rarely, the nerve palsy may be the result of congenital absence or affected by infection, infarction, hemorrhage, or demyelinating lesions.[4,24,25,27,28]

Isolated abducens nerve palsy causes a horizontal diplopia. Syndromes that cause elevated intracranial pressures may cause abducens palsy with compression of the nerve as it travels over sharp ridges of the clivus and petrous temporal bone. Similarly to the other oculomotor nerves, isolated abducens palsy may be caused by infection, infarction, hemorrhage, tumors, or demyelinating lesions.[4,24,25,27]

Patients who present with multiple CN palsies, specifically CNs III, IV, V, and VI should draw high suspicion for involvement of the cavernous sinus. Lesions in this region may affect any one of these ocular nerves but commonly involve all three. The differential for cavernous sinus lesion is broad and may include carotid aneurysms, carotid dissection, carotid-cavernous fistula, cavernous sinus thrombosis, infarction, infection, tumor, and idiopathic orbital inflammatory disease (IOID). Less commonly, patients may have pituitary adenoma or lesions from the paranasal sinuses or nasopharynx that may invade the cavernous sinus.[4,24,25,27] Patients with cavernous sinus thrombosis typically exhibit symptoms of eyelid edema, conjunctival injection, orbital pain, and proptosis. With high clinical suspicion, the best initial imaging study is contrasted

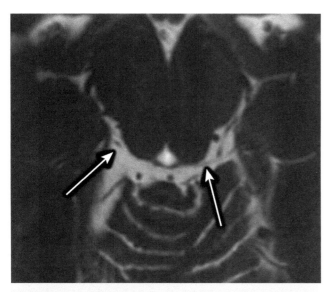

**Fig. 12.13** Axial thin-section T2-weighted MR image demonstrates the bilateral small trochlear nerves (*arrows*) arising from the posterior midbrain.

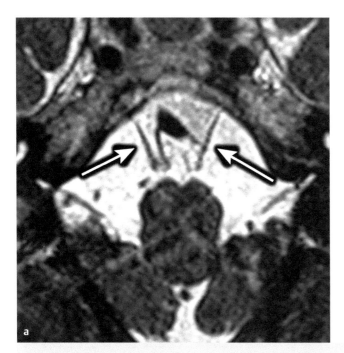
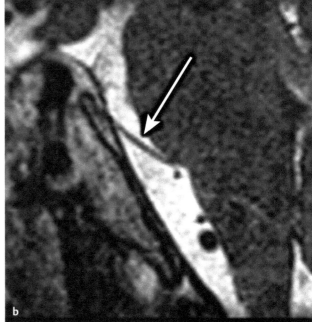

**Fig. 12.14** Axial steep oblique thin-section T2-weighted section (**a**) and sagittal off-midline MR images demonstrate the abducens nerves, arising from the anterior off-midline pontomedullary junction (**a**; *arrows*) and extending superiorly through the prepontine cistern (**b**; *arrow*) to enter the cavernous sinus.

MR with MR venogram as it will show absence of enhancement within the cavernous sinus (▶ Fig. 12.16).[4,24,25,27] A rare but often cited cause of cavernous sinus lesion is IOID (or Tolosa–Hunt syndrome). Patients characteristically present with severe unilateral headaches, orbital pain, and ophthalmoplegia. The classic imaging finding in this syndrome is asymmetric cavernous sinus enhancement from inflammation of the cavernous sinus. Patients exhibit characteristic MR imaging findings and often require serial imaging to assess for response to steroids (▶ Fig. 12.17).[24,25,27,29]

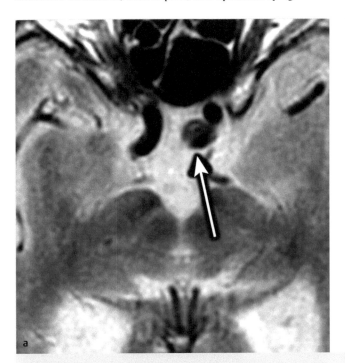
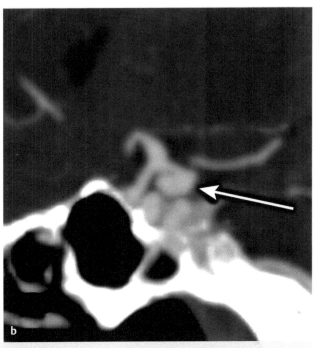

**Fig. 12.15** Axial thin-section T2-weighted MR image (**a**) demonstrates a left posterior communicating artery (PCOM) aneurysm (*arrow*) at the left anterior circle of Willis. Sagittal reconstruction (**b**) image from a CT angiography study shows the PCOM aneurysm arising from the posterior left internal carotid artery (*arrow*).

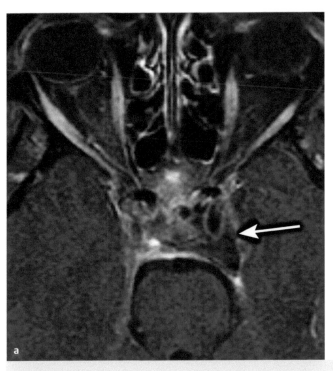
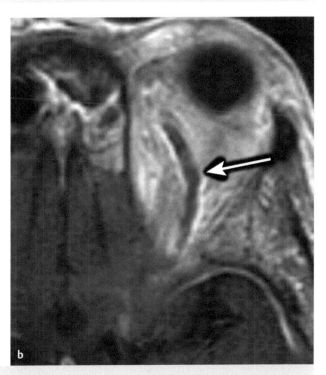

**Fig. 12.16** Axial thin-section T1-weighted postcontrasted fat-saturated image (**a**) demonstrates abnormal lack of contrast enhancement within the left cavernous sinus (*arrow*), consistent with cavernous sinus thrombosis. Axial T1-weighted postcontrasted image (**b**) shows abnormal enlargement of the left superior ophthalmic vein (*arrow*).

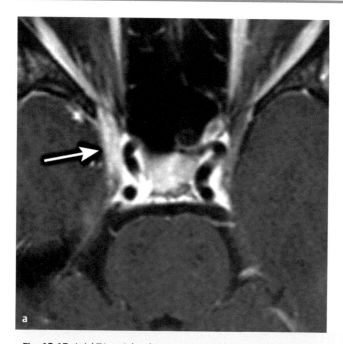
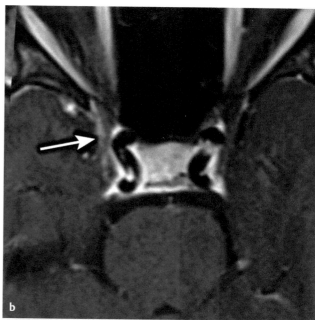

**Fig. 12.17** Axial T1-weighted postcontrasted fat saturated MR image (**a**) in a patient with abnormal enhancement within the right cavernous sinus (*arrow*), consistent with orbital inflammatory disease (IOID) or Tolosa-Hunt syndrome. (**b**) Follow-up similar axial thin-section postcontrasted T1-weighted MR image with fat saturation a year later demonstrated resolution of the prior right cavernous sinus enhancement (*arrow*).

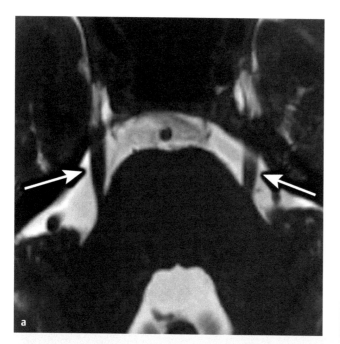
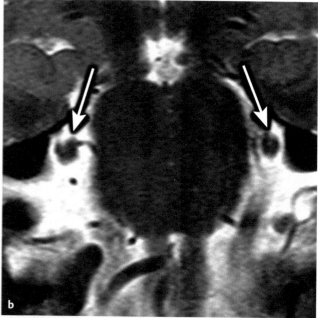

**Fig. 12.18** Axial thin-section T2-weighted MR image (**a**) through the mid-pons demonstrates the large nerve bundle fibers of the bilateral trigeminal nerves (*arrows*). Coronal thin-section T2-weighted image (**b**) demonstrates the large nerve bundles in cross-section (*arrows*) lateral to the pons.

## 12.5 Cranial Nerve V: Trigeminal Nerve

The trigeminal nerve is the primary sensory nerve of the face and provides motor innervation to the muscles of mastication. It is the largest of all the CNs and has three divisions: ophthalmic (CN $V_1$), maxillary (CN $V_2$), and mandibular (CN $V_3$). Briefly, the trigeminal nerve arises from the lateral pons, enters the trigeminal cistern (Meckel's cave) in the middle cranial fossa and forms the trigeminal ganglion, and splits into three divisions (▶Fig. 12.18). The ophthalmic division passes through cavernous sinus and then the superior orbital fissure to exit at the supraorbital foramen, and receives sensory information from the tip of the nose and the skin of the face above the orbit.

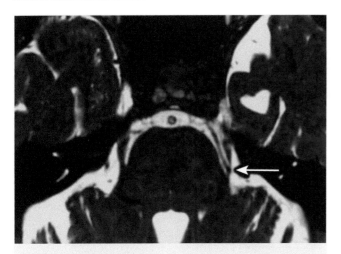

**Fig. 12.19** Axial thin-section T2-weighted MR image through the mid-pons shows a left-sided vascular loop (*arrow*) significantly displacing the left trigeminal nerve root entry zone, in a patient with left-sided trigeminal neuralgia, consistent with a trigeminal vascular loop syndrome.

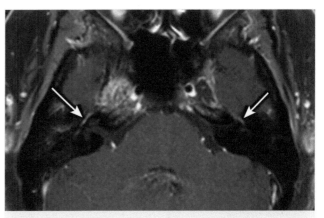

**Fig. 12.20** Axial thin-section T1-weighted postcontrasted MR image with fat saturation demonstrates bilateral normal enhancement along the facial nerves (*arrows*), with the left geniculate ganglion and slight enhancement along the left greater superficial petrosal nerve.

It also supplies sensory information from the cornea, paranasal sinuses, and nasal mucosa. The maxillary division passes through the cavernous sinus, then through foramen rotundum, into the pterygopalatine fossa. It then extends laterally through the pterygomaxillary fissure, into the retromaxillary fat pad, and turns anteriorly in the sagittal plane to exit at the infraorbital foramen. It receives sensory information from the skin between the inferior eyelid and the superior lip, maxillary teeth, paranasal sinuses, and nasal mucosa. The mandibular division passes inferiorly from the trigeminal cistern through the foramen ovale. It receives sensory information from the skin of the mandible, mandibular teeth, oral mucous membranes, and the anterior two-thirds of the tongue. It also supplies motor innervation to the muscles of mastication including the medial and lateral pterygoids, temporalis, and masseter.[15,16,17]

MR imaging is the best modality for evaluating the trigeminal nerve due to its superior tissue contrast and multiplanar capability. Often the entire nerve must be imaged, and MR captures the distal and proximal nerve divisions as well as the trigeminal ganglion most accurately. MR or CT angiography may be obtained to evaluate neurovascular pathology. CT is often required in conjunction to MRI to provide a detailed map of the bony anatomy of the skull base and foramina. In cases of trauma, CT should be the first-choice modality.[30,31,32,33,34]

Clinically, patients with trigeminal nerve dysfunction will present with facial pain or numbness, or disorders of the muscles of mastication. In patients with idiopathic trigeminal neuralgia, electrophysiological studies should be normal. When abnormal, this should make the clinician question if there may be some underlying anatomic pathology, and the patient should undergo MR imaging evaluation. The most common cause of trigeminal neuralgia is due to compression by a vascular loop displacing the root entry zone of the trigeminal nerve. Criteria for confirmation of neurovascular compression include contact of a vessel with the nerve, perpendicular course to the nerve axis, and subsequent indentation, deviation, atrophy and/or encasement of the nerve. The relationship between nerve and blood vessel is best demonstrated by thin-section T2-weighted or CSF bright

MR sequences and MR angiography (▶Fig. 12.19). Similar to the other CNs, the trigeminal nerve may be affected by infarcts, hemorrhages, demyelinating diseases, tumors, or metastasis, and these pathologies are best investigated by MR imaging.[4,30,32,35,36,37]

## 12.6 Cranial Nerve VII: Facial Nerve

The facial nerve is the primary motor nerve of the voluntary and involuntary muscles of facial expression. It arises from the inferolateral pons and passes with the vestibulocochlear nerve through the cerebellopontine angle (CPA) cistern and internal auditory canal (IAC). It then takes a serpiginous course through temporal bone and exits the skull in the stylomastoid foramen. The nerve then pierces the parotid gland and sends terminal branches to the facial muscles.[4,15,16,17]

In contrast to the other CNs, a variety of settings exist in which CT is the primary imaging modality of the facial nerve. For example, CT is preferred for lesions of the labyrinthine, temporal, and mastoid segment osseous borders. It is favored in osseous abnormalities that may affect the nerve such as fibrous dysplasia, Paget's disease, or osteoporosis. More specifically, CT temporal bone is the most appropriate modality in the setting of congenital malformation, temporal bone fracture, and middle ear pathologies. On the other hand, lesions of the intracanalicular, cisternal, or intra-axial segments are best imaged on MR. It is normal with modern thin-section MR imaging to see segmental enhancement along the intratemporal facial nerve, especially at the tympanic segment (▶Fig. 12.20). MR imaging is also preferred for evaluation of perineural tumor spread, hemifacial spasm, and herpetic (Bell's) palsy (though routine imaging is not recommended for a typical herpetic palsy).[38] CT and MR imaging are complimentary for evaluation of facial nerve tumors (▶Fig. 12.21).[39,40,41]

Clinically, patients with facial nerve dysfunction typically present with facial paralysis. While the etiology is broad, there are a variety of common conditions that are most appropriately diagnosed clinically rather than by imaging. Selected topics for discussion will include herpetic palsy, otitis media, and herpes zoster oticus (Ramsay–Hunt syndrome).

Herpetic palsy is the most common cause of peripheral facial nerve injury. Given that the diagnosis is straightforward,

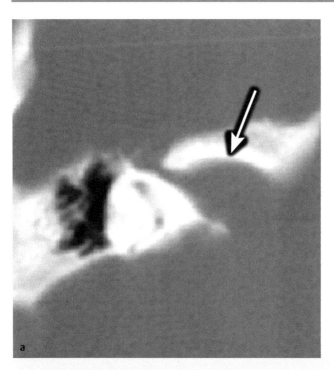
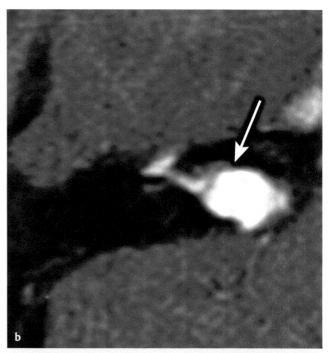

**Fig. 12.21** Axial thin-section bone algorithm CT (**a**) and correlating axial thin-section T1-weighted postcontrasted MR image (**b**) demonstrate enlargement of the right internal auditory canal (**a**; *arrow*) with avid enhancement (**b**; *arrow*) extending along the labyrinthine segment of the facial nerve anteriorly and laterally to the geniculate ganglion, consistent with a facial nerve schwannoma.

imaging is rarely recommended. MR imaging may be recommended in selected atypical cases in which paralysis persists for a prolonged period of time (>3 months), the palsy is slowly progressive, there is a clinical history suggesting a specific etiology, for example, a cutaneous malignancy, or if there is recurrent palsy. In these cases, MR imaging may show abnormal enhancement of the entire intratemporal segments of the facial nerve, as well as a tuft of nodular enhancement within the lateral IAC at the opening of the labyrinthine segment of the facial nerve.

Herpes zoster oticus is another well-known inflammatory disorder of the facial nerve that is caused by the varicella-zoster virus. There is a clinical triad of otalgia, vesicles in the external auditory canal, and ipsilateral facial paralysis. The clinical diagnosis is straightforward and imaging is reserved for unusual cases. Herpes zoster oticus will often involve the inner ear. In the cases present with asymmetric sensorineural hearing loss, imaging may be indicated to rule out retrocochlear pathology. Similarly to a herpetic palsy, MR imaging demonstrates abnormal enhancement of the facial nerve segments within the temporal bone, but with linear enhancement along the facial nerve in the IAC.

Otitis media is another cause of facial nerve dysfunction that is more appropriately diagnosed clinically than by imaging. The signs and symptoms of otitis media are generally obvious to the clinician. In addition, it is known that approximately 50% of patients have a congenital dehiscence of the inferior wall of the tympanic segment of the facial nerve, making it particularly susceptible to infection and inflammation that may extend into the otic capsule. In equivocal cases, CT may demonstrate middle ear opacification that abuts the facial nerve canal. MR imaging may be useful to determine the extent of infectious spread.[39,40,42]

Other conditions in which imaging of the facial nerve is appropriate and often necessary for diagnosis include neoplasms, vascular, congenital, and traumatic etiologies. Overall, primary tumors of the facial nerve are rare with facial nerve schwannoma being the most common type. Patients with schwannoma typically have some element of facial paralysis combined with hearing loss. MR imaging demonstrates an enhancing lesion usually involving multiple segments of the nerve. Characteristically, facial nerve schwannomas are often dumbbell shaped with extension from the IAC to the geniculate ganglion. They are typically isointense to hypointense on T1-weighted images prior to contrast administration and hyperintense on T2-weighted images, with avid enhancement following contrast. CT is complimentary and commonly demonstrates smooth osseous expansion without bony erosion or destruction. There may be evidence of destruction of the ossicular chain if the schwannoma arises from the mastoid or tympanic segment (▶Fig. 12.21).[39,41,43,44]

As in other traumatic cases, imaging is often needed to assess facial nerve injury, and a thin-section bone algorithm (maximum edge enhancement algorithm) CT is the best modality for evaluation of the intratemporal bone segments. Specifically, temporal bone CT with submillimeter cuts is used to evaluate possible temporal bone fractures that may extend into the facial nerve canal and/or otic capsule. While most temporal bone fractures are longitudinal, transverse fractures are more likely to result in facial paralysis. Imaging is often important in cases of trauma because facial paralysis is often delayed and incomplete. High suspicion for nerve involvement based on imaging studies may tailor the clinician's use of serial monitoring or steroids (▶Fig. 12.22 and ▶Fig. 12.23).[39,40,41]

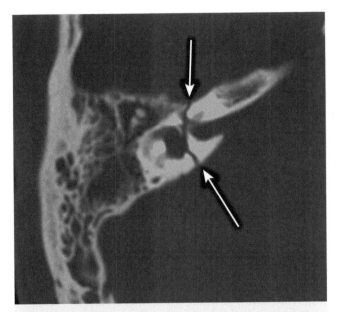

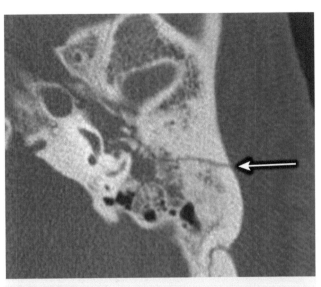

**Fig. 12.22** Axial thin-section bone algorithm CT of the right temporal bone demonstrates a transverse fracture (*arrows*) extending through the right labyrinthine segment of the facial nerve anteriorly and superior vestibular canal and medial vestibule posteriorly.

**Fig. 12.23** Axial thin-section bone algorithm CT of the left temporal bone shows a longitudinal fracture (*arrow*) extending toward the middle ear cavity with separation of the malleus and incus.

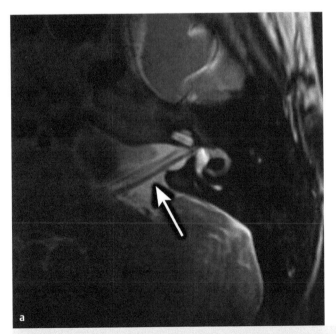

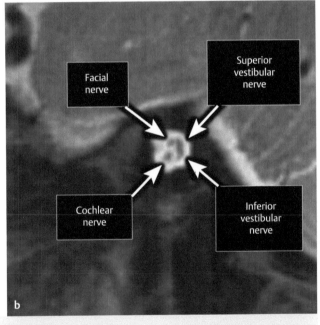

Facial nerve

Superior vestibular nerve

Cochlear nerve

Inferior vestibular nerve

**Fig. 12.24** Axial thin-section T2-weighted MR image (**a**) demonstrates the normal larger vestibulocochlear nerve (*arrow*) posterior to the facial nerve within the cerebellopontine angle and the internal auditory canal (IAC). Thin-section oblique sagittal T2-weighted MR image (**b**) obtained perpendicular to the long axis of the IAC demonstrates the nerves within the midportion of the IAC (*labeled arrows*), with the anterior and superior facial nerves, anterior and inferior cochlear nerves, and the posterior combined superior and inferior vestibular nerves.

# 12.7 Cranial Nerve VIII: Vestibulocochlear Nerve

The vestibulocochlear nerve is a special sensory nerve involved in hearing and balance. It arises from the inferolateral pons, and transverses the CPA and IAC parallel to the facial nerve. At the midportion of the IAC, it divides into the vestibular nerve and the cochlear nerve (▶ Fig. 12.24). The vestibular nerve then divides into a superior and inferior division within the lateral IAC and receives sensory information from the vestibule (saccule and utricle) and three semicircular canals. The superior vestibular nerve extends through the superior vestibular canal posterior to the labyrinthine segment of the facial nerve, dividing into the utricular nerve, the superior ampullary nerve, and the lateral ampullary nerve. The inferior vestibular nerve divides into the posterior ampullary nerve, which courses through the singular canal to the posterior semicircular canal ampulla, and the saccular nerve, which passes through the inferior vestibular canal to the saccule. Fibers from the spiral ganglia populating the modiolus coalesce to form the cochlear nerve and receive sensory information from the basilar membrane; the cochlear nerve then leaves the posterior modiolus and extends through the cochlear nerve canal into the IAC to reach the CPA and pons.[15,16,17]

Like most other CNs, the vestibulocochlear nerve is best visualized on MR imaging. MR is used to evaluate the CPA, IAC, and brain. MR is particularly sensitive for identifying the labyrinthine and cochlear structures, and potentially enlarged endolymphatic duct and sac, and perilymphatic fluid. CT is complementary to better visualize the osseous structures of the dense otic capsule. Likewise, CT is important in evaluation of the middle ear bones and in cases of trauma.

Lesions of the vestibulocochlear nerve often present clinically with hearing loss, tinnitus, or vertigo. The vestibulocochlear nerve and important ear structures may be afflicted by infection, inflammation, vasculopathies, demyelinating diseases, tumors, and metastasis. One of the more common presentations of audiovestibular neuropathy is vestibular neuritis. Patients generally present with an acute onset of severe vertigo with associated nausea, vomiting, and balance issues. In most cases, a diagnosis can be reached with a complete history and physical examination. However, CT of the temporal bone may be indicated in patients who are suspected to have intracranial pathology of otologic origin in patients who have known chronic ear disease. Likewise, MR imaging may be indicated to identify a central cause in patients who display other neurological abnormalities.[45,46]

Imaging is particularly helpful in defining retrocochlear pathology, such as acoustic neuromas. Patients with an acoustic neuroma most often present with unilateral hearing loss, and MR imaging is a key component of the workup. Acoustic neuromas are rounded masses that almost always arise from within the IAC. These tumors exhibit mass effect on surrounding structures including erosion and widening of the IAC. They are most commonly hypointense on T1-weighted images before contrast and hypointense on T2-weighted images, presenting as a filling defect on CSF bright sequences. Smaller tumors are most often homogenously enhancing, but larger tumors may enhance heterogeneously with cystic regions and/or areas of hemorrhage (▶ Fig. 12.25).[47,48,49,50] There is much debate among clinicians about the role of surgical management, radiation, or observation with serial imaging of acoustic neuromas. Suggested growth rate per year of acoustic neuromas is about 1 to 2 mm. While a faster rate of tumor growth often predicts accelerated hearing loss, there currently are no reliable indicators for which patients are more at risk for rapid growth of their tumors. Given the variable pattern in growth behavior, there is no definitive recommendation for frequency of follow-up visits or length of observation periods. However, it is generally recommended that if the chosen management strategy is observation, the first follow-up MR imaging should occur at 6 to 12 months. If no growth is detected at that point, future visits can be scheduled at yearly intervals, until a history of dormancy is established. It is important to note that tumor growth of 2.5 mm per year or greater has been associated with higher rates of hearing loss.[51] Treatment of patients with acoustic neuromas is very individualized. In general, younger patients with large tumors are often treated surgically. Older patients with small tumors tend to be recommended for stereotactic radiation. Hearing preservation has been described in the surgical management of patients with small tumors.[52,53,54,55]

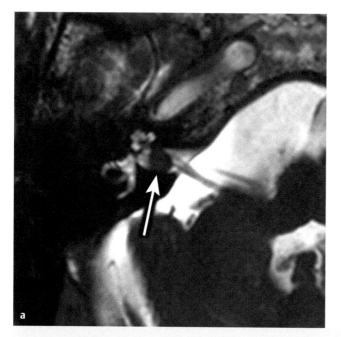 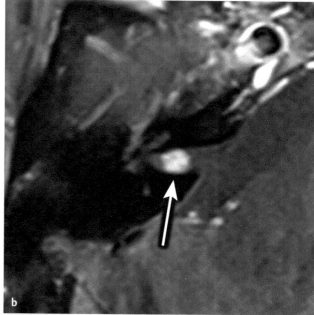

**Fig. 12.25** Axial thin-section T2-weighted MR image (**a**) and correlating axial thin-section T1-weighted postcontrasted fat-saturated image (**b**) demonstrates a T2 filling defect within the mid-IAC (**a**; *arrow*), with avid enhancement following contrast administration (**b**; *arrow*), most likely representing a vestibulocochlear schwannoma.

## 12.8 Cranial Nerves IX, X, and XI: Glossopharyngeal, Vagus, and Spinal Accessory Nerves

For the purposes of this chapter, the glossopharyngeal, vagus, and spinal accessory nerves will be discussed together. While these lower CNs do have their own intrinsic pathologies, often these nerves are affected together where they pass through the jugular foramen (▶Fig. 12.26).

The glossopharyngeal nerve provides motor and sensory innervation to the pharynx and parasympathetic fibers for taste and salivation. This nerve arises from the medulla oblongata, runs through the jugular foramen pars nervosa, and then passes through vasculature and musculature before diving into branches.[4,15,17] The vagus nerve likewise supplies motor and sensory innervation to the pharynx as well as the larynx, parasympathetic fibers for taste and salivation, and parasympathetic innervation to the gastrointestinal tract. It arises from the medulla, passes through the jugular foramen pars vascularis, and then descends into the suprahyoid neck carotid space. The right vagus nerve gives off the recurrent laryngeal nerve branch, which wraps around the subclavian artery. The left vagus nerve gives off branches to the esophagus, lungs, and heart, and then the recurrent laryngeal nerve branch wraps around the aorta. Both nerve branches innervate the intrinsic muscles of the larynx.[4,15,17] The spinal accessory nerve is an interesting CN in that it has both a cranial root and a spinal root. The cranial component arises from the vagus nerve, and the spinal component arises from the first five to six cervical spinal nerves. These spinal branches come together to form a nerve root, ascend through the foramen magnum, and

join with the cranial root. After joining, the nerve then passes through the jugular foramen pars vascularis with the vagus nerve. It then splits to send branches along with the vagus nerve and branches to supply the sternocleidomastoid and trapezius muscles.[4,15,17]

The mainstay for assessing these nerves is MR imaging of the skull base and neck. MR imaging has the capability to demonstrate pathologies of the brainstem and cervical spinal cord, skull base, carotid sheath, neck, and mediastinum. The multiplanar capabilities of MR imaging allow for visualization of the nerves throughout their length and in cross-section. MR imaging also can assess end-organ denervation, which can manifest as atrophy and fatty infiltration of pharyngeal, soft palate, sternocleidomastoid, and trapezius muscles. CT is commonly the first imaging modality to assess neck and chest pathologies. Otherwise, it is complementary to demonstrate changes in bony anatomy, especially when imaging the jugular foramen. Ultrasound is less commonly used to evaluate gross lesions along the course of the nerves through the neck but may be helpful in guiding biopsy procedures.[56,57,58,59]

Clinically, disorders affecting the glossopharyngeal and vagus nerves present with dysphagia and hoarseness. Neurofibromas and schwannomas may affect these nerves; however, lesions intrinsic to the nerves are rare. More often, they are injured iatrogenically as with cardiac procedures near the carotid arteries. However, the recurrent laryngeal nerve branch of the vagus nerve may suffer consequences of inflammation or viral illness, and patients will present with unilateral vocal fold paralysis. The recurrent laryngeal nerve likewise may be injured iatrogenically or may be involved in apical lung tumors or thyroid neoplasms.[4,56,57]

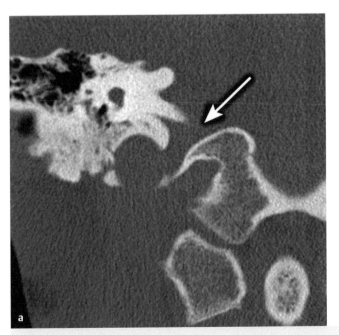 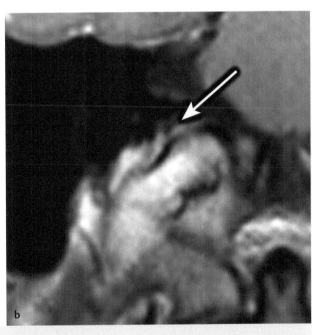

**Fig. 12.26** Thin-section bone algorithm CT (**a**) and correlating coronal thin-section postcontrasted T1-weighted MR image (**b**) demonstrate the jugular foramen (*arrows*) containing the internal jugular vein and cranial nerves IX, X, and XI.

Disorders affecting the spinal accessory nerve present with shoulder dysfunction, specifically winging of the scapula and weakness in shoulder shrug. Patients may also have weak head turn to the affected side. Most often, this nerve is injured iatrogenically in procedures like neck dissections, those which involve the branchial plexus, or lymph node biopsies in the posterior neck.[15,56]

Lesions at the jugular foramen may affect all three of these nerves. The differential predominantly includes paragangliomas and nerve sheath tumors, trauma at the skull base, infections, or vascular compression. Paragangliomas (historically glomus tumors) typically compress the glossopharyngeal, vagus, and spinal accessory nerves within the jugular foramen. On MR imaging, jugular paragangliomas that are highly vascular usually display contrast enhancement, flow voids, and a salt-and-pepper appearance (▶Fig. 12.27). On CT, they may demonstrate bony infiltration or destruction like moth-eaten permeative destructive erosion of the jugular foramen and loss of the caroticojugular spine (▶Fig. 12.28). Angiography may be useful to assess vascularity of these tumors and to perform preoperative embolization.[56,57,59]

## 12.9 Cranial Nerve XII: Hypoglossal Nerve

The hypoglossal nerve is the primary motor nerve of the tongue. It arises from the medulla and passes through the hypoglossal canal. The nerve receives some somatic and motor sensory fibers from C1 and C2 and then takes a somewhat tumultuous course through the face and neck, traversing between and around other important neurovascular structures, then sends off branches to the tongue and suprahyoid muscles.[4,15,17]

Like most other CNs, the hypoglossal nerve is best imaged with MR studies. MR can be used to evaluate the nerve at the skull base and along its cisternal length with thin T2-weighted

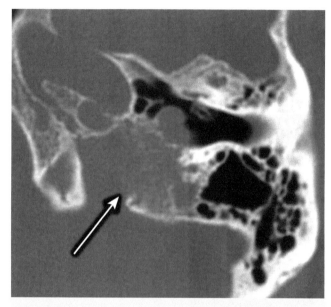

**Fig. 12.28** Axial thin-section bone algorithm CT image through the jugular foramen demonstrates the permeative destructive osseous changes (*arrow*) consistent with a left jugular paraganglioma.

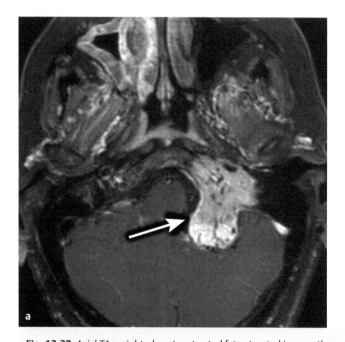
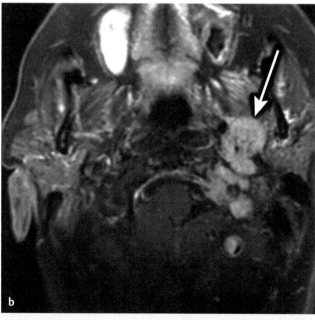

**Fig. 12.27** Axial T1-weighted postcontrasted fat-saturated images through the level of the jugular foramen (**a**) demonstrate a large left jugular foramen mass (*arrow*) with multiple flow voids ("pepper") often described with a jugular foramen paraganglioma. The second image (**b**) demonstrates the inferior extension of the mass into the suprahyoid neck carotid space (*arrow*).

or CSF bright MRI sequences (►Fig. 12.29). CT is a useful complementary study to evaluate related bony structures and the hypoglossal canal and foramina and is often used to evaluate the suprahyoid neck and oral cavity as the hypoglossal nerve fibers extend through the sublingual spaces (►Fig. 12.30).[60,61]

Clinically, peripheral lesions of the hypoglossal nerve present with tongue weakness, dysarthria, and/or difficulty eating.

On examination, the tongue will deviate toward the side of the lesion and may exhibit atrophy. Injury to the hypoglossal nerve at the skull base may be caused by fractures, anatomic variabilities of nearby blood vessels, dissection of the internal carotid artery, paragangliomas, neural sheath tumors, metastases, or extension of extracranial neoplasms (►Fig. 12.31). In the sublingual space, injury to the hypoglossal nerve may be caused by local malignancies, for example, oral cavity squamous cell carcinomas or salivary gland malignancies (►Fig. 12.32). Other etiologies include infections and iatrogenic complications such as following neckdissection.[60,61]

## 12.10 Multiple Cranial Neuropathies

Rather than presenting with isolated nerve dysfunction, many patients exhibit multiple cranial neuropathies. This can be distressing to both the patient and the clinician. However, there is an intimate association among many CNs as they course through the skull base and throughout the head and neck. If the clinician has a solid foundation of CN anatomy, specific patterns of CN injury may be useful in guiding diagnosis and treatment planning. As mentioned throughout this chapter, MR is often the most useful imaging study for evaluating cranial neuropathies. Depending on the scenario, CT, angiography, and ultrasound may be additional useful diagnostic tools.[62,63]

## 12.11 Conclusion

Imaging plays a critical role in defining CN anatomy and pathology related to the CNs. MRI and CT imaging provide complementary imaging information. A discerning clinician will know when to order appropriate imaging to aid in the clinical evaluation and treatment of patients with cranial neuropathies.

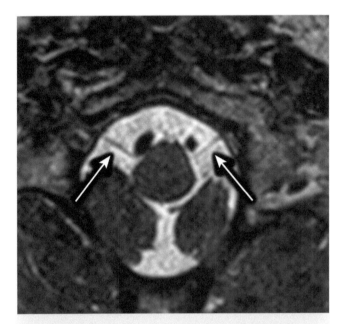

**Fig. 12.29** Axial thin-section T2-weighted MR image through the level of the hypoglossal canals demonstrates the normal linear hypoglossal nerves (*arrows*), extending from the medulla laterally and anteriorly toward the hypoglossal canals, immediately lateral to the vertebral artery flow voids.

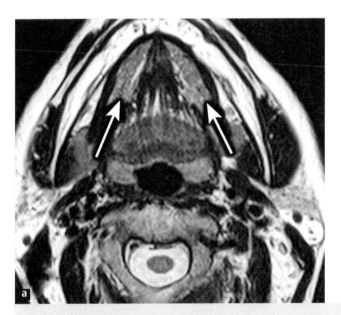
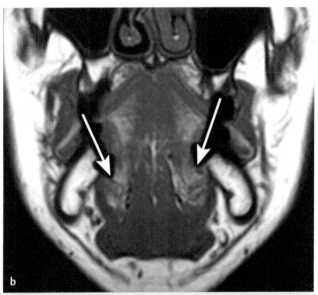

**Fig. 12.30** Axial T2-weighted (**a**) and coronal T1-weighted precontrasted (**b**) MR images demonstrate the normal bright T1 and T2 signal intensity of the fat of the sublingual spaces (*arrows*), medial to the mylohyoid muscle and lateral to the root of the tongue, containing the lingual and hypoglossal nerves laterally and the glossopharyngeal nerves medially.

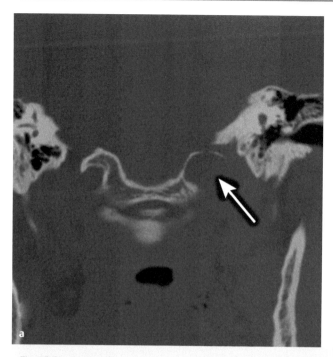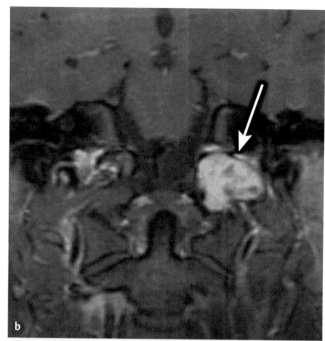

**Fig. 12.31** Coronal thin-section bone algorithm (**a**) and correlating coronal T1-weighted postcontrasted fat-saturated MR image (**b**) through the level of the jugular foramen demonstrate left hypoglossal canal enlargement with benign osseous borders (**a**; *arrow*), with well-circumscribed heterogeneous avid enhancement (**b**; *arrow*), consistent with a hypoglossal nerve schwannoma.

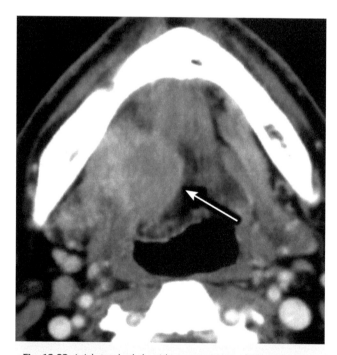

**Fig. 12.32** Axial standard algorithm postcontrasted CT through the level of the oral cavity demonstrates a right high-density mass (*arrow*) consistent with a squamous cell carcinoma invading the sublingual space with mass effect on the low-density midline fatty lingual septum displaced toward the left side.

# References

[1] Blitz AM, Choudhri AF, Chonka ZD, et al. Anatomic considerations, nomenclature, and advanced cross-sectional imaging techniques for visualization of the cranial nerve segments by MR imaging. Neuroimaging Clin N Am 2014; 24(1):1–15

[2] Policeni B, Corey AS, Burns J, et al; Expert Panel on Neurologic Imaging. ACR Appropriateness Criteria® Cranial Neuropathy. J Am Coll Radiol 2017; 14(11S):S406–S420

[3] Morani AC, Ramani NS, Wesolowski JR. Skull base, orbits, temporal bone, and cranial nerves: anatomy on MR imaging. Magn Reson Imaging Clin N Am 2011;19(3):439–456

[4] Jha RM, Klein JP. Clinical anatomy and imaging of the cranial nerves and skull base. Semin Neurol 2012;32(4):332–346

[5] Raut AA, Naphade PS, Chawla A. Imaging of skull base: pictorial essay. Indian J Radiol Imaging 2012;22(4):305–316

[6] Mathur A, Jain N, Kesavadas C, Thomas B, Kapilamoorthy TR. Imaging of skull base pathologies: role of advanced magnetic resonance imaging techniques. Neuroradiol J 2015;28(4):426–437

[7] Paul AB, Oklu R, Saini S, Prabhakar AM. How much is that head CT? Price transparency and variability in radiology. J Am Coll Radiol 2015;12(5): 453–457

[8] The 2007 Recommendations of the International Commission on Radiological Protection. ICRP publication 103. Ann ICRP 2007;37(2–4):1–332

[9] McCollough CH, Christner JA, Kofler JM. How effective is effective dose as a predictor of radiation risk? AJR Am J Roentgenol 2010;194(4):890–896

[10] McCollough CH, Bushberg JT, Fletcher JG, Eckel LJ. Answers to common questions about the use and safety of CT scans. Mayo Clin Proc 2015;90(10): 1380–1392

[11] US Food and Drug Administration. What are the Radiation Risks from CT? Silver Spring, MD: FDA; 2017

[12] Fraum TJ, Ludwig DR, Bashir MR, Fowler KJ. Gadolinium-based contrast agents: a comprehensive risk assessment. J Magn Reson Imaging 2017;46(2):338–353

[13] Kay J. Nephrogenic systemic fibrosis: a gadolinium-associated fibrosing disorder in patients with renal dysfunction. Ann Rheum Dis 2008;67(Suppl 3): iii66–iii69

[14] Schlaudecker JD, Bernheisel CR. Gadolinium-associated nephrogenic systemic fibrosis. Am Fam Physician 2009;80(7):711–714

[15] Rea P. Clinical Anatomy of the Cranial Nerves. San Diego, CA: Academic Press; 2014

[16] Borden N, Forseen S, Stefan C, Moore A. Imaging anatomy of the human brain: a comprehensive atlas including adjacent structures. New York, NY: Demos Medical; 2016

[17] Parry AT, Volk HA. Imaging the cranial nerves. Vet Radiol Ultrasound 2011;52(1, Suppl 1):S32–S41

[18] Duprez TP, Rombaux P. Imaging the olfactory tract (cranial nerve #1). Eur J Radiol 2010;74(2):288–298

[19] Castillo M, Mukherji SK. Magnetic resonance imaging of the olfactory apparatus. Top Magn Reson Imaging 1996;8(2):80–86

[20] Becker M, Masterson K, Delavelle J, Viallon M, Vargas M-I, Becker CD. Imaging of the optic nerve. Eur J Radiol 2010;74(2):299–313

[21] Mallery RM, Prasad S. Neuroimaging of the afferent visual system. Semin Neurol 2012;32(4):273–319

[22] Fadzli F, Ramli N, Ramli NM. MRI of optic tract lesions: review and correlation with visual field defects. Clin Radiol 2013;68(10):e538–e551

[23] Menjot de Champfleur N, Lebocq N, Menjot de Champfleur S, Bonafé A. Imaging of the pre-chiasmatic optic nerve. Diagn Interv Imaging 2013;94(10): 973–984

[24] Ferreira T, Verbist B, van Buchem M, van Osch T, Webb A. Imaging the ocular motor nerves. Eur J Radiol 2010;74(2):314–322

[25] Mark AS. Oculomotor motion disorders: current imaging of cranial nerves 3, 4, and 6. Semin Ultrasound CT MR 1998;19(3):240–256

[26] Tantiwongkosi B, Hesselink JR. Imaging of ocular motor pathway. Neuroimaging Clin N Am 2015;25(3):425–438

[27] Eisenkraft B, Ortiz AO. Imaging evaluation of cranial nerves 3, 4, and 6. Semin Ultrasound CT MR 2001;22(6):488–501

[28] Choi BS, Kim JH, Jung C, Hwang JM. High-resolution 3D MR imaging of the trochlear nerve. AJNR Am J Neuroradiol 2010;31(6):1076–1079

[29] Schuknecht B, Sturm V, Huisman TA, Landau K. Tolosa–Hunt syndrome: MR imaging features in 15 patients with 20 episodes of painful ophthalmoplegia. Eur J Radiol 2009;69(3):445–453

[30] Bathla G, Hegde AN. The trigeminal nerve: an illustrated review of its imaging anatomy and pathology. Clin Radiol 2013;68(2):203–213

[31] Cassetta M, Pranno N, Pompa V, Barchetti F, Pompa G. High resolution 3-T MR imaging in the evaluation of the trigeminal nerve course. Eur Rev Med Pharmacol Sci 2014;18(2):257–264

[32] Borges A, Casselman J. Imaging the trigeminal nerve. Eur J Radiol 2010;74(2):323–340

[33] Rubinstein D, Stears RL, Stears JC. Trigeminal nerve and ganglion in the Meckel cave: appearance at CT and MR imaging. Radiology 1994;193(1):155–159

[34] Williams LS, Schmalfuss IM, Sistrom CL, et al. MR imaging of the trigeminal ganglion, nerve, and the perineural vascular plexus: normal appearance and variants with correlation to cadaver specimens. AJNR Am J Neuroradiol 2003;24(7):1317–1323

[35] Peschillo S, Delfini R. Trigeminal neuralgia: a new neuroimaging perspective. World Neurosurg 2013;80(3–4):293–295

[36] Leclercq D, Thiebaut JB, Héran F. Trigeminal neuralgia. Diagn Interv Imaging 2013;94(10):993–1001

[37] Harsha KJ, Kesavadas C, Chinchure S, Thomas B, Jagtap S. Imaging of vascular causes of trigeminal neuralgia. J Neuroradiol 2012;39(5):281–289

[38] Baugh RF, Basura GJ, Ishii LE, et al. Clinical practice guideline: Bell's palsy. Otolaryngol Head Neck Surg 2013;149(3, Suppl):S1–S27

[39] Singh AK, Bathla G, Altmeyer W, et al. Imaging spectrum of facial nerve lesions. Curr Probl Diagn Radiol 2015;44(1):60–75

[40] Veillona F, Ramos-Taboada L, Abu-Eid M, Charpiot A, Riehm S. Imaging of the facial nerve. Eur J Radiol 2010;74(2):341–348

[41] Jäger L, Reiser M. CT and MR imaging of the normal and pathologic conditions of the facial nerve. Eur J Radiol 2001;40(2):133–146

[42] Kumar A, Mafee MF, Mason T. Value of imaging in disorders of the facial nerve. Top Magn Reson Imaging 2000;11(1):38–51

[43] Mundada P, Purohit BS, Kumar TS, Tan TY. Imaging of facial nerve schwannomas: diagnostic pearls and potential pitfalls. Diagn Interv Radiol 2016;22(1):40–46

[44] McRackan TR, Wilkinson EP, Rivas A. Primary tumors of the facial nerve. Otolaryngol Clin North Am 2015;48(3):491–500

[45] Jeong SH, Kim HJ, Kim JS. Vestibular neuritis. Semin Neurol 2013;33(3): 185–194

[46] Goddard JC, Fayad JN. Vestibular neuritis. Otolaryngol Clin North Am 2011;44(2):361–365, viii

[47] Haque S, Hossain A, Quddus MA, Jahan MU. Role of MRI in the evaluation of acoustic schwannoma and its comparison to histopathological findings. Bangladesh Med Res Counc Bull 2011;37(3):92–96

[48] Smirniotopoulos JG, Yue NC, Rushing EJ. Cerebellopontine angle masses: radiologic-pathologic correlation. Radiographics 1993;13(5):1131–1147

[49] Tsunoda A, Komatsuzaki A, Suzuki Y, Muraoka H. Three-dimensional imaging of the internal auditory canal in patients with acoustic neuroma. Acta Otolaryngol Suppl 2000;542:6–8

[50] Stucken EZ, Brown K, Selesnick SH. Clinical and diagnostic evaluation of acoustic neuromas. Otolaryngol Clin North Am 2012;45(2):269–284, vii

[51] von Kirschbaum C, Gürkov R. Audiovestibular function deficits in vestibular schwannoma. BioMed Res Int 2016;2016:4980562

[52] Lin EP, Crane BT. The management and imaging of vestibular schwannomas. AJNR Am J Neuroradiol 2017;38(11):2034–2043

[53] Jethanamest D, Rivera AM, Ji H, Chokkalingam V, Telischi FF, Angeli SI. Conservative management of vestibular schwannoma: predictors of growth and hearing. Laryngoscope 2015;125(9):2163–2168

[54] Quist TS, Givens DJ, Gurgel RK, Chamoun R, Shelton C. Hearing preservation after middle fossa vestibular schwannoma removal: are the results durable? Otolaryngol Head Neck Surg 2015;152(4):706–711

[55] Raheja A, Bowers CA, MacDonald JD, et al. Middle fossa approach for vestibular schwannoma: good hearing and facial nerve outcomes with low morbidity. World Neurosurg 2016;92:37–46

[56] Larson TC III, Aulino JM, Laine FJ. Imaging of the glossopharyngeal, vagus, and accessory nerves. Semin Ultrasound CT MR 2002;23(3):238–255

[57] Castillo M, Mukherji SK. Magnetic resonance imaging of cranial nerves IX, X, XI, and XII. Top Magn Reson Imaging 1996;8(3):180–186

[58] Li AE, Greditzer HG IV, Melisaratos DP, Wolfe SW, Feinberg JH, Sneag DB. MRI findings of spinal accessory neuropathy. Clin Radiol 2016;71(4):316–320

[59] Ong CK, Chong VF. The glossopharyngeal, vagus and spinal accessory nerves. Eur J Radiol 2010;74(2):359–367

[60] Loh C, Maya MM, Go JL. Cranial nerve XII: the hypoglossal nerve. Semin Ultrasound CT MR 2002;23(3):256–265

[61] Alves P. Imaging the hypoglossal nerve. Eur J Radiol 2010;74(2):368–377

[62] Carroll CG, Campbell WW. Multiple cranial neuropathies. Semin Neurol 2009;29(1):53–65

[63] Keane JR. Multiple cranial nerve palsies: analysis of 979 cases. Arch Neurol 2005;62(11):1714–1717

# 13  Conclusion and Discussion Points

*Seilesh C. Babu and Neal M. Jackson*

As the previous chapters have demonstrated, cranial nerve disorders can be very complex to diagnose and treat. While there are dozens of diagnostic modalities available, the best approach to diagnosis begins with a detailed history and physical examination. A correct diagnosis is paramount and may require extensive testing. Oftentimes, a specialist with specific testing or tools (e.g., laryngeal endoscopy, audiogram, electroneuronography) is called upon to carry out the next steps in the diagnostic evaluation. Radiologic imaging plays a large role in many situations to confirm the diagnosis or to rule out life-threatening pathology such as intracranial masses or malignancy.

Treatment options also range from observation to surgery. For some self-limited benign conditions for which a spontaneous recovery is anticipated (e.g., a unilateral acute facial nerve paralysis), the medically appropriate decision to observe for recovery is also cost-effective. However, for certain conditions that manifest as a cranial neuropathy (e.g., slow-onset, progressive facial nerve weakness from a growing tumor in the cerebellopontine angle), the medically appropriate decision is surgical resection, which is costly. In this example, both situations involve unilateral facial nerve weakness. The details and time course of the clinical history are key differentiating factors that ultimately lead to correct diagnosis and appropriate treatment.

Obviously, an accurate diagnosis is necessary for cost-effective management decisions. The opposite is true: the least cost-effective action is a wrong treatment due to misdiagnosis. This is both costly and potentially harmful to the patient.

Finally, as discussed previously, despite the increased focus on minimizing cost, one must remain vigilant of being too cost conscientious when human lives are at risk.

# Index

Note: Page numbers set in **bold** indicate headings.